OXFORD HISTORICAL MONOGRAPHS

MEDICINE AND RELIGION *c.*1300

The Case of
Arnau de Vilanova

JOSEPH ZIEGLER

CLARENDON PRESS · OXFORD

1998

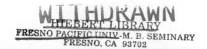

Oxford University Press, Great Clarendon Street, Oxford OX2 6DP

Oxford New York
Athens Auckland Bangkok Bombay
Buenos Aires Calcutta Cape Town Dar es Salaam
Delhi Florence Hong Kong Istanbul Karachi
Kuala Lumpur Madras Madrid Melbourne
Mexico City Nairobi Paris Singapore
Taipei Tokyo Toronto Warsaw
and associated companies in
Berlin Ibadan

Oxford is a registered trade mark of Oxford University Press

Published in the United States by
Oxford University Press Inc., New York

British Library Cataloguing in Publication Data
Data available

Library of Congress Cataloging in Publication Data
Data applied for

ISBN 0–19–820726–3

1 3 5 7 9 10 8 6 4 2

Typeset by Cambrian Typesetters, Frimley, Surrey
Printed in Great Britain by
Bookcraft Ltd., Midsomer-Norton
Nr. Bath, Somerset

PREFACE

This book is a revised version of a D.Phil. thesis, which was submitted in 1994 to the Faculty of Modern History, Oxford University, but whose origins lie further back in time. A brief history of its evolution will explain its present form and illuminate the odd, unexpected ways in which ideas develop. Aware of my particular interest in scholastic culture, it was the late Amos Funkenstein who in 1989 first suggested that I concentrate my research on academic heresy and more specifically on Masters' trials. 'Academic condemnations c.1280–c.1350' was the research topic which brought me to Oxford in 1990. I wanted to examine the procedure of the condemnations, to uncover the characteristics and intellectual profiles common to the condemned masters, and to analyse the impact of the condemnations on scholastic culture. Soon after plunging into extensive reading on the various cases of university masters whose ideas were suppressed, I realized that the topic I had chosen was far too ambitious if it were to be completed within three to four years. I had to narrow it down, despite the disappointment which such a change would cause: for this meant abandoning my attempt to engage the general phenomenon of condemnation. Four of the fifteen cases of condemned university masters who were on my list (Arnau de Vilanova, Pietro d'Abano, Cecco d'Ascoli and Marsilio da Padova) had a medical background—a fact which drew my attention. This sub-group introduced an intriguing question: what role, if at all, did their medical background play when they produced ideas inimical to Christian orthodoxy? Was there around 1300 a direct relationship between medicine and academic heresy? Or, more generally, what was the relationship between medicine and religion at that time?

It is widely accepted that there are parallels between medicine and religion today. Hospitals to some degree are the churches of modernity. Medical vocabulary is, like the liturgy, exclusive, invocatory, monopolistic, and often incomprehensible to the lay audience. Hospitals are now those places where individuals from all classes and walks of life gather together, united by fear of death and hope of salvation. Not for nothing did Philip Larkin in 'The Building' paint a hospital in specifically hieratic tones, calling the patients 'congregations'.[1] The blind, sheep-like

[1] P. Larkin, *Collected Poems*, ed. A. Thwaite (London and Boston, 1990), 191–3.

trust which people are enjoined to have for their doctors is precisely the same as that which they were once enjoined to have for their priests. The patients buy their cure/salvation through an act of confession in which they tell a story about their symptoms to their doctor: similarly, telling one's sins to one's priest was necessary for expiation.[2] In many respects medicine has assumed religion's traditional role as the guardian of human morals. The priest and the physician thus share grounds, tools, techniques, and clients. Again, Philip Larkin says it much better in 'Days':

> What are the days for?
> Days are where we live.
> They come, they wake us
> Time and time over.
> They are to be happy in:
> Where can we live but days?
>
> Ah, solving that question
> Brings the priest and the doctor
> In their long coats
> Running over the fields.[3]

How exactly did medicine and religion coexist in the traditional society of late thirteenth- and early fourteenth-century Europe, dominated by Christian values yet undergoing dramatic intellectual changes? I chose to follow up this topic by looking at the first of the four masters mentioned above, Arnau de Vilanova, and by putting his work within a wider context. The results of this research will unfold in the following pages. This is by no means a definitive study. It leaves unanswered questions; it invites differing interpretations; it demands more proofs and further examples. But I hope it will stimulate others to improve upon it and to increase and refine our understanding of this aspect of medieval culture.

Personal names provided an irritating problem. In the end, I decided to use the English form for popes, kings, saints, and Classical sources. For all the rest I usually kept the Catalan name for the Catalan, the French for the Frenchmen, the Italian for the Italians, and so forth. I am sure that many inconsistencies remain, but I found no better solution. Biblical citations are rendered into English according to the King James Version. In case of a discrepancy between the reference from the Vulgate and that of

---

[2] S. Poole, 'Whoa! I gotta pumper', *TLS*, Feb. 2 (1996), 18.
[3] Larkin, *Collected Poems*, 67.

the translation I indicate both and put the latter in square brackets. The translation of Ecclesiasticus 38 is the Anchor Bible translation (vol. 39) which I occasionally modified to regain the literal meaning of the text.

I am very conscious of the extent to which this book has been made possible by the help and advice of others. My chief academic debt is to Jean Dunbabin and Richard Smith, my supervisors. Their constructive suggestions, intellectual stimulation, care, and encouragement were invaluable. Jean Dunbabin even courageously undertook to lead me through the production of this book. I am immensely grateful to her. Other people read and amended drafts of this work. I have been encouraged, helped, taught, and corrected by them. I would like to thank Luis García-Ballester and Michael McVaugh, who have made my first encounter with medieval medicine an exciting experience, and whose friendship I cherish as much as I do their intellectual insight. Peter Biller and Alexander Murray, who examined my thesis, enriched me tremendously. This revised version of it is largely a reflection of their penetrating remarks and critique. David D'Avray was very helpful on the preaching literature, and the thoughtful comments of Maurice Keen were highly productive. Lesley Smith was always there to give crucial advice. Many others answered my questions and added their own imprint on my work, from my teachers at the Department of History in the Hebrew University of Jerusalem to my Catalan tutor in Oxford, Silvia Coll-Vinent. I am grateful to them all. Two conferences ('Medicine as Cultural System', Tel-Aviv and Jerusalem, 1993, organized by the Van Leer Foundation, and 'The First International Workshop on Arnau de Vilanova', Barcelona, 1994, organized by J. Perarnau and L. García-Ballester) substantially contributed to the formation and clarification of my thoughts. I met with kind assistance in the Bodleian Library and in particular I am grateful to Martin Kauffmann and the staff of Duke Humphrey's Library. I would like to thank Humaira Erfan Ahmed for getting the book ready for press. The research for this book would not have been possible without the financial and logistic support of the University of Oxford, the Faculty of Modern History, Merton and Green Colleges, the Wellcome Trust, and in particular its Oxford Unit, the Lothian Fund, the Anglo-Jewish Association, and Yad Hanadiv Foundation. The University of Haifa—my present home—was extremely helpful in the later stages of the work. I am grateful to them all.

Finally, I would like to express my gratitude and admiration to all members of my family, whose manifold support renders this book theirs too.

CONTENTS

LIST OF ABBREVIATIONS

AFH	*Archivum Franciscanum Historicum*
AFP	*Archivum Fratrum Praedicatorum*
AST	*Analecta Sacra Tarraconensia*
Astesana	Astesano di Asti, *Summa de casibus* (Strasbourg, 1474)
ATCA	*Arxiu de Textos Catalans Antics*
ATIEAV	*Actes de la I Trobada Internacional d'Estudis sobre Arnau de Vilanova*, ed. J. Perarnau, 2 vols. (Barcelona, 1995)
AVOMO	Arnau de Vilanova, *Opera Medica Omnia*, ed. L. García-Ballester, J. A. Paniagua, and M. R. McVaugh (Barcelona, 1975–)
Cart. Mont.	*Cartulaire de l'Université de Montpellier*, i. ed. A. Germain (Montpellier, 1890)
CCCM	*Corpus Christianorum Continuatio Mediaevalis*
CCSL	*Corpus Christianorum Series Latina*
Chart. Univ. Par.	*Chartularium Universitatis Parisiensis*
CSEL	*Corpus Scriptorum Ecclesiasticorum Latinorum*
DS	*Dictionnaire de Spiritualité Ascétique et Mystique Doctrine et Histoire*
DTC	*Dictionnaire de Théologie Catholique*
Glossa Ordinaria	*Biblia sacra, cum glossa ordinaria . . . et postilla Nicolai Lyrani*, 6 vols. (Lyons, 1589)
LPM	Llull, *Liber principiorum medicine*
PL	J. P. Migne (ed.), *Patrologie cursus completus. Series Latina* (Paris, 1844–63)
RTAM	*Recherches de Théologie Ancienne et Médiévale*
Sde	Giovanni da San Gimignano, *Summa de exemplis et rerum similitudinibus locuplentissima*
TRE	*Theologische Realenzyklopädie* (Berlin and New York, 1976–)

I

Introduction

Patterns of Relationship between Religion and Medicine

Humbert de Romans (d. 1277), in a model sermon directed at students of medicine, taught that the liberal arts, medicine, and law emerged as the result of the deterioration of human condition after Adam's Sin.[1] The sermon is included in Humbert's collection of *ad status* sermons[2] compiled between 1266 and 1277. These model sermons, directed to a variety of sorts and conditions of men, have already proved to be valuable for religious history and for highlighting social reality in the thirteenth century.[3] Humbert, a Paris-educated cleric who joined the Dominican Order in 1224 and became Master General of the Order from 1254 to 1263, reveals in this sermon his perception of the nature of the relationship which exists between medicine and religion. The liberal arts illuminate human reason which Original Sin has obscured. The science of law was invented to protect the right of possession in the postlapsarian world, which is no longer characterized by common ownership. The art of medicine is necessary to oppose bodily corruptibility which is revealed by sickness. But medicine stands first among these three sciences, says Humbert, and he confirms that the status of medicine was rising at that time within the academic world. As a science (*scientia*), medicine is better (*melior*) than the liberal arts, which are lacking in utility. Medicine is better than law, which is useful, because the object of its dealings—the body—is more valuable than the things (*res*) which the science of law regulates.

---

[1] Humbert de Romans, *Sermones ad diuersos status* (Hagenau, 1508), tr. I, 66, 'Ad studentes in medicina' (see Appendix III). On Humbert de Romans, see T. Kaeppeli, *Scriptores Ordinis Praedicatorum Medii Aevi*, ii (Rome, 1975), 283–95; *Lexikon des Mittelalters* (Zurich and Munich, 1977–), v. 209; *DS* 7/1 (1969), 1112.

[2] D. L. D'Avray, *The Preaching of the Friars* (Oxford, 1985), 80 ; D. L. D'Avray and M. Tausche, 'Marriage Sermons in *ad status* Collections of the Central Middle Ages', in *Modern Questions about Medieval Sermons: Essays on Marriage, Death, History and Sanctity*, ed. N. Bériou and D. L. D'Avray (Spoleto, 1994), 77–134 at 77–84: an introduction to the genre.

[3] A. Murray, 'Religion among the Poor in Thirteenth Century France: The Testimony of Humbert de Romans', *Traditio*, 30 (1974), 285–324.

Yet according to Humbert the usefulness of medicine to the body is not its sole merit. The science of medicine has a religious significance which rightly allows it to be valued more highly than the liberal arts and law. The religious usefulness of medicine entails three aspects. First, the examination and the knowledge of the body's natural constitution (*natura corporis humani*) teaches how wretched and fragile it is. Second, medical practice enables the practitioner to perform frequent acts of mercy (*opera misericordie*) when treating patients who are subject to misery. Third, medical practice is useful for spiritual medicine of souls (*medicina spiritualis animarum*). The art of medical science produces excellent guidance with respect to spiritual medicine.[4]

Humbert thus holds that the boundaries between corporeal and spiritual medicine are far from impermeable. Moreover, both practical and theoretical medicine enhance spiritual speculation. Humbert's sermon thus clearly calls for a refinement of our judgement of the status, cultural role, image, and self-image of medicine and physicians in the later middle ages.

There is some evidence to indicate that physicians interested themselves in the soul of their patients in late antiquity, and that the awareness of medicine's spiritual aspects was not unique to the thirteenth century.[5] The author of a letter from 374 or early 375, printed today in the compilations of letters of St Basil (*c.*329–379) but also occasionally attributed to St Gregory of Nyssa (*c.*335–394), praises Eustathius, a chief physician (*archiatrus*) thus: 'But in your hands the science is especially expert and you extend the boundaries of your philanthropy not limiting the favour of your profession to bodies but taking thought also for the correction of spiritual infirmities'.[6] Together with the author, Eustathius the physician dispels the 'heavy inflammation of the heart' caused by those who hate orthodox Christians and accuse them of polytheism on account of their Trinitarian dogma. Hence when we engage the spiritual dimension of medicine around 1300 we must be aware of its past expressions. In this respect, the Bible is a powerful core text which clearly suggests that medicine and religion converge.

---

[4] For a later version of a similar theme, see Jean Gerson's sermon from 1406, 'Pro licentiandis in medicina', in Jean Gerson, *Oeuvres complètes*, v. ed. P. Glorieux (Paris, 1963), 144–51 and esp. 148–50 where he discusses medicine as a source of metaphors and its spiritual value for preachers.

[5] D. W. Amundsen and G. B. Ferngren, 'The Early Christian Tradition', in R. L. Numbers and D. W. Amundsen (eds.), *Caring and Curing: Health and Medicine in the Western Religious Traditions* (New York and London, 1986), 58.

[6] Saint Basil, *The Letters*, tr. R. J. Deferrari, iii (London and Cambridge, Mass., 1961), 49, 189.

According to Scripture, neither medicine nor the physician were religiously neutral. On the contrary, both derived their high status from their divine origin. 'Honour the physician because of his essential function', exclaims Ecclesiasticus 38 in its opening verse. Medical cure and its suppliers are part of the divinely ordained cosmos. The physician of Ecclesiasticus is a divine creation, which derives his knowledge and healing capacities directly from God.[7] As a divine agent he deserves respect from his clients; as a divine agent he practises medicine both by using the knowledge acquired from God and by communicating through prayer with God during his practice. While the fifteen verses in Ecclesiasticus 38 dealing with medicine and the physician received varied interpretations (as we shall see in Chapter 5), one conclusion is clear: Scripture precluded a sharp separation between medicine and religion.

There are quantitative indicators which hint that academic medicine and religion were intertwined at the turn of the thirteenth century. We know that 33.6 per cent of practitioners from the French medical milieu studied by Danielle Jacquart belonged to the clergy (25.9 per cent secular and 5.7 per cent regular); 15.6 per cent of medical practitioners in Jacquart's analysis were prebend-holding clerics, and 44.5 per cent of these went on to be priests.[8] Another interesting statistic (albeit disappointingly low) reveals that 4.7 per cent of the physicians surveyed by Jacquart wrote a medical treatise which has survived.[9]

Papal circles established close ties with Salernitan physicians and natural philosophers already in the twelfth century. The papal court at Viterbo of the late thirteenth century has recently been described as a centre for the production, circulation and transmission of scientific knowledge in general and medical knowledge in particular. Late-thirteenth-century Popes were highly aware of the benefits of caring for the body and of environmental, hygienic, and climatic influences on the physical condition of mankind in general. They also actively and enthusiastically took care of their own health and the well-being of their body. The concentration of physicians in the pontifical *familia* or in households of individual cardinals, their role as important cultural agents, and their frequent promotion to ecclesiastical office illuminate one relationship

---

[7] 'Honora medicum propter necessitatem; etenim illum creavit Altissimus. A Deo est enim omnis medela, et a rege accipiet donationem. Disciplina medici exaltabit caput illius, et in conspectu magnatorum collaudabitur. Altissimus creavit de terra medicamenta, et vir prudens non abhorrebit illam' (Ecclus. 38: 1–4).

[8] D. Jacquart, *Le Milieu médical en France du XIIe au XVe siècle* (Geneva, 1981), 155–56, 380, 386.   [9] Ibid. 199–200.

between the ecclesiastical hierarchy and the medical profession,[10] totally refuting old-fashioned, erroneous, and superficial assertions concerning ecclesiastical hostility to medicine and its practitioners.

The examination of the role of miracles and magic in the curing process suggests that fourteenth-century physicians and patients recognized and employed routes to health other than the strictly medical. Thus, for example, miracles of physical healing constitute 45 to 60 per cent of the items in medieval collections of miracles related to the cult of St Martial in Limoges.[11] Similiar patterns appear in trials of canonization, where between 80 and 90 per cent of the attested miracles in the thirteenth and fourteenth centuries are therapeutic.[12] But recent studies have shown that, irrespective of their social class and status, patients looked first to practitioners when ill. Prayer for heavenly intervention in times of acute disease was a last resort when standard treatment had failed. Sometimes, the agonizing patient opted for the Saint's healing powers at the instigation of his physician who had given up his efforts to cure and his hope in the feasibility of natural cure.[13] Physicians even appeared as witnesses in trials of canonization, where their scientific expertise was sought in order to enhance the extraordinary healing powers of the venerated saint.[14] Thus the religious medicine of the Church acted not as a rival to professional medicine but as its supplement and complement.[15]

But convergence is not the only form of relationship between medicine

---

[10] A. Paravicini-Bagliani, *Medicina e scienze della natura alla corte dei papi nel Duecento* (Spoleto, 1991) esp. 119–40, 235–66, and 393–408, and *Il corpo del Papa* (Turin, 1994), esp. 263–316 and 334–48.

[11] A. Carion, 'Miracles de Saint-Martial', in J. Gelis and O. Redon (eds.), *Les Miracles miroirs des corps* (Paris, 1983), 89–124 at 116, 118.

[12] A. Vauchez, *La Sainteté en Occident aux derniers siècles du Moyen Âge* (Rome and Paris, 1981), 543–56 at 547.

[13] See e.g. miracle 7 in the Life of St Louis, composed in 1302/3 by Guillaume de Saint-Pathus and quoted in S. Chennaf and O. Redon, 'Les Miracles de Saint Louis', in Gelis and Redon (eds.), *Les Miracles*, 55–85 at 80.

[14] See *Acta Sanctorum* (Paris, 1877), 2 Iul. I, 525F–27A, for the case of Jean de Tournemire, master of medicine and physician to Pope Clement VII, who testified in 1390 in the canonization process of Pierre de Luxembourg; Vauchez, *La Sainteté*, 549; F. Antonelli, *De inquisitione medico-legali super miraculis in causis beatificationis et canonizationis* (Studia Antoniana, 18; Rome, 1962), 21–30.

[15] N. G. Siraisi, *Medieval and Early Renaissance Medicine* (Chicago and London, 1990), 39–42; M. R. McVaugh, *Medicine before the Plague: Practitioners and their Patients in the Crown of Aragon 1285–1345* (Cambridge, 1993), 136–8; K. Park, *Doctors and Medicine in Early Renaissance Florence* (Princeton, 1985), 50–1; R. Finucane, *Miracles and Pilgrims: Popular Beliefs in Medieval England* (London, 1995), 59–82, and *The Rescue of the Innocents: Endangered Children in Medieval Miracles* (New York and London, 1997), ch. 3.

and religion in the thirteenth century. Two decades before Humbert composed his sermon, another prominent Dominican, Albertus Magnus, acknowledged that theology, medicine, and natural philosophy were clearly separate. In his commentary on the second book of Petrus Lombardus's *Sentences* Albertus discusses the nature of 'that light of which it is said *and God divided the light from the darkness'* (Genesis, 1: 4). His answer that light is a corporeal form *(forma corporis)* rather than a simple body or a bright confusion relies on the philosophers Aristotle and Avicenna, and contradicts Augustine. This induces Albertus to justify his method of reasoning; he declares his adherence to the principle that the topic of the debated question should determine the authorities one uses for its solution. Thus, on questions concerning faith and morals, Augustine rather than the philosophers should determine the solution; if the problem belongs to medicine, one should follow Galen and Hippocrates; and when one deals with the nature of things *(natura rerum)* Aristotle is the preferable authority.[16]

Albertus maintains here the existence of clear disciplinary boundaries which allow medicine an autonomous place next to theology and natural philosophy. His view has buttressed the conviction of some historians that the second half of the thirteenth and the beginning of the fourteenth centuries mark a radical change in the ways physicians perceived themselves and the way medicine was perceived by society.[17] One of the hallmarks of this change was a growing interest and confidence in the efficacy of academic medicine and its practitioners. This was the product of the incorporation of medicine into scholastic culture and its consequent exposure to recent developments in natural philosophy. One of the expressions of this change was a gradual withdrawal of the clergy from medical practice. Furthermore, the growing disjunction between the medical and clerical domains became apparent in the content of learned medicine, which became more and more religiously neutral and devoid of a spiritual dimension.[18]

The fact that, throughout Europe, the regular clergy was losing ground as suppliers of medical care is one of the indicators for the

[16] Albertus Magnus, *Super II Sententiarum*, d.13, a.2, in *Opera Omnia*, ed. A. Borgnet (Paris, 1894), 27: 247[a].
[17] L. García-Ballester, 'Introduction', in *Practical Medicine from Salerno to the Black Death*, ed. L. García-Ballester, R. French, J. Arrizabalaga, and A. Cunningham (Cambridge, 1994), 1–29 at 23; id., 'The Construction of a New Form of Learning and Practising Medicine in Medieval Latin Europe', *Science in Context*, 8 (1995), 75–102.
[18] The notion of a growing disjunction is implicit in McVaugh, *Medicine before the Plague*, esp. 72–5.

growing separation between medicine and religion. Since the little detailed evidence we have concerning individual physicians until this period suggests that ecclesiastics continued to practise medicine, this change apparently took place in the twelfth century. In monasteries, monks who were physicians treated their brethren and possibly also some lay patients.[19] But in the twelfth century they met with a growing criticism which was expressed in ecclesiastical legislation. Canon 9 promulgated by the Second Lateran Council (1139) forbade monks and canons regular to learn civil law and medicine with a view to temporal gain.[20] The canon, which did not apply to the whole clergy, was never incorporated into any official collection of canon law. A weakened version of it enacted in 1163 by Pope Alexander III at the Council of Tours, and later included in the *Decretales* of Gregory IX (1234), simply forbade monks and regular clergy to leave their religious houses for the study of medicine and civil law.[21] A similar rule was adopted by the Cistercian Order shortly after Bernard of Clairvaux's death in 1153. It forbade the Order's physicians to practise outside their monasteries or to treat laymen, and expressed the fear that the *stabilitas loci* of monastic life was in danger.

The declining number of regular clergy among French physicians from the thirteenth century fortifies the view that a clearer divide between the medical and the religious professions was emerging. The fact that relatively few physicians produced theological writings and that few took a theology degree after completing their medical course of study provides further support for the notion of the growing separation between academic medicine and the clerical world.[22] This hypothesis is confirmed by recent statistics from the Crown of Aragon showing that only one per cent of the identified Christian physicians between 1300 and 1345 were clerics.

[19] A. F. Dowtry, 'The *Modus Medendi* and the Benedictine Order in Anglo-Norman England', in *The Church and Healing*, ed. W. J. Sheils (Studies in Church History, 19; Oxford, 1982), 25–38 at 31–3. For the monastic ideology of medical care, see the treatise in defence of medicine which opens the 8th-century manuscript of the 'Lorscher Arzneibuch' in U. Stoll (ed.), *Das 'Lorscher Arzneibuch'* (Sudhoffs Archiv, Beiheft 28; Stuttgart, 1992), 48–62 and Cassiodorus's praise of medical men among the brothers in 6th century Vivatium, in: *Cassiodori senatoris institutiones*, ed. R. A. B. Mynors (Oxford, 1963) I. 31, pp. 78–9.
[20] *Decrees of the Ecumenical Councils*, ed. N. P. Tanner, i (London, 1990), 198–9.
[21] D. W. Amundsen, 'The Medieval Catholic Tradition', in Numbers and Amundsen (ed.) *Caring and Curing*, 84–5.
[22] Jacquart, *Le Milieu médical*, 383 n. 18 (for the decline in numbers of regular clergy among the physicians), 388 n. 24, 392 n. 31 (for the prolific extra-medical activities in astrology, diplomacy, government, and commerce), 389 n. 26 (for the non-medical works produced by physicians), 393 n. 34 (for the 5.7 per cent of the total number of physicians who over the four centuries took a degree in theology, and the growing weight of the secular clergy).

The virtual disappearance of clerics as medical practitioners is explained by their displacement by a gradually increasing pool of secular physicians.[23] This development, however, was not universal. Whereas throughout parts of southern and northern Europe there was a sharp decline in the number of regular clergy studying or practising medicine, England and northern France showed no such decline among the secular clergy. For example, eight out of the forty known medical scholars in fourteenth-century Oxford also studied theology. For them at least, medicine was still a preamble to the ultimate degree, the doctorate in theology.[24]

There are occasional signs of opposition to the involvement of clerics in medical practice. Thus, for example, in 1219 Honorius III extended to clerics whose major functions were spiritual and to those who possessed ecclesiastical benefices Alexander III's prohibition (1163) on studying medicine, originally directed only to the regular clergy. Then in 1294 Celestine V substantially enlarged this. He prohibited all clerics (including those in minor orders who held ecclesiastical benefices) from practising medicine (*physica*), exempting clerics from the prohibition, however, if they did so without charge, for charity, and in order to assist relations and friends.[25] However, Darrel Amundsen has already shown that the prohibitions in canon law on medical practice by clerics were not as restrictive as has sometimes been alleged and that there is no evidence that the papacy opposed the teaching and study of medicine at the universities under ecclesiastical control.[26] The relatively large number of medical students holding prebends proves that the letter of the prohibition was not fully observed, and that the broadly formulated exemption at the end of Celestine's text did, in practice, legitimize medical treatment by all clerics, since every case treated without charge could be defined as *pro Deo*.

The fact that little attention was devoted by canon law to medicine and its practitioners within lay society is another indication of a separation

[23] McVaugh, *Medicine before the Plague*, 72 n. 1, 75.

[24] F. Getz, 'The Faculty of Medicine before 1500', in *The History of the University of Oxford*, ii. *Late Medieval Oxford*, eds. J. I. Catto and R. Evans (Oxford, 1992), 381–2, 388.

[25] 'Non licet clericis qui in sacris ordinibus sunt constituti vel etiam in minoribus dum tamen sint beneficiati nisi gratis pro Deo vel parentibus vel amicis nec etiam tunc si posset esse ibi periculum. Chirurgia autem, que adustionem vel abscissionem inducit, est penitus eis interdicta.' *Maxima Bibliotheca Veterum Patrum*, xxv (Lyons, 1677), 822.

[26] D. W. Amundsen, 'Medieval Canon Law on Medical and Surgical Practice by the Clergy', *Bulletin of the History of Medicine*, 52 (1978), 22–44; also in id., *Medicine, Society, and Faith in the Ancient and Medieval Worlds* (Baltimore and London, 1996), 222–47. For a summary of canons relating to medicine see also J. Shatzmiller, *Jews, Medicine and Medieval Society* (Berkeley, 1994), 8–10.

between medicine and religion. For example, in the context of the legal discussion of the just-price theory, canonists were not inclined to impose limits on medical fees, but contented themselves with exhorting physicians to restrain their greed, and predicting dire consequences *post mortem* for medical profiteers. This they did despite the physician's ability to exploit his patients—a relationship which led them in another field to the conclusion that government was entitled to cap charges and honoraria due to lawyers by imposing maximum fees for legal services.[27]

The confessors' manual, *Summa de casibus conscientie* of the Franciscan Astesano di Asti, which was completed by 1317 and offered a practical and systematic treatment of doctrinal and canonical matters of interest to confessors, clearly illustrates both clerical lack of interest in medical practice among the laity and its intense preoccupation with the effect of medical practice on the clerical order.[28] *Astesana* categorically rejects the use of magical or superstitious therapies. It is, however, prepared to acknowledge that sometimes the physical and the spiritual fuse and interact. It accepts the possible influence of the evil eye, and backs this belief with authorities like Avicenna, Algazel (al-Ghazali), and Galen.[29] *Astesana* allows the amputation of a putrefied organ when the health of the body depends on it. However, it strictly forbids any bodily mutilation simply to avoid sin or reduce temptation; it implicitly rejects any form of castration.[30] It frees the sick from the obligation to take the Eucharist before they have eaten. Medical emergency thus creates an exception to the religious rule.[31] The place devoted to these medical cases in *Astesana* is at best marginal.

But the article in *Astesana* most packed with references to medical practice is that which deals with ordination.[32] It devotes a long discussion to the impediments which prevent promotion to higher orders, such as the shedding of blood. An entire section of the article discusses the question of a cleric who, either as a medical practitioner or as a mere attendant and

---

[27] J. Brundage, *Medieval Canon Law* (London and New York, 1995), 77.

[28] *Astesana*; L. Wadding, *Scriptores ordinis minorum* (Rome, 1650), 42–3; L. E. Boyle, *Pastoral Care, Clerical Education and Canon Law, 1200–1400* (London, 1981), iii. 261–2. Later *summe conscientie*, particularly in the fifteenth century, evince wider interests in and more detailed analysis of medical topics. D. W. Amundsen, 'Casuistry and Professional Obligations: The Regulation of Physicians by the Court of Conscience in the Late Middle Ages', *Transactions and Studies of the College of Physicians of Philadelphia*, n.s., 3 (1981), 22–39, 93–112 (also in id., *Medicine, Society and Faith*, 248–88).

[29] *Astesana*, i. 15, 'De multipliciis observanciis supersticionis'.

[30] Ibid. 26, 'De iniuriis corporalibus aliis ab homicidio'.

[31] Ibid. iv. 18, 'De impedimento eucharistie'.

[32] Ibid. vi. 14/8, 'De modestia ordinandi'.

custodian of a sick person, was allegedly involved in a case of malpractice which ended in the death of the patient. Can he be promoted to higher orders? What about physicians (*Quid est de medicis?*), asks *Astesana*, thereby implying that at the beginning of the fourteenth century some physicians were also clerics. *Astesana* rules that if the death cannot be shown to have been the fault of the physician or the attendant, it does not create an impediment to ecclesiastical promotion. A sudden traumatic shock caused by an unpredictable complexional fluctuation fatally affecting the patient in the midst of surgery or phlebotomy is one of the clinical scenarios discussed by *Astesana*. It adds 'sensible advice' (*sanum consilium*), though, attributed to the canonist Bernardus (probably Bernard of Parma) and acclaimed by Hostiensis, suggesting that those who have been ordained or anticipate ordination should refrain from practising surgery. Bernardus specifically allows clerics to perfom cauterization because it does not necessarily lead to the spilling of blood; but Ramon de Penyafort differs on this issue. He forbids all clerics to practise medicine (*phisica*) as long as they are beneficed. While he strictly forbids surgery under any circumstances, clerics are allowed to provide medical care for the poor without any monetary remuneration, for their brethren, and for their family.

Evidence for the existence of ambivalence towards medicine, and in extreme cases rejection of human medical care, suggests that a third pattern of relationship between medicine and religion—that of rivalry—must also be taken into account. The prohibitions on monks studying and practising medicine imply a fear that theology and the monastic lifestyle may be undermined by a preoccupation with medicine. The rivalry between medicine and religion can be seen among some monastic writers, who criticize corporeal medical cure which comes at the expense of the far more important cure of souls. But the main text which communicates this sense of rivalry between medicine and religion is clearly Canon 22 of Lateran IV (1215), which cautions physicians who are treating severely ill patients to summon the priest and thus ensure that the patient has confessed before the actual treatment starts.[33] The canon creates distinct boundaries between the physicians of the body and those of the soul. Its underlying assumption is that bodily disease is

---

[33] The text of Canon 22 is in A. García y García (ed.), *Constitutiones Concilii quarti Lateranensis una cum commentariis glossatorum* (Vatican City, 1981), 68–9. The English version is in *Decrees of the Ecumenical Councils*, i. 245–6. Cf. *Astesana*, v. 16, 'Qualis debet esse Confessor', which adds the adverb *districte* to Innocent's prohibition and quotes Hostiensis and the gloss of Johannes Teutonicus as well.

sometimes (*nonnunquam*) caused by sin and therefore it is necessary first
to provide for the health of the soul before proceeding to physical cure.
The penal clause (anathema) is followed by a more general prohibition of
any treatment which would endanger the soul of the patient. This is
based on the belief that the soul is much more precious than the body.
The commentaries of Johannes Teutonicus, Vincentius Hispanus,
Damasus, Casus Parisienses and Casus Fuldenses add little to its content,
but all stress the absolute priority of health of the soul over that of the
body. The canonist Henry of Susa (Hostiensis, 1200–79) is the only glos-
sator who makes a substantial addition in his commentary, when he labels
transgression against the canon as a mortal sin.[34]

Convergence, separation, rivalry: which of the three was dominant
around 1300?

Why 1300?

The role of medicine and medical practitioners in a divinely ordained society strictly governed by Christian ethical mores and a powerful clerical
order can be discussed in relation to every century in the middle ages, if not
to every period in the history of any traditional society.[35] But the years
around 1300 in the West have special interest for the historical researcher,
as has been shown by recent scholarship in the history of medicine.

According to Luis García-Ballester,[36] this is the period in which a new
form of medicine resting on new concepts and a new understanding of
desirable ways and methods of medical training was finally introduced
and accepted in the Latin West. It was the culmination of a process, starting in the late eleventh century in southern Europe, of basing medicine
on natural philosophy. The translation into Latin of a set of Arabic medical texts (particularly the *Isagoge* of Johannitius and the *Pantegni* of
Haly Abbas) by Constantinus Africanus (d. 1087) in Monte Cassino
required in their reader an understanding of Aristotle's cosmological and
biological ideas to render intelligible their Galenic foundation.

[34] García y García (ed.), *Constitutiones*, 209, 316–17, 429, and 469. Hostiensis, *In quin-
tum Decretalium Librum Commentaria* (Venice, 1581), 103va (*De penitentiis et remissionibus*, c.
xiii).
[35] *Health/Medicine and the Faith Traditions: An Inquiry into Religion and Medicine*, ed.
M. E. Marty and K. L. Vaux (Philadelphia, 1982); R. Porter, 'Religion and Medicine', in
Companion Encyclopedia of the History of Medicine, ed. W. F. Bynum and R. Porter (London
and New York, 1993), ii. 1449–68.
[36] García-Ballester, 'The Construction of a New Form of Learning and Practicing
Medicine in Medieval Latin Europe'.

Henceforth, a physician who wished to approach his profession with a certain degree of competence and produce rationally founded explanations for pathological conditions needed to master a new and ever-growing corpus of medical and natural philosophical knowledge. The Constantinian corpus of medical texts was only minimally adapted to its new ethical environment and to the moral dictates of the Church.[37]

Constantinus was only one of several translators in southern Italy and Sicily in the eleventh century who introduced hitherto unknown medical texts of Greek origin and a new model of Arabic medicine. The medical school at Salerno became an important centre for the diffusion of works of Aristotle and of newly recovered medical texts. *De urinis* by Theophilus Protospatharius, a treatise on pulses attributed to Philaretus, Galen's *Tegni*, and the *Aphorisms* and *Prognosis* of Hippocrates are some of these new treatises which, in the twelfth century, came to provide the basis for the training of physicians in southern Italy. By the second half of the twelfth century the *Isagoge*, 'On Urines', 'On Pulses', 'Aphorisms', and 'Prognosis' were being commented on with glosses and scholastic questions.[38] These commentaries suggest a growing tendency to fuse the empiricist tradition of medicine with the theoretical tradition, a hitherto unknown phenomenon amongst Latin medical authors. The empiricist tradition stressed the cure of the disease rather than its causes, and rejected medicine based on reasoning from the hidden causes of disease in favour of that based solely on experience.

Another important centre for the diffusion of medical knowledge in the twelfth century was Toledo, which is more renowned for its role in reintroducing Aristotle's *libri naturales* to the Latin West. There, Gerard of Cremona (d. 1187) translated Avicenna's *Canon*, which played a decisive role in the Aristotelizing Galenism that was implanted in the university medical schools from the first third of the thirteenth century. For medicine to appear on an equal footing with other academic disciplines, it was first necessary to apply the new logic to medical instruction. New technical language had to be invented and accepted in the universities so that medical scholars could begin to appreciate the full sophistication of

---

[37] D. Jacquart, 'Aristotelian Thought in Salerno', in *A History of Twelfth-Century Western Philosophy*, ed. P. Dronke (Cambridge, 1988), 407–28; id., 'The Influence of Arabic Medicine in the Medieval West', in *Encyclopedia of the History of Arabic Science*, iii, ed. R. Rashed (London and New York, 1996), 963–84; D. Jacquart and F. Micheau, *La Médecine arabe et l'Occident médiéval* (Paris, 1990), 118–29; M. H. Green, '*Constantinus Africanus* and the Conflict between Religion and Science', in G. R. Dunstan (ed.), *The Human Embryo: Aristotle and the Arabic and European Traditions* (Exeter, 1990), 47– 69.

[38] B. Lawn, *The Prose Salernitan Questions* (London, 1979).

Greco-Arabic traditions, assimilate them, and develop them. This was a lengthy process: it was not until 40 years after Gerard of Cremona's death that the systematic use of Avicenna's *Canon* in Europe began. From the second third of the thirteenth century onwards, the energy of physicians articulated and extended their theoretical knowledge along Avicennan lines. The success of their efforts gave learned medicine the intellectual sophistication necessary to break away from its sources and create a distinctive Latin medical tradition.[39]

By the end of the thirteenth century, there had developed a new method of inquiry and communication (the scholastic *lectio–questio–disputatio* scheme) and a new institution for the transmission of knowledge (the university). The medical faculty was not only a shrine of knowledge which served the particular interests of those engaged in the medical profession: through examinations and licensing policies, it enabled the civil power to establish and develop a system of medical care. An employment market linking the world of knowledge to that of practice gradually emerged.

What was the concept of health which emerged from the new medical writings of physicians well-versed in Aristotelian natural philosophy? According to most modern historians of medicine, the medical system that emerged was religiously neutral.[40] Learned medical practitioners came to understand health according to the intellectual criteria formulated in Aristotle's *libri naturales*. The physician was expected to be concerned with bodily health defined in terms of a balance of the basic qualities of heat, cold, dampness, and dryness. Health was also defined with the help of other concepts introduced into western medicine through the translations of Arabic works and the Galenic corpus. The quantitative and qualitative balance of the body as a whole and of each of its parts (*complexio*) became a key concept for defining and explaining healthy or pathological conditions. A balanced complexion (*equalis complexio*) meant health, whereas an imbalanced complexion (*inequalis complexio, discrasia*) indicated the presence of a disease. The concept of the 'radical moisture' (*humidum radicale*) was used to explain the natural process of ageing and death and certain pathological processes related to fevers.[41] It came to

---

[39] M. R. McVaugh, 'Medical Knowledge at the Time of Frederick II', *Micrologus*, 2 (1994), 3–17; Jacquart and Micheau, *La Médecine arabe et l'Occident Médiéval*, 147–65; D. Jacquart, 'Les traductions médicales de Gérard de Crémone', in P. Pizzamiglio (ed.), *Gerardo da Cremona* (Cremona, 1992), 57–70.

[40] García-Ballester, 'The Construction of a New Form of Learning', 86–91.

[41] On this concept which was developed in classical antiquity and the Middle Ages see M. R. McVaugh, 'The *Humidum Radicale* in Thirteenth-Century Medicine', *Traditio*, 30 (1974), 259–83.

define medicine's boundaries: although the physician cannot stop the ageing process or prevent death, he can slow down the process of desiccation which is at the root of man's physical decline. Once the physician has identified the patient's individual complexion, he can devise a regimen for preserving his health.

Galenism endeavoured to regulate human life to guarantee a healthy balance between the individual's body and the environment in which he lived. A man's health was thus also the product of the 'six non-natural things', necessary for life and affecting the condition of the body, though not part of his natural endowments. Making up the physical, social, and moral environment, they were: air and environment, food and drink, sleep and wakefulness, motion and rest, evacuation and repletion, and the passions of the soul. A substantial part of the causal and therapeutic explanation of Galenic pathology, as well as the entire doctrine of the preservation and maintenance of health, were based on the six non-natural things.[42]

The fuller assimilation of Greek medical theory in the Latin West from the second half of the thirteenth century onwards had practical implications; it divested disease of its social and moral meanings and helped to change social attitudes towards it. This is particularly visible in the case of leprosy. The difference in attitudes towards lepers in medieval Islamic societies and Christian societies reflected the morally neutral aetiology based on Greek medical theory adopted by the Arabs and the moral or religious meaning attached to the disease by Christians. But the gradual assimilation of Greek medical theory into Western medical tradition brought about a change of attitudes towards the disease. As it came under the authority of the physicians it lost its moral meaning and came to be treated on the basis of its natural aetiology: the writing of learned physicians who offered preservative, curative, and palliative treatments of leprosy suggest that they did not call on supernatural help to cure this disease.[43]

[42] L. García-Ballester, 'Dietetic and Pharmacological Therapy: A Dilemma Among Fourteenth-Century Jewish Practitioners in the Montpellier Area', *Clio Medica*, 22 (1991), 24. On the Hippocratic origin of that notion see O. Temkin, *Hippocrates in a World of Pagans and Christians* (Baltimore and London, 1991), 190, and L. García-Ballester, 'On the Origin of the "six non-natural things" in Galen', in *Galen und das Hellenistische Erbe*, ed. K. Kollesch and D. Nickel (Stuttgart, 1993), 105–15.

[43] M. W. Dols, *The Black Death in the Middle East* (Princeton, 1977), 284–301; id., 'The Leper in Medieval Islamic Society', *Speculum*, 58 (1984), 891–916; McVaugh, *Medicine before the Plague*, 218–25; L. E. Demaitre, 'The Description and Diagnosis of Leprosy by Fourteenth-Century Physicians', *Bulletin of the History of Medicine*, 59 (1985), 327–44; id., 'The Relevance of Futility: Jordanus de Turre (fl. 1313–1335) on the Treatment of Leprosy', *Bulletin of the History of Medicine*, 70 (1996), 26–81 at 35–6.

Physicians won growing social acceptance as health was increasingly perceived as a community objective.[44] They started appearing as professional witnesses in lawsuits concerning environmental pollution. Ecclesiastical courts could ask physicians to appear as experts. In Aragon, physicians could overrule the decision of a lay jury which confirmed cases of suspected leprosy. City councils endeavoured to confront the health problems of the community and individuals within it by hiring academically trained medical professionals. A new market was opened up in which health was conceived as something to be bought and therefore subject to legal control. A dense network of physicians emerged in many regions of Italy from the mid-thirteenth century onwards, and in Provence and the Crown of Aragon from the closing years of that century. By supporting these men, the urban bourgeoisie provided physicians with the backing of their own social position and prestige and expressed a growing satisfaction with their effectiveness as dispensers of health. The vibrant medical market supplied the physicians with higher salaries and more lucrative contracts.

References to medical authors were very rare in the universities in the first half of the thirteenth century. This was the formative stage of medieval universities; but, for academic medicine, it was marked by the decline of the medical school at Salerno and the prominence of just three *studia*: Bologna, Montpellier, and Paris. Medicine was none the less taught in other schools in the thirteenth century. For example, the study of medicine was certainly part of the curriculum of the Paduan school by 1262,[45] and there is some evidence that medical degrees were granted in Naples. However, the size of these schools, their literary output, and the scope of medical activity they show relegate them to a position of insignificance in comparison with Bologna, Montpellier, and Paris. Although Padua's insignificance was soon to be reversed, by 1300 it already enjoyed a certain modest distinction and was well within the mainstream of European medical development.

The medical university at Montpellier received its first statutes in 1220; they were revised in 1240. We know of no statutes for the Parisian medical faculty before 1270, the year in which the first formal medical degrees were granted by the University of Bologna.[46] By 1300 the medical

[44] García-Ballester, 'The Construction of a New Form of Learning', 90–1.

[45] N. G. Siraisi, *Arts and Sciences at Padua: The Studium of Padua before 1350* (Toronto, 1973), 145.

[46] McVaugh, 'Medical Knowledge at the Time of Frederik II', 3; N. G. Siraisi, 'The Faculty of Medicine', in *A History of the University in Europe*, i. *Universities in the Middle Ages*, ed. H. De Ridder-Symoens (Cambridge, 1992), 360–87 at 364–9.

schools in Montpellier, Bologna, Padua, and Paris produced the new academically trained practitioner. This physician, increasingly likely to be a layman, had acquired certain knowledge about the constitution of matter and the cosmos in general which was essential to his trade. The major sources of this knowledge were Aristotelian natural philosophy and Galenism. They were revived and renewed during the thirteenth century, and established a close causal relationship between the components of living matter (elements, qualities, humours) and health. The Salernitan commentators had already discovered the link between medicine and natural philosophy through the *Pantegni*, the *Isagoge*, and Aristotle himself. But the university system institutionalized it. From now on, the libraries of university-trained physicians would testify to the existence of this link. For this 'new' physician, diagnosis of disease came before the aspiration to cure it. Versed in Aristotelian biological and physical knowledge and in Aristotle's rules of logic, the physician was expected to reflect upon the causes of health and disease and to produce an efficient therapy. Yet this did not mean erasure of the disciplinary boundaries between medicine and natural philosophy. Where the lines should be drawn was a topic discussed among academic physicians from the 1240s, thus suggesting that the disciplines were entrenched well before the statutes appeared.[47]

By 1300 Italian physicians came to employ a new channel for improving their anatomical knowledge, performing anatomical dissections and medical post-mortems. The first unambiguous record for an autopsy performed by a Cremonese physician curious to determine the cause of death in times of an epidemic dates from 1286. The forensic context provided Bolognese physicians with ample opportunities to dissect bodies in order to look for hidden and internal causes of death. By the early fourteenth century, the university of Bologna had introduced the practice of dissecting human corpses into the study and teaching of anatomy; the first unambiguous account of such a dissection, performed by Taddeo Alderotti, refers to 1316 and appears in the anatomy textbook of his student, Mondino de' Liuzzi.[48] For various reasons dissection remained infrequent before the fifteenth century, and its objective was instruction more than investigation. But the reintroduction of human dissection on

---

[47] García-Ballester, 'The Construction of a New Form of Medical Learning', 92.

[48] K. Park, 'The Criminal and the Saintly Body: Autopsy and Dissection in Renaissance Italy', *Renaissance Quarterly*, 47 (1994), 1–33, esp. 4–13, and 'The Life of the Corpse: Division and Dissection in Late Medieval Europe', *The Journal of the History of Medicine and Allied Sciences*, 50 (1995), 111–32; Siraisi, *Medieval and Early Renaissance Medicine*, 86–97.

a regular basis is an evidence for the growing commitment of the new physician to first-hand knowledge and understanding of the internal organs.

Full social acceptance of the new type of physician and the new way of conceiving medicine would eventually take place only when the new physician was able to offer specific strategies for the maintenance and restoration of good health. Meanwhile, the ratio of university-trained physicians to inhabitants even in the most privileged regions of southern Europe is estimated to be no more than between 1 and 6 per 10,000.[49] Medical practitioners emerging from the academic world were a new phenomenon, and hence constituted a small minority (albeit a growing one) among the medical community, and an even smaller one among the people as a whole.

This concise summary of the history of western learned medicine between the eleventh and fourteenth centuries entirely ignores its religious aspects. It is my contention that this omission is serious. The layman or cleric studying medicine in the schools was exposed during his training to various forms of ecclesiastical control and influence. For example, the statutes of the medical school at Montpellier (where Arnau de Vilanova taught between 1289 and 1300 and perhaps also between 1305 and 1308) reveal the extent of the Church's absolute institutional control.[50] The statutes were issued by papal authority, and they regulated every aspect in the school's activities.[51] They enjoined religious duties such as funeral attendance, weekly mass,[52] taking oaths to observe the statutes upon inception, the obligation for all holders of ecclesiastical benefices or those in holy orders to receive the tonsure, and punishment by anathema in case of a breach of the statutes.

The administration of the medical university of Montpellier was closely monitored and controlled by the ecclesiastical authority. Its chancellor could be elected only with episcopal agreement: according to the

[49] L. García-Ballester, M. R. McVaugh, and A. Rubio-Vela, 'Medical Licensing and Learning in Fourteenth-Century Valencia', *Transactions of the American Philosophical Society*, 79/6 (1989), 54.
[50] All the following references to the Montpellier statutes are from *Cart. Mont.* On the school of medicine at Montpellier see L. Dulieu, *La Médecine à Montpellier*, i (Montpellier, 1975).
[51] For 1220 *Cart. Mont.*, 180–3—Cardinal Conrad of Urach; for 1239, ibid., 185–6—bishop Guido Soranus, legate of Gregory IX; for 1289 ibid., 210–12—apostolic letter of Nicholas IV decreeing the establishment of a *studium generale* in Montpellier; for 1309, ibid., 219–21—Clement V's decision.
[52] This duty was added in the statutes of 1340: *Cart. Mont.*, 341. Attendance was obligatory and fines for failing to attend were imposed according to status.

statutes from 1240, he would be required to perform his oath in front of the bishop of Maguelonne. In 1309 Clement V changed the procedure of electing a chancellor. The new procedure, which demanded a two-thirds majority of the masters, retained the bishop's right of veto and was reconfirmed in 1324. A copy of the statutes was to be kept by the chancellor of the school, the bishop, and the prior of the church of St Firmin.[53] As early as 1239 the bishop acquired a key position in licensing graduates. He would select two masters (in consultation with the guild of physicians) to assist him in deciding whether a bachelor was worthy to practise. It was his prerogative to exempt the bachelor from two more years of study after taking the bachelor's oath.[54] The bishop was to act as judge of appeal in civil cases, as sole judge in criminal cases, and would intervene whenever institutional upheavals occurred.[55] He would also receive complaints and appeals by the medical university against his judicial vicar (*officialis*) if he violated the statutes or overstretched his authority, or against any university procedure which harmed one of its members.[56] The medical university or individual masters could appeal to the Pope whenever they felt that the bishop (directly or through the *officialis*) or the university had violated the statutes. An unconstitutional interference by the bishop or his (*officialis*) in the university's licensing policy, desire to secure medical licence to a protégé found unsuitable by the university, or a need to defend the bishop from a violent and undisciplined master would instigate papal intervention in the activities of the medical university. Pope John XXII was particularly active in this respect.[57] The Papacy also could set the academic curriculum. In a papal decision of 1309 Clement V, advised by Arnau de Vilanova, introduced a new medical curriculum based mainly on Galenic texts (some of them newly introduced to the West).[58]

Did these strong institutional ties between the medical school and the Church affect the content of the medicine taught and the scholars' grounding in medical ethics and religious education? The religious and cultural context of academic medicine throughout the middle ages included powerful traditions linking physical cure with religious charity and/or miraculous intervention. How did these traditions and the imperative that gave at least lip-service to the priority of the cure of the soul over that of the body affect the content of learned medicine? What influence did the

---

[53] Ibid. 181, 222–3, 224–5, 252–3.
[54] Ibid. 188. On the licensing procedures at Montpellier in the fourteenth century, see ibid., 217–19 and García-Ballester *et al.*, 'Medical Licensing', 12–13.
[55] *Cart. Mont.*, 186.   [56] Ibid. 203–6 (for 1281), 238.
[57] Ibid. 213–15, 235–6, 249, 278–80, 280–1.   [58] Ibid. 219–21.

presence of theological institutions (whether as faculties of theology within the university or as independent *studia* run by the Orders) have on the relations between theologians and medicine or physicians? The immediate outcome of the incorporation of medicine into the university system north of the Alps was the clericalization of the profession,[59] and some exchange of knowledge between theologians and physicians who were studying in the same towns (and sometimes in the same institutions) is therefore predictable. Nancy Siraisi suggests that although metaphysics was certainly thought to be a necessary part of the training in arts given to future physicians, it is conceivable that this subject may have been somewhat neglected by teachers whose orientation was towards medical practice. In the case of the medical school in Padua, Pietro d'Abano, who had a special interest in metaphysical questions, was unique. In Paris and other northern *studia* the influence of theology on medicine was only indirect and came via the impact of the faculty of theology on the faculty of arts. At the same time, the absence of faculties of theology in the formative years of the Italian medical schools had the effect of leaving philosophy free to develop a particularly close association with medicine.[60]

In the particular case of Montpellier, which did not have a faculty of theology until 1421, did the scholars or the masters in the faculty of medicine have any contacts with formal theological studies? We know too little about such specific contacts, but the infrastructure which would make them plausible was there. Arnau de Vilanova's career reveals one such possible channel of influence through the Dominican *studium* at Montpellier which, together with the Dominican schools at Barcelona and Cologne, acquired the status of a *studium generale* at the general chapter convened in 1303 in Besançon.[61] From 1263 a Cistercian *studium theologie* around the monastery of Valmagne also permitted interested outsiders to gain theological knowledge, though little is known about it. By 1281 it had to face competition from the newly founded *studium* in Toulouse. The Franciscan convent in Montpellier acquired the status of *studium generale* in 1281 and provided yet another place of possible encounter between scholars of medicine and of theology.[62]

[59] Jacquart, *Le Milieu médical*, 380, table 15, and Getz, 'The Faculty of Medicine', 388, for the clerical character of Oxford.

[60] Siraisi, 'The Faculty of Medicine', 374, and *Arts and Sciences at Padua*, 135.

[61] A. Germain, *Histoire de la Commune de Montpellier*, iii (Montpellier, 1851), 323; cf. p. 22 below.

[62] *Cart. Mont.*, 197–8; A. Gouron, 'Deux universités pour une ville', in G. Cholvy (ed.), *Histoire de Montpellier* (Montpellier, 1985), 114–16.

Let us now examine the image of this 'new physician' using medieval sources. The image of the perfect physician who is a model of moral uprightness is a commonplace in late medieval literature. For example, the Dominican Jacopo de Cessole (Jacobus de Cessolis), a member of the Dominican house in Genoa between 1318 and 1322, introduced chess as a poetic metaphor for social and political analysis, in his *Solacium ludi schaccorum*.[63] By identifying the castles, rooks, and knights with the representatives of the higher estates (*nobiles*) and comparing the pawns to members of the lower social classes (*populares*) he criticized his own society. Each of the eight pawns represents one to three different members of the lower social class (peasant; smith, bricklayer or carpenter; notary or cloth-maker; merchant or money-changer; innkeepers; town custodians; gamblers, wastrels, or vagabond) and receives a specific moralization. The fifth pawn, standing in front of the queen, represents the physician, the apothecary, and the surgeon.[64] Jacopo, who depicts the physician as holding a book in his right hand, an apothecary's mortar in his left and carrying iron tools on his belt for treating wounds and ulcers, stresses that the perfect physician should be acquainted with the relevant literature of medical science (Hippocrates, Galen, Avicenna, and Rhazes) as well as all the liberal arts. This portrayal of the learned physician reflects the growing prestige of medicine in the first half of the fourteenth century and the strong links between natural philosophy and medicine. The perfect physician exhibits moral propriety (*humanitas morum*), refined eloquence (*urbanitas verborum*), and chastity (*castitas corporis*). The physician's position on the chessboard before the queen hints at the chastity expected from him when treating women and examining their private parts. The perfect physician promises a cure and visits his patients frequently. Yet the *Solacium ludi schaccorum* criticizes both the surgeons, who have acquired the reputation of pitiless butchers, and the apothecaries, who constantly make mistakes in concocting medicines and who irresponsibly sell poisonous medicines to simple people. The emergence of scholastic medicine also has a price, and Jacopo condemns the excessive litigiousness of physicians, their indulgence in hair-splitting, and their futile discussions, in which they assess each other's competence

---

[63] H. J. R. Murray, *A History of Chess* (Oxford, 1913), 529–63 and esp. 537–45; E. Köpke, *Iacobus de Cessolis* (Brandenburg a. d. Havel, 1879); R. A. Müller, *Der Arzt im Schachspiel bei Jakob von Cessolis* (Munich, 1981); Kaeppeli, *Scriptores Ordinis Praedicatorum* ii. 311–18; J.-Th. Welter, *L'Exemplum dans la littérature religieuse et didactique du Moyen Âge* (Paris, 1927), 351–4.

[64] Müller, *Der Arzt im Schachspiel*, 34–5.

by their ability to argue, not by the efficacy of their treatments. He does not hint at any possible spiritual implications of medical practice and knowledge; nor does he suggest that some form of tension prevailed between physicians and the clergy.

Other invectives against medical men in that period revolved around the greediness of the physicians, their barren scholastic approach, their presumption, and their incompetence. Petrarch in his *Invectivarum contra medicum quendam libri IV* (*c.*1352/3) rebuked physicians for preferring a socially profitable and lucrative profession to the cultivation of their moral integrity. He reproached them for their tendency to indulge in dialectic and rhetoric, and to confuse curing with persuasion. He hinted at their inclination to breach the limits of their discipline by behaving as if they were philosophers, and criticized the unfounded arrogance of those who pretended to a monopoly on health and even claimed to resurrect the dead, thus usurping the glory due to God.[65]

Finally, let us return to Humbert de Romans's sermon. After praising the physicians and their academic discipline, Humbert also discusses the moral dangers involved in medical practice and focuses the second part of the sermon on the religious significance of medical malpractice. He openly condemns ignorant physicians who harm rather than cure; avaricious practitioners who exploit the distress of the patient's family for private gain and charge excessive fees; and those who neglect to fulfil the religious duties imposed on a Christian physician. The first are guilty of homicide; the second are traitors; the last are religious rebels. Physicians are expected above all to refrain from any medical practice which contravenes divine commands or endangers the patient's soul. They should also have faith in God rather than in the absolute efficacy of their art when it comes to treating their patients. Prayer is thus the proper reaction to disease, for does not Ecclesiasticus 38 speak of physicians who should pray for the sick?[66] Medical practitioners thus constitute a potential danger to their patients' souls, and are branded as prone to laxity in faith. It would

---

[65] 'Miseri qui sub auxilii vestri fiducia egrotant! Christus autem, in cuius manu salus hominum sita est, salvum illum, ignorantibus omnibus vobis, fecit—et faciat precor quantum sibi, quantum ecclesie, cui presidet, est necesse!—; vos, Dei beneficium et complexionis ac nature sue laudem usurpantes videri vultis illum a mortuis suscitasse, et nunc laudem, transacto periculo concordatis'. Petrarch, *Contra medicum objurgantem invectivarum libri IV*, i. 105–14, in F. Petrarca, *Invective contra medicum*, ed. P. G. Ricci and B. Martinelli (Rome, 1978); B. Martinelli, 'Il Petrarca e la Medicina', ibid. 201–49; K. Bergdolt, *Arzt, Krankheit und Therapie bei Petrarca* (Darmstadt, 1992), esp. ch. 40; Park, *Doctors and Medicine*, 221–4.

[66] Humbert de Romans, *Sermones ad diuersos status*, tr. I, 66. Cf. Appendix III, pp. 318–19.

be rash simply to tie physicians with heresy;[67] but Humbert's warnings to them induce us to explore the form assumed by the traditional tensions between medicine's physical and spiritual aspects. Was his concern about the religious reliability of physicians the result of the actual behaviour of medical practitioners? This is the second theme discussed in this book, which attempts to explore the spiritual aspects of learned medicine around 1300 and to re-examine the notion of a growing separation between the medical and the clerical functions. The focus of this study is a parallel analysis of religious attitudes in medical writings and of the medical impact on the spiritual writings of learned physicians.[68] This will clarify Humbert's praise for medicine as a vehicle for religious specula-tion and his anxieties over the physician's moral and religious behaviour.

Arnau de Vilanova: a Biographical Note

I have chosen to focus my discussion on Arnau de Vilanova (*c.*1240–1311) because he produced a large corpus of medical as well as spiritual works, which give us access to his mind, and because he exem-plifies the shortcomings of the historiographical approach that sharply separates medical careers from religious and spiritual interests. Arnau was, and still is, recognized as a leading academic physician at the turn of the thirteenth and fourteenth centuries. In his lifetime and beyond, he was constantly attacked by Church authorities. This loaded relationship with the Church initially triggered my research. In what follows I shall offer a short biography of Arnau and then use him to illustrate the fun-damental argument of this book: namely, that medicine in this period had a cultural and spiritual/religious role which went far beyond its thera-peutic function.

More is known about Arnau's spiritual than his medical career, but from at least the late 1280s they were intertwined. The last decade of his life was dominated by his spiritual interests and political activities, though even then he produced some important medical texts and par-ticipated in the reform and regularization of medical education at Montpellier. In the 1290s, while he was teaching at Montpellier and was

---

[67] For the scant evidence concerning medical practitioners among thirteenth-century Cathars and Waldensians see P. Biller, '*Curate infirmos*: The Medieval Waldensian Practice of Medicine', in *The Church and Healing*, ed. Sheils, 55–77; W. L. Wakefield, 'Heretics as Physicians in the Thirteenth Century', *Speculum*, 57 (1982), 328–31.

[68] Cf. Jacquart, *Le Milieu médical*, 223 n. 1 for a list of all medical practitioners con-nected with the medieval French intellectual milieu who produced philosophical and theo-logical writings.

fully immersed in scholastic medicine, he produced some of his longest and more influential spiritual texts. I shall therefore describe the parallel development of Arnau's two careers. Only a few details are known with certainty about Arnau's early years.[69] A Catalan by birth, he spent his childhood in Valencia where he received his primary education and was tonsured (probably between 1250 and 1255). In the 1260s he was a student at the *studium* of Montpellier, where during that decade he completed his Arts course and eventually acquired the title of Master of Medicine. There are two contradictory pieces of evidence for his study of theology from his later life. His opponents held that Arnau, as a physician with no theological training, could not speak with authority about theological matters. When the issue came up in the polemic of Girona in 1303, Arnau declared that he had not only heard (*audivit*) theology but also solemnly read (*legit*) it at the Dominican school in Montpellier. To read theology meant to lecture on it; nevertheless, all historians who studied Arnau interpreted the expression as denoting his having being taught by the Dominicans.[70] The second piece of evidence appears in a letter which Arnau wrote in 1304 to Pope Benedict XI. There he did not deny an allegation that, except for six months of theology, all his studies were based on the secular sciences.[71] Whether Arnau only listened for six months to lectures in theology or participated in a more structured course at the Dominican school in Montpellier, he certainly never acquired a degree in theology, which would have authorized him to speak publicly on theological matters.

At an unknown time and prior to his departure to Barcelona, Arnau married Agnès Blasi in Valencia. The couple had a daughter called Maria

[69] For the vast bibliography on Arnau see J. Mensa i Valls, *Arnau de Vilanova, espiritu-al: Guia bibliogràfica* (Barcelona, 1994). The most recent biographical summary of Arnau is J. Perarnau and F. Santi, 'Villeneuve (Vilanova, Arnaud de)', in *DS* 16 (1994), 785–97, and J. A. Paniagua, 'Cronología de los hechos conocidos de la vida de Arnau de Vilanova' in id., *Studia Arnaldiana: Trabajos en torno a la obra médica de Arnau de Vilanova, c.*1240–1311 (Barcelona, 1994), 465–81. See also M. R. McVaugh, 'Arnald of Vilanova', in *Dictionary of Scientific Biography*, i (New York, 1970), 289–91; M. Gerwing, *Vom Ende der Zeit: Der Traktat des Arnald von Villanova über die Ankunft des Antichrist in der akademischen Auseinandersetzung zu Beginn des 14 Jahrhunderts* (Münster, 1996), 26–75.

[70] *Tertia denunciatio gerundensis*, in J. Carreras i Artau, 'La polémica gerundense sobre el Anticristo entre Arnau de Vilanova y los dominicos', *Anales del Instituto de Estudios Gerundenses*, 5/6 (1950/1), 55; cf. Arnau de Vilanova, *Obres Catalanes* i, ed. M. Batllori (Barcelona, 1947), 16, and F. Santi, *Arnau de Vilanova: L'obra espiritual* (Valencia, 1987), 84.

[71] *De morte Bonifatii*, MS Vat.lat. fol.213^{va-b}; cf. H. Finke, *Aus den Tagen Bonifaz VIII* (Münster, 1902), p. cxc. 'semper in scientiis secularibus ab infantia quasi vel puericia studui et nunquam scolas theologicorum nisi sex mensibus aut circiter frequentavi'.

who would end her life in a Dominican nunnery. In 1312 Pope Clement V, who was looking for a medical book allegedly written for him by the deceased physician, referred to Arnau as a cleric of the diocese of Valencia (*clericus Valentine diocesis*).[72] This reinforces the view that Arnau was a married clerk (*clericus coniugatus*). Yet his lifestyle suggests full assimilation into the laity; it induced Paul Diepgen to regard him as a lay theologian.[73] By 1280 he was a physician at the Aragonese royal court and acquired in 1281 an annual rent of 2,000 écus of Barcelona from Peter III of Aragon, in recognition of his services and on condition that he reside in Barcelona. During his stay in Barcelona in the early 1280s he improved his theological knowledge by attending the Dominican school where Ramon Martí was the most prominent master. Here he also learned Arabic and possibly rudimentary Hebrew, and in 1282 he concluded (alone or with collaborators) his translation from Arabic of the Galenic treatise *De rigore et tremore et iectigatione et spasmo*.[74] He also translated Avicenna's *De viribus cordis*.

James II, king of Aragon from 1285, and his brother Frederick III, king of Trinacria (Sicily) (1296–1337), entrusted Arnau with the well-being of the royal family (including giving medical advice during the pregnancy of the Aragonese queen, Blanche of Anjou) as well as with various state affairs. It is likely that as early as 1288, Arnau started to work on the controversial eschatological treatise *De tempore adventus Antichristi*, which would place him at the end of the century on a collision course with the theologians of Paris.

From 1289 or 1290 Arnau was again based in Montpellier where he launched his academic career as a Professor of Medicine. It is possible that during this time he was exposed to the spiritual, apocalyptic mood which engulfed Franciscan circles in Montpellier.[75] It is also possible that during these years he actually met Peter of John (Olivi) who lectured at the Franciscan *studium generale* in Montpellier from 1289. Apart from ideological affinities, no direct link between the two can be established.

---

[72] A. Rubió i Lluch, *Documents per l'història de la cultura catalana mig-eval*, i (Barcelona, 1908), 56–7, no. xliv.

[73] P. Diepgen, *Arnald von Villanova als Politiker und Laientheologe* (Berlin and Leipzig, 1909), 15.

[74] *AVOMO*, xvi, ed. M. R. McVaugh (Barcelona, 1981). *AVOMO* is the critical edition of Arnau's medical texts. The publication, which started in 1975, is still continuing and its general editors are L. García-Ballester, M. R. McVaugh and J. A. Paniagua.

[75] Santi, *Arnau de Vilanova*, 109; R. Manselli, *Spirituali e Beghini in Provenza* (Rome, 1959), 55–80, and 'La religiosità d'Arnaldo da Villanova', *Bullettino dell'Istituto Storico Italiano per il Medio Evo e Archivio Muratoriano*, 63 (1951), 1–100, at 23–42.

During this period he produced both medical and spiritual texts. Among the spiritual works we find didactic treatises such as _Alphabetum catholicorum ad inclitum regem Aragonum pro filiis erudiendis_[76] and _De prudentia catholicorum scholarium_[77] (composed for the royal house of Aragon between 1295 and 1297); anti-Jewish apologetics (_Allocutio super significatione nominis tetragrammaton_,[78] c.1292); and prophecy and reform (_Introductio in librum Ioachim De semine scripturarum_,[79] c.1292). His medical corpus during this period probably included _De intentione medicorum_, a commentary on Galen's _De malitia complexionis diverse_, _De dosi tyriacali_, _De consideracionibus operis medicine_, _Aphorismi de gradibus_, _De humido radicali_, _Repetitio super canone 'Vita brevis'_, and _De parte operativa_.[80] This miscellaneous corpus reflects Arnau's contribution to medieval Western medicine; he fused the Western empirical tradition with the systematic medical philosophy of the Greeks and Arabs.

After 1300, when he resigned his professorial chair at the University of Montpellier, he was associated with the court of King James II of the Crown of Aragon and with the papal curia of Boniface VIII and his successors, Benedict XI and Clement V. Arnau's appointment as a physician to the papal court allowed him to recruit help from Boniface VIII during the first stage of his clash with the theologians of Paris. Arnau's medical output between 1300 and 1305 declined, but did not cease. In 1300, according to some manuscript versions of the _Medicationis parabole_, he may have dedicated this compilation of aphorisms to Philip IV, possibly to win the king's support against the Paris theologians. In July 1301 he finished a practical book on health (_regimen sanitatis_, possibly the treatise known as _Contra calculum_) which he dedicated to Boniface VIII. Yet during this tumultuous period he focused most of his intellectual efforts on trying to change the attitude of the Church to his eschatological message.

Arnau's collision with the Church occurred in three stages. The first was the Paris controversy and its repercussions in 1300 and 1301; the second,

---

[76] _Dyalogus de elementis catholice fidei_ (_Alphabetum catholicorum_) in W. Burger, 'Beiträge zur Geschichte der Katechese im Mittelalter', _Römische Quartalschrift_ (Geschichte), 21/4 (1907), 173–94.

[77] Graziano di Santa Teresa, 'Il _Tractatus de prudentia catholicorum scolarium_ di Arnaldo da Villanova', in _Miscellanea André Combes_, ii (Rome and Paris, 1967), 425–48.

[78] J. Carreras i Artau, 'La _Allocutio super Tetragrammaton_ de Arnaldo de Vilanova', _Sefarad_, 9 (1949), 75–105.

[79] Manselli, 'La religiosità', 43–59. Here Arnau used the pseudo-Joachimite text _De semine scripturarum_ as the basis for his analysis of Scripture.

[80] For a tentative hypothesis of the development of Arnau's medical corpus, see Michael McVaugh's introduction to Arnau's _Aphorismi de gradibus_ in _AVOMO_, ii. 77–81.

the struggle with local Church authorities in Aragon, and in particular with the Dominicans, between 1302 and 1305. Lastly came the posthumous sentential condemnation of thirteen of his works in 1316. In July 1300 he was sent to Paris on a diplomatic mission on behalf of James II. The purpose of the mission was to negotiate the territorial dispute between France and Aragon over the Perenese valley *Val d'Aran*. On this mission Arnau published his controversial eschatological treatise, *Tractatus de tempore adventus Antichristi*,[81] in which he determined the exact date of the appearance of the Antichrist who would unfold the apocalyptic events that would lead to the consummation of time and Christ's ultimate victory. Arnau's fusion of Daniel 12: 11 ('And from the time that the daily sacrifice shall be taken away and the abomination that maketh desolate set up, there shall be a thousand two hundred and ninety days') and Ezekiel 4: 6 ('I have appointed thee each day for a year') lay at the basis of the date (1376–8) which he fixed for the advent of the Antichrist. In September 1300, after having successfully completed his diplomatic mission, Arnau was arrested in Paris through the combined action of the Paris theologians, the chancellor, the *officialis*, and the bishop of Paris. Under pressure, he renounced his *Tractatus de tempore adventus Antichristi*.[82] Was this a typical case of policing academic orthodoxy as described by William Courtenay?[83] According to Courtenay, who used the earlier studies of Josef Koch, from the beginning of the thirteenth century to *c.*1280 the corporation of masters, specifically those of theology, took over the task of directing and controlling academic orthodoxy. The masters acted through the authority of the local bishop, and in Paris under the leadership and the direction of the chancellor, mainly targeting masters of arts and/or students in theology. Courtenay regards Peter of John Olivi's first trial (1283–5) as precedent-setting; it created

[81] J. Perarnau, 'El text primitiu del *De mysterio cymbalorum ecclesiae* d'Arnau de Vilanova', *ATCA*, 7/8 (1988/9), 134–69; Gerwing, *Vom Ende der Zeit*, 76–253.

[82] The main sources for this episode are Arnau's letter of protest directed to the King of France in M. Menéndez y Pelayo, *Historia de los heterodoxos españoles*, iii (Buenos Aires, 1951), pp. lxxviii–lxxxiii, and Arnau's appeal to the Pope in *Chartularium Universitatis Parisiensis*, ed. H. Denifle and E. Chatelain (Paris, 1891), ii. 87–90. Later versions of the affair appear in his protestation at Perugia in 1304. For a description of the episode of 1300–1 see R. E. Lerner, 'The Pope and the Doctor', *The Yale Review*, 78 (1988–9), 62–79.

[83] W. J. Courtenay, 'Inquiry and Inquisition: Academic Freedom in Medieval Universities', *Church History*, 58 (1989), 168–81; R. W. Southern, 'The Changing Role of Universities in Medieval Europe', *Historical Research*, 60 (1987), 134–46; J. M. M. H. Thijssen, 'Academic Heresy and Intellectual Freedom at the University of Paris, 1200–1378', in *Centres of Learning: Learning and Location in Pre-Modern Europe and the Near East*, ed. J. W. Drijvers and A. A. MacDonald (Leiden, 1995), 217–28.

the structure and the procedure for all future trials of 'academic heresy', including those of Jean de Paris (1304), Meister Eckhart (1326–9), William Ockham (1324–6), and Marsilio da Padova (1327). The trials were all internal actions of the university, without recourse to bishop or Pope. A subcommission, separate from those who brought the accusation and composed of distinguished and respected masters of theology, was entrusted with the task of examining the suspect proposition or work and assessing the degree of its error, if any.

Arnau was not a member of the University of Paris when the masters of theology decided to condemn his book. But as a master of medicine and a recently active professor at Montpellier, he was part of the academic world.[84] Six characteristics are common to the judicial process involving Arnau and to the academic trials of the thirteenth century.

First, the open conflict began over a book. Arnau started working on a first draft of the text as early as 1288 and the final version of *Tractatus de tempore adventus Antichristi* appeared in 1297. The immediate cause for the intervention of the Paris theologians was not so much the ideas elucidated by the text as Arnau's attempt to diffuse the book in Paris during the autumn months of 1300. The interval between the completion of the text and its condemnation suggests that had Arnau been more discreet and kept his opinions to himself, a modus vivendi between his ideas and ecclesiastical authority might have been found. His bold attempt to disseminate the text in Paris, of all places, ignited the conflict.

Second, the episode highlights the overwhelming importance of the faculty of theology in Paris. The corporation of masters of theology (acting through the authority of the bishop and under the leadership of the chancellor) took over the task of policing orthodoxy. According to Arnau, four or five *doctores* schemed against him, manipulated the chancellor as well as the bishop, and worked in close contact with the *officialis* to bring about his arrest. Arnau complained that the theologians not only evaluated his ideas, but were also judges and executors of the sentence.

Third, the procedure employed in Arnau's case reflects the belief that an offending teacher was redeemable provided he, and preferably others too, were made fully aware of the evil nature of his opinions. The accused per-

---

[84] For the penetration into scholastic debates of Arnau's eschatological ideas and his portrayal as a theologian see H. Pelster, 'Die Quaestio Heinrichs von Harclay über die zweite Ankunft Christi und die Erwartung des baldigen Weltendes zu Anfang des XIV Jahrhunderts', *Archivio Italiano per la storia della Pietà*, 1 (1951), 25–82 at 58–61; Gerwing, *Vom Ende der Zeit*, 254 ff.

son was expected to recant in public. The disputed book was not considered redeemable, and was destroyed. The main purpose of the inquest was to demonstrate how the apparent errors extracted from a certain text were to be understood within the context of the text as a whole, and the procedure aimed at extracting a quick and decisive recantation by the accused of his errors through a process called *temperamentum* (moderation or qualification). This gave the accused the opportunity to read to the judges a preconcocted document containing a revised and corrected version of the text. Arnau accepted the procedure under stress of what he later called unfair physical and psychological pressure; but he alleged that the procedure was misused and he was forced to read a text with which he did not agree.

Fourth, the Pope participated in the process after the condemnation. Arnau appealed to Boniface VIII, who played a conciliatory role. He reprimanded Arnau in private, forced him to deny the problematic propositions extracted from the book, and ratified the condemnation of the Paris theologians. Yet he did not anathematize the work and contended that Arnau's main error lay in not having presented the treatise to him first.[85] His apparent ambivalence towards the disputed work would appear in the list of accusations made by Guillaume de Plaisian on behalf of Philip IV in 1303 against Boniface.[86]

Fifth, the trial, followed by Arnau's intensive search for self-vindication and compensation for the injustice done to him, simply made the issue more controversial and further encouraged his opponents to attack him.

Finally, Arnau's case reveals the importance of political protection. It is possible that his quick release from jail in 1300 was due to his contacts with the French royal court (Guillaume de Nogaret, *miles domini regis Francie*, is mentioned among the seven persons who intervened on his behalf), and the relatively quiet years between 1305 and 1308 were the result of the combined protection of James II of Aragon and of Clement V, who was more favourably disposed towards Arnau's religious ideas than his two predecessors. It has recently been suggested that Arnau's medical skills and prominence as a court figure may explain the relative

---

[85] 'ego in nullo fefelleram nisi quia prius eidem non presentaueram dictum opus.' MS Vat. lat. 3824, fol. 216va.

[86] B. Hauréau, 'Arnauld de Villeneuve', in *Histoire littéraire de la France*, xxviii (Paris, 1881), 39; E. C. Du Boulay, *Historia universitatis parisiensis*, iv (Paris, 1668), 42 nr. 8; *Chart. Univ. Paris.* ii. 90; P. Dupuy, *Histoire du différend d'entre le pape Boniface VIII et Philippes le bel roy de France* (Paris, 1655), 103 no. viii.

tolerance with which he was treated by the papacy. Furthermore, the fact that he strongly championed the absolute authority of the ecclesiastical hierarchy to guard man's spiritual life also strengthened his position at the curia.[87]

The second phase of Arnau's struggle with the Church began in the Province of Tarragona, where local Dominicans kept up the attack on him. In this phase, which embraced also the Provençal Church authorities, local church assembly became an increasingly important venue for investigation and clarification of questions of orthodoxy. There was no particular prohibition against Arnau's text(s) until 1316, yet ecclesiastical dissatisfaction with his spiritual activities was simmering. In late 1302 Arnau was forced to engage with the Dominicans of Girona, who were savaging his eschatological theories from the pulpits. Both parties attempted to induce the bishop to intervene on their behalf; Arnau has described the ensuing polemic in four texts.[88] In 1303 he read a summary of his ideas to the synod at Lleida (presided over by the Archbishop of Tarragona), including a fierce attack on the regular clergy.[89] In 1304 he faced similar attacks from the Dominicans in Provence. His appearance before the episcopal court in Marseilles provides us with detailed information concerning the content of the debate.[90] At the same time he made a constant effort to obtain support and patronage from the Aragonese royal court and papal curia. In 1304 he appeared at the papal conclave in Perugia; in July 1305 he was given the chance to explain his ideas to the royal assembly in Barcelona; and in August 1305 he submitted a compilation of his writings to the scrutiny of Pope Clement V, who did not reject them outright.[91] All this did not deter local Church officials from acting independently. In December 1305 King James II (Arnau's patron at that stage) intervened on behalf of Gombaldus de Pilis, a member of his household who had been excommunicated by the inquisitor of Valencia for possessing texts compiled by Arnau. In a letter to the

---

[87] C. R. Backman, 'The Reception of Arnau de Vilanova's Religious Ideas', in S. L. Waugh and P. D. Diehl (ed.), *Christendom and its Discontents: Exclusion, Persecution and Rebellion, 1000–1500* (Cambridge, 1996), 112–31 at 115–18.

[88] J. Carreras i Artau, 'La polémica gerundense sobre el Anticristo entre Arnau de Vilanova y los dominicos', *Anales de Instituto de Estudios Gerundenses*, 5/6 (1950/1), 5–58 at 33–58.

[89] *Confessio Ilerdensis*, in MS Vat. lat. 3824, fols. 175ra–80ra.

[90] *Denunciatio facta Massilie*, in MS Vat. lat. 3824, fols. 180ra–181rb, 192rb–193rb, 202vb–204rb.

[91] J. Perarnau, 'Problemes i criteris d'autenticitat d'obres espirituals atribuïdes a Arnau de Vilanova', in *ATIEAV*, i. 29–31.

Dominican inquisitor Nicholas Eymeric, James asked him to revoke the decision because everyone, including the royal family, possessed and read these books.[92]

The years 1305 to 1308 mark a period of relative calm in this stormy decade. During this period Arnau produced his final synthesis of theoretical medicine, *Speculum medicine*, and a widely popular *regimen sanitatis* which he wrote for James II. He also produced two books for Pope Clement V, *Liber de confortatione visus* and *De medicina practica*. It was his advice that shaped the papal decree of 8 September 1309 which regularized medical education at Montpellier, establishing a corpus of fifteen Greek and Arabic texts as the basis of future study at the school. He thus played an important role in the assimilation of the newly discovered Galenic corpus (the so-called 'New Galenism') into the academic curriculum.[93] Whether he wrote the commentary of 1306 on the Apocalypse ascribed to him is now a subject of controversy.[94]

Arnau's Sicilian link materialized in 1304/5, when he found refuge at the court of Frederick III, king of Trinacria (Sicily) and James II's brother. At that time Sicily was undergoing an ambitious programme to revitalize religious observance and hence was sympathetic to Arnau's preaching. Arnau's prophetic mysticism won an eager following, especially among members of the royal family and court. When he fell out with James II in 1309, Arnau became Frederick III's religious mentor and guided him on his path to reform. He exhorted him to lead a crusade against Islam and to administer his realm in a spirit consonant with the duties of the perfect Christian king. In 1310 Arnau composed the *Informació espiritual per al rei Frederic*, which laid out a number of reforms for instant implementation, ordering the public reading of Scripture in the vernacular; completing the restoration of churches; expelling all divines, sorcerers, and superstitious peddlers from the island; reforming the practice of slavery by offering religious instruction to all Muslims; appointing all the prelates in the realm, or at least confirming and certifying their qualifications; urging all Sicilian Jews to convert within one year or face expulsion; and building hospitals and hostels

---

[92] Menéndez y Pelayo, *Historia de los heterodoxos* iii. pp. cxxiv–cxxv; Paniagua, 'Cronología', 473.

[93] *Cart. Mont.*, 219–21; *AVOMO*, xv. 17–36; L. García-Ballester, 'Arnau de Vilanova (*c.*1240–1311) y la reforma de los estudios médicos en Montpellier (1309); El Hipòcrates latino y la introducciòn del nuevo Galeno', *Dynamis*, 2 (1982), 97–158.

[94] Arnau de Vilanova, *Expositio super Apocalypsi*, ed. J. Carreras i Artau (Barcelona, 1971); Perarnau, 'Problemes i criteris', 48–70.

for the poor in all major cities.[95] Some of these recommendations on the conversion of Sicily's Jews and Muslims were subsequently incorporated into the new legislation of Sicily, *Ordinationes Regni Sicilie*.[96] Encouraged by the apparent application of his plans, Arnau extracted a public vow from Frederick that he would never withdraw his offer of protection to all observers of evangelical poverty. While Arnau's spiritual writings did not create the growing interest in eschatological mysticism which existed in Sicily, they may have contributed to focusing and clarifying it, and giving it a direction more closely related to that of the Spirituals.[97] The link between the Spiritual Franciscans, who disdained the Scholastic method and learning, and Arnau, who was part of the scholastic world, was their shared belief in an impending apocalypse and its concomitant need for reform and repentance. Ultimately, Arnau's activity in Sicily prepared the way for the reception of the Tuscan Spirituals proscribed by the Council of Vienne.

During the last decade of his life, when his spiritual zeal dramatically increased and overshadowed his medical career, Arnau came to be associated with various groups of 'Poor Brethren of Penitence', called Beguins by the inquisitors. He composed and propagated vernacular writings for these Beguins, male and female Franciscan tertiaries of Languedoc and Catalonia under religious guidance from spiritual Franciscans. Some lived communally, others lived at home, but all sought to follow Franciscan ideals of poverty and humility while living in the world and without taking monastic vows. The *Confessió de Barcelona* (1305) and the *Raonament d'Avinyó* (c.1310) were declarations of faith which laid out the ideals and the practices which Arnau came to share with these groups of lay spirituals.[98] His *Informatio beguinorum seu lectio narbone*, written between 1302 and 1311 and directed to the Beguins of Narbonne, and the *Alia informatio beguinorum*, written between 1305 and 1311, apparently for a Beguin community in Barcelona, were manuals of pastoral guidance designed expressly for Beguin communities.[99]

---

[95] *Informació espiritual per al rei Frederic*, in Arnau de Vilanova, *Obres Catalanes* i. 223–43.

[96] *Capitula Regni Sicilie*, ed. Francesco Testa, i (Palermo, 1741), 65–88.

[97] C. R. Backman, 'Arnau de Vilanova and the Franciscan Spirituals in Sicily', *Franciscan Studies*, 50 (1990), 7–15, and *The Decline and Fall of Medieval Sicily: Politics, Religion, and Economy in the Reign of Frederick III, 1296–1337* (Cambridge, 1995), 200–9.

[98] *Confessió de Barcelona*, in Arnau de Vilanova, *Obres Catalanes* i. 101–39; *Raonament d'Avinyó*, ibid. 167–221.

[99] *Lliçó de Narbona*, ibid. 141–66; J. Perarnau, L' "*Alia Informatio Beguinorum*" d'Arnau de Vilanova (Barcelona, 1978).

In these treatises Arnau stated his belief that God's chosen are those who renounce individual and communal property. Ecclesiastical carnality was the manifestation of the Antichrist's imminent reign. Until the earthly Sabbath which would follow the evil accompanying the Antichrist's reign, the laity should pursue lives of humility, charity, poverty, self-mortification, and endurance, imitating Christ's suffering.[100] Hence, for Arnau, the movement for the reform of the Church was the sole antidote against the machinations of the Antichrist. It was the rediscovery and the incorporation of the 'Truth of Christianity' or the 'evangelical Truth' hidden in Scripture and particularly in the New Testament which was the key to this reform. Arnau shared with the Tertiary Franciscans in particular the belief in the necessity of absolute poverty—personal and communal—as the best defence of the spiritual person in the approaching times of vicissitudes. In order to defend his evangelical views, Arnau promoted the translation of the Bible into Catalan, with the purpose of exposing the poor to the evangelical truth. Scripture should be accessible to all, without ecclesiastical mediation.

Probably by 1305 Arnau had set up a *Scriptorium* in Barcelona.[101] At his death it contained seventeen manuscript volumes of his spiritual works. They were collected by his two executors, who assigned them to 'various people of penitence'. This *Scriptorium* probably produced books meant mainly for the communal house of Beguins in Barcelona, but it also supplied written material to several other Beguin houses in Catalonia. Arnau also produced *summae* of his writings in Latin and in various Romance languages here, some of which were even translated into Greek. These *summae* then circulated: the Latin *summae* (like the *summa* of MS Vat. lat. 3824) were directed to cultivated readers; the vernacular *summae* were directed at various Beguin communities.

During the last decade of his life Arnau was deeply involved with the Aragonese courts and entertained friendly relations with their Angevin rivals. A seventeenth-century tradition places him at the court of Robert of Anjou in 1309 seeking the bestowal on Frederick III of the title 'King of Jerusalem'. But there is no direct documentary evidence for this visit, and the two medical treatises attributed to Arnau and in

---

[100] R. E. Lerner, 'Writing and Resistance among Beguins of Languedoc and Catalonia', in *Heresy and Literacy 1000–1530*, ed. P. Biller and A. Hudson (Cambridge, 1994), 191–6.

[101] R. Chabàs, 'Inventario de los libros, ropas y demás efectos de Arnaldo de Villanueva', *Revista de Archivos, Bibliotecas y Museos*, 9 (1903), 189–203; Perarnau, *L' "Alia informatio"*, 111–26; H. Lee, M. Reeves, and G. Silano, *Western Mediterranean Prophecy: The School of Joachim of Fiore and the Fourteenth-Century Breviloquium* (Toronto, 1989), 55–8.

some manuscripts dedicated to Robert of Anjou are of doubtful author-ship.[102] For Arnau, who believed the royal House of Aragon and then of Trinacria to be the likely source of the God-elected King who would purge Christendom, restore its apostolic past, and lead it to its last phase according to the apocalyptic scheme, politics and prophecy were linked.

In 1311, en route to the papal court on a diplomatic mission on behalf of Frederick III, Arnau died off the coast of Genoa, where he may have been buried. But his imprint on the intellectual life of medieval Europe did not end with his death. On 9 November 1316 the Synod of Tarragona issued a posthumous and public condemnation of most of his spiritual writings. The intensifying anti-spiritual attitudes of the papal court since the Council of Vienne (1311), and its increased activity in guarding orthodoxy during the pontificate of John XXII, are the background for this condemnation. The synod forbade men to possess the controversial writings and ordered that they be collected for burning.[103] In spite of uproar and protestation by Arnau's friends and associates, who opted for an appeal to the papal court, the letter of the condemnation was strictly enforced, with the result that only a few manuscripts of his writings actu-ally survive. That the Synod of Tarragona was acting uncanonically in 1316 when it deliberated on and then judged works which the Holy See should have examined, was one of the main planks in the protest of Ramon Conesa (the executor of Arnau's will). The growing anti-Arnaldian sentiments of the Aragonese court, which distanced itself from radical ideas of social and religious reform, did not contribute to the preservation of Arnau's œuvre. In 1346 his writings, together with those of Peter of John Olivi, were burnt in front of the cathedral of Girona.

The sentence of Tarragona stresses the careful scrutiny and examina-tion of the suspect treatises that was performed by a commission espe-cially created for that purpose. As in many academic trials after 1280, a subcommission, which was separate from those who brought the accusa-tions and those who would render the final judgement, was responsible for evaluating the disputed texts.[104] In Arnau's case the Provost of Tarragona (the archiepiscopal see being vacant), in consultation with the

---

[102] J. Perarnau, 'Noves dades biogràfiques de mestre Arnau de Vilanova, *ATCA*, 7–8 (1988–9), 281–2. The treatises are *Liber de vinis* and *De conservanda iuventute*.

[103] For the text of the condemnation of Tarragona see Santi, *Arnau de Vilanova*, 283–9. See also C. Du Plessis D'Argentré, *Collectio judiciorum de novis erroribus qui ab initio duodec-imi saeculi ad annum 1735 in Ecclesia proscripti sunt et notati*, pt. 1/1 (Paris, 1728), 268–9; Nicolaus Eymericus, *Directorium Inquisitorum* II (Rome, 1578), 198¹–199¹. On the con-demnation see Perarnau, 'Problemes i criteris', 32–4.

[104] Courtenay, 'Inquiry and Inquisition', 174.

Inquisitor, assembled eight learned men to serve on this commission. It is obvious that its members (described as *viri venerabiles, discreti et litterati*) were carefully chosen. They all belonged to the regular clergy; there were three Dominicans, three Franciscans, and two Cistercians representing the two great abbeys in the Archdiocese, Poblet and St Creus. There was an attempt to create full congruence between the Dominicans and the Franciscans; thus a *lector* of the Barcelona Preachers was followed by a *lector* of the Barcelona Franciscans. This pattern similarly applies to members of the commission who came from Tarragona and partly also to those who came from Lleida. The report of the commission was then presented to the general Chapter of the Church of Tarragona, where it was discussed again with the participation of more people (among whom were the Dominican Prior of the Province of Aragon together with four canons from the Church of Tarragona and the abbots of Poblet and St Creus). The Chapter then issued the condemnation (*sententialiter condempnare*) which encompassed fourteen propositions, and ordered that thirteen books be collected within ten days and destroyed.

The sentence of Tarragona reveals another feature common to many academic trials of the late thirteenth and fourteenth centuries, namely that of the categorization of the condemned propositions according to the degree or type of censure. The text uses four categories: heresies (*hereses*), errors (*errores*), rash words (*temeritates*), and false and dubious words (*falsa et dubia*). Some of the propositions are simply condemned. 'Erroneous' is the most frequently used label, and it may be combined with others, namely *temerarium et etiam erroneum,* or even have additional adjectives, like *temerarium et periculosum* (rash and dangerous). Only once, regarding Arnau's preference for good deeds (alms-giving) over performing Mass in his *De helemosina et sacrificio*, did the committee label a proposition as heretical. Nine of the thirteen treatises condemned to be burned were in Catalan. At the beginning of the condemnation the authors expressed fear of the danger to which simple men and women were exposed through them, suggesting the possibility of a link between these largely vernacular treatises and the Beguins of Provence, whom the Church authorities of Tarragona were attempting to control.

Doubtless, Arnau's last decade was dominated by his spiritual and political activities. But was Arnau of 1300–11 a different person from Arnau of the 1280s and 1290s? The fact that in both periods he concomitantly produced spiritual and medical texts suggests that he never clearly separated his spiritual from his medical interests. The purpose of this book is to explore the nature of this coexistence between the medical profession and strong spiritual inclination.

Outline of the Book

One of the characteristics of modern life is a sharp functional differentiation between professional groups in society. This is particularly visible in the academic world, which preaches the idea of interdisciplinary studies yet is often reluctant to accept actual professional movement between the disciplines. This differentiation, which is a result of the explosion of knowledge and the inbuilt demands of modern science, was absent in the middle ages. The harmony impressed upon medieval learning by the medieval university fostered a universally common and more or less cohesive structure for education. Since the methods of investigation which were used to elucidate doctrinal statements about the Christian religion were equally applicable for elucidating statements on every other subject, anyone who had mastered the scholastic method could move from one subject to another with relatively little difficulty. Consequently, leading scientists and leading theologians were often one and the same men, and the union of science and theology arose from the familiarity of theologians with all the basic forms of secular learning.[105] All this calls for the united study of Arnau de Vilanova's medical and spiritual careers.

Arnau de Vilanova has been a special victim of the tendency among modern historians to regard medicine at the turn of the thirteenth century as a perfectly demarcated field. In a small but important book, which is still the authoritative source for determining the authenticity of the medical treatises attributed to Arnau, Juan Antonio Paniagua created a distinctive portrait of the Catalan physician as a rational, systematic, Galenic physician who stressed reason, experiment, and scientific sources, rejecting magic and utterly absorbed in the medico-scholastic world of Montpellier at the end of the thirteenth century.[106] This portrait, still upheld by many Arnau scholars today, led Paniagua to reject as

[105] R. W. Southern, *Scholastic Humanism and the Unification of Europe*, i (Oxford, 1995), 8–9; J. E. Murdoch, 'From Social into Intellectual Factors: An Aspect of the Unitary Character of Late Medieval Learning', in *The Cultural Context of Medieval Learning*, ed. J. E. Murdoch and E. D. Sylla (Dordrecht and Boston, 1975), 271–339, and 'Philosophy and the Enterprise of Science in the Later Middle Ages', in *The Interaction between Science and Philosophy*, ed. Y. Elkana (Atlantic Highlands, NJ, 1974), 51–74 and esp. 62 ff.

[106] J. A. Paniagua, *El Maestro Arnau de Vilanova médico* (Valencia, 1969) [revised edition in Paniagua, *Studia Arnaldiana*, 49–143], and 'Abstinencia de carnes y medicina', *Scripta Theologica*, 16 (1984), 323–4.

doubtful, or even apocryphal, treatises which were tainted with magic or which were foreign to the rational frame of mind characteristic of what he believed to be a thirteenth-century Galenic scientist. When confronted with the apparent contradiction between his image of a rational, stable, and highly conservative medical master and that of a radical, prophetic vision-ary and eschatological reformist, Paniagua emphatically stated that these two patterns of behaviour fitted well into the same personality. Medicine, grounded on a solid, scholastic, and scientific basis was Arnau's profession, and it fully occupied his mind. On the other hand, the religious activity that filled the last years of his life emerged rather from his heart, and, lack-ing a solid basis in theological studies, it was more passionate and so more audacious and novel. This dichotomic approach, between medicine, which is in the realm of the mind, and religious thought, which is in the disor-dered realm of the heart, has relieved most historians of the task of looking at both facets in order to find the relationship between them. Arnau's reli-gious radicalism is relegated to the latter part of his life, after he had aban-doned his chair at Montpellier, and can thus be dismissed as an aberration. But how can we explain Arnau's five major spiritual writings which were produced during the prime of his scientific activity at Montpellier in the 1290s? Paniagua mentioned the religiosity which sometimes creeps into the medical texts, the vivacious polemical tone of some of the treatises so rem-iniscent of scholastic debates, and the simple methods of exposition and explanation common to medical discourse and scholastic debates. He made no systematic attempt to discover whether other relationships existed between medicine and religious thought in Arnau's writings.

This 'split-personality' approach to Arnau holds a self-imposed com-partmentalization of the medical and spiritual activities responsible for his double career. It has been adopted by most intellectual historians, who have studied his religious ideas but have disregarded possible connections with his medical background. In a valuable discussion of Arnau's spiritu-ality, Robert Lerner has recently described him as an example of a new intellectual development in the late thirteenth century, in which laymen repeatedly claimed to apprehend and reach the highest truths,[107] ignoring possible connections with Arnau's medical background. Francesco Santi has mentioned the apparent conflict between Arnau's spiritual output and his medical persona,[108] but refrained from further elaboration.

It is not my intention to deny the accepted notion that Arnau was a

---

[107] R. E. Lerner, 'Ecstatic Dissent', *Speculum*, 67 (1992), 33–57 and esp. 42–6.

[108] F. Santi, 'Arnaldo da Villanova. Dal potere medico al non potere profetico', in *Poteri carismatici e informali: chiesa e società medioevali* (Palermo, 1993/4), 261–86 at 267.

transmitter of Joachimite eschatological ideas and was possibly influenced by Peter of John Olivi, and perhaps also by cabbalistic ideas or methods, or later by various Beguin groups.[109] Yet Arnau, whose name was always preceded by the titles *magister* or *medicus*, and whose verifiable academic training was based exclusively on his medical course of studies taken at the *studium* of Montpellier in the 1260s, was regarded by all contemporaries as a physician first and foremost. I do not suggest that there were any links between the specific spiritual content of his writing and his medical texts or vice versa. Paniagua reached the conclusion that Arnau almost never projected his religious views into his medical writings; I propose both to re-examine this proposition and to check whether he also projected his medical thought into his spiritual writings.

The invocations for divine aid which open many medieval medical texts are the most natural targets for investigation when one looks for religious imprints on the author. They can add to our knowledge of the author's religious attitudes and philosophical frame of mind.[110] But little can be learned about the religious imprint on Arnau the physician from the short, casual, and often formulaic invocations of God which frequently appear in the *proemia* or conclusions of his medical treatises.[111]

---

[109] From the vast literature on each topic I mention only the most recent publications which include specific bibliographies. For the cabbala connection: Santi, *Arnau de Vilanova*, 58, 95–7; M. Idel, 'Ramon Lull and Ecstatic Kabbalah', *Journal of the Warburg and Courtauld Institutes*, 51 (1988), 170–4 at 174. For the Joachimite link: M. Reeves, *The Influence of Prophecy in the Later Middle Ages* (Oxford, 1969), 219, 221, 314–17; H. Lee, 'Scrutamini Scripturas: Joachimist Themes and *figurae* in the Early Religious Writing of Arnold of Vilanova', *Journal of the Warburg and Courtauld Institutes*, 37 (1974), 33–56. For the prophetic context and links between Arnau and Beguins: Lee, Reeves, and Silano, *Western Mediterranean Prophecy*, 27–46, 55–7; Perarnau, *L' "Alia informatio beguinorum"*, 103–84; Lerner, 'Writing and Resistance', 191–6.

[110] C. O'Boyle, 'Medicine, God and Aristotle in the Early Universities: Prefatory Prayers in Late Medieval Medical Commentaries', *Bulletin of the History of Medicine*, 66 (1992), 185–209.

[111] See the pious dedicatory paragraph to *Liber de vinis*, fol. 262va (ascribed to Arnau with some plausibility according to McVaugh, *Medicine before the Plague*, 148, n. 54); the invocation of the eternal wisdom and the True Teacher who illuminate all those who believe in them with the Truth at the beginning of Arnau's *Speculum medicine*, fol. 1ra; the declaration in the *Aphorismi de gradibus* that only the lovers of the heavenly Lamb can attain the fullness of truth in any useful thing, *AVOMO*, ii. 145; the introductory notes to *Contra calculum*, fol. 305va and *De venenis*, fol. 216vb which accept the divine origin of medicine and the causal connection between sin and disease. *De venenis* is now believed to have been largely compiled by Arnau; it was assembled and edited by his disciple, Pedro Cellerer. M. R. McVaugh, 'Two Texts, One Problem: The Authorship of the *Antidotarium* and *De venenis* Attributed to Arnau de Vilanova', in *ATIEAV*, ii. 75–94; also in *ATCA* 14 (1995). All the references to Arnau's medical texts and those attributed to him are, unless otherwise noted, from his *Opera* (Lyons, 1520).

Arnau's medical texts themselves are devoid of any allusions to a moralistic interpretation of disease as the consequence of sin, and rely solely on a natural explanation. Diseases in Arnau's medical writings are neither the results of a direct divine intervention nor of the flawed moral behaviour of a patient. According to the Hippocratic concept (shared by Arnau) which was diffused in the West via Johannitius's *Isagoge*, medicine was an art needed for regulating the non-natural aspects of the human life *(res non naturales)*. Thus it might seem that, by definition, learned medicine had little to do with religion or theology either in theory or in practice. However, a more detailed analysis of the medical works and their juxtaposition with Arnau's spiritual texts opens new paths towards understanding the person himself and the patterns in which medicine and spirituality interact.

Three studies which treated Arnau's medical and spiritual texts as a whole provide a starting-point for the present work, and I take them as a source for useful references despite my reservations concerning their arguments. In a series of studies at the beginning of this century, Paul Diepgen tried to recreate Arnau's world-view (*Weltanschauung*). His conclusion was that Arnau had consciously combined his religious and medical views and created a grand synthesis of Christian mysticism, scholastic natural philosophy, medicine, and Neoplatonic views of nature.[112] According to Diepgen, a common philosophical basis (Augustinian Neoplatonism) is the explanation for Arnau's prolific interests. Diepgen neither systematically studied Arnau's spiritual writings nor tried to see his particular case in a broader historical context. Yet his observation that Arnau's medical and spiritual works had sprung from the same root makes him the first modern scholar who attempted to create a coherent picture of this enigmatic physician. Later, Salvador de les Borges tried to show the convergence of Arnau's religious and medical writings on the moral ethical level. His study, based on many medical texts which today are believed to be apocryphal, led to the conclusion that Arnau's medicine was subordinate to his religious beliefs. Salvador de los Borges's attempt to Christianize Arnau's medicine is unsatisfactory, yet he deserves credit for being the first to have attempted an integrated study of Arnau's spiritual and medical writings. His observation that some key

[112] P. Diepgen, *Studien zur Geschichte der Beziehungen zwischen Theologie und Medizin im Mittelalter: Die Theologie und der ärztliche Stand* (Berlin, 1922), and *Medizin und Kultur: Gesammelte Aufsätze*, ed. W. Artelt, E. Heischkel, and J. Schuster (Stuttgart, 1938), 108–85, esp. the article entitled 'Die Weltanschuung Arnalds von Villanova und seine Medizin' at 176–85.

moral rules and characteristics were common to medical and Christian ethics must be taken into consideration when analysing Arnau's thought.[113] A more recent attempt to link Arnau's medical and spiritual writings was made by Chiara Crisciani, who also relied on texts now thought to be apocryphal.

Her views on possible relationships between Arnau's perception of medical epistemology and his particular ideas about the *usus pauper*, or between his ideas of perfection in medicine and the *vita evangelica*, should be handled with caution.[114] If there was a direct relationship between Arnau's medical thought and radical Franciscan ideas of poverty, other medical men in large numbers might be expected to have contributed to the heated debate which enveloped the Franciscans at that period.

But Crisciani's allusion to a broader scheme of fall and salvation, common to both medicine and theology, offers a better starting-point than the Franciscan link for examining the relationship between Arnau's medical and spiritual writings. Crisciani suggests that the physician's daily contact with signs of physical decay and corruption, which were associated in the medieval mind with sin, could easily impel the pious physician towards offering his diagnostic and curative skills to spiritual diseases as well.[115] I intend to follow this line of thought, and treat Arnau's writings not in the narrow context of his own peculiar religious ideas, but rather as representing general trends linking academic medical practitioners with religious speculation at the turn of the thirteenth and fourteenth centuries. I shall argue that the very fact that Arnau expressed himself so openly in the fields of biblical exegesis, spirituality, and Christian morals, as if he were qualified to do so, may have been directly related to his perception of the role of the physician and the place which the science of medicine occupied.

The larger question of the extent to which Arnau's experience as a medical practitioner and as an academic physician affected the character of his spiritual writings should be broken down into smaller questions. What medical information did Arnau use in his spiritual discourse? How did he justify a physician's right to discuss theological matters? Did the language he used indicate that he was a physician? Did his medical background cause him to introduce any specific approaches or attitudes to

---

[113] Salvador de les Borges, *Arnau de Vilanova moralista* (Barcelona, 1957).

[114] C. Crisciani, '*Exemplum Christi* e sapere. Sull'epistemologia di Arnaldo da Villanova', *Archives Internationales d'Histoire des Sciences*, 28 (1978), 245–92; at 247 n. 9 a bibliographical note on older studies.

[115] Ibid. 274, 276, and esp. 284–5.

religious and philosophical questions? And, more generally, did the apparent disjunction between Arnau's medical and spiritual careers really exist? How can his movement between the two vocations be explained, at a time in which, according to some historians, the barriers separating various scientific disciplines were being raised within the Aristotelian and scholastic traditions?[116]

In order to contextualize Arnau, I have chosen to compare him with two other south European thinkers of his period with similar interests. This is essential in order to determine whether a certain thought or mode of expression of Arnau's should be ascribed specifically to his medical background. These two thinkers will serve as 'controls', a concept I have borrowed from the natural sciences. The choice of control is crucial to its efficacy as a basis for comparison; it must be either similar to the main object of the study, or diametrically opposed to it. The first control is the Genoese physician Galvano da Levanto, who like Arnau was a theologizing physician active at the same period. If Arnau's characteristics are typical of a wider circle of physicians, we should detect them also in the writings of Galvano. The second control is the Dominican Giovanni da San Gimignano, who represents clerics with no medical background yet who extensively employed medical language and medical subject-matter in their writings. If Arnau's characteristics are present in Giovanni's texts, then they cannot be simply the consequence of Arnau's medical education.

The first part of my discussion is largely based on language analysis. Chapter 2 deals with the use of religious language in medical texts and with the use of medical language in religious texts. Chapter 3 considers how Arnau's thought processes were affected by his medical background and elucidates the phenomenon of theologizing physician. Chapter 4 discusses the use of the medical model, medical language, and medical subject-matter by preachers of that period. Finally, in Chapter 5, I discuss in the context of the traditional tensions between medicine and religion in Christian society, points of potential friction between medical and religious practice as they appear in Arnau's medical and spiritual texts. Thus I seek to employ Arnau as a means of contributing to a broader debate on the place of medicine and its practitioners in late-medieval culture, and I shall try to show that medicine in Arnau's time had a cultural role, in addition to its main function as a therapeutic art for curing physical ailments.

---

[116] A. Funkenstein, *Theology and Scientific Imagination from the Middle Ages to the Seventeenth Century* (Princeton, 1986), 6, 307–17; García-Ballester, 'Introduction', in *Practical Medicine from Salerno to the Black Death*, 12–13, 23.

A Note on the Sources

Whenever a medical treatise by Arnau had not yet been critically edited, I have used the 1520 Lyons edition.[117] Using Renaissance editions of medieval texts is always problematic: they are fraught with printing errors and editors' alterations to the text and punctuation.[118] They also portray the Renaissance image of Arnau, and hence include many works (such as treatises on alchemy) which are doubtful, non-authentic, or apocryphal. Arnau's Renaissance image is reflected in Johann Weyer's *De praestigiis daemonum*. Weyer, a sixteenth-century physician, depicted Arnau as one of the practitioners of infamous magic who followed the follies of earlier magicians and duly suffered an unhappy end. According to Weyer, these men merely compiled raving nonsense and superstitions unworthy of all pious men.[119] The Renaissance editors therefore attributed various treatises related to magic and alchemy to Arnau, a recognized physician who was also branded a heretic. They did so despite the hostility to alchemy he expressed in *Speculum medicine*, where he spoke of the 'silly alchemists' (*fatui alchimiste*).[120]

I accept Paniagua's determination of authenticity (updated to the state of present research),[121] and exclude from my investigation those texts which he has described as definitively spurious, except where they provide corroborative evidence for a notion already expressed in one of Arnau's authentic texts. Elsewhere I sometimes use the printed edition as a compendium of useful texts which, although coming from a large variety of sources chronologically far apart, and in some cases of obscure authorship, seem to be representative of physicians' thought in the later middle ages.

My study of Arnau's spiritual writings is based on the corpus of texts listed by Francesco Santi and Josep Perarnau.[122] Whenever there is a

[117] Paniagua, *El Maestro*, 24–5.

[118] L. García-Ballester, E. Sánchez-Salor, M. R. McVaugh, and A. Trías, 'Las ediciónes Renacentistas de Arnau de Vilanova: su valor para la edición crítica de sus obras médicas', *Asclepio*, 37 (1985), 39–66.

[119] G. Mora (ed.), *Witches, Devils and Doctors in the Renaissance: Johann Weyer, 'De praestigiis daemonum'* (New York, 1991), 106.

[120] *Speculum medicine*, fol. 16rb. In *Liber de vinis*, fol. 264vb–65ra, the alchemists are under attack for pretending to endow gold with specific virtues.

[121] Paniagua, *El Maestro*, and 'En torno a la problemática del corpus científico arnaldiano', *ATIEAV*, ii. 9–22 at 20–2; also in *ATCA* 14 (1995).

[122] F. Santi, 'Gli *Scripta spiritualia* di Arnau de Vilanova', *Studi Medievali*, 26 (1985), 977–1014 (also in his *Arnau de Vilanova*, 245–77). For a recent discussion of problems of authenticity in the spiritual works attributed to Arnau see Perarnau, 'Problemes i criteris'; at 41–5 Perarnau compiles a list of the 77 treatises he regards as authentic.

printed edition, I use it, bearing in mind that most of the printed texts cannot be regarded as critical editions. When there is no available printed edition I have consulted MS Vat. lat. 3824, the major manuscript that includes all of Arnau's spiritual texts produced by August 1305. It was written under Arnau's direct supervision and was handed to the newly elected Pope Clement V for his assessment.[123] I have also examined two treatises in MS Rome, Archivio Generale dei Carmelitani, III, Varia 1—*Tractatus quidam* and a commentary on Matthew 24—whose authorship is today a matter of controversy.[124] From Santi's list I did not look at *Expositio super Apocalypsi*, whose authorship is disputed today,[125] and nrs. 53–54, which are Greek versions of now lost works.[126] I have also excluded from my study two texts recently attributed with some doubt by Josep Perarnau to Arnau, *Conflictus iudeorum* and *Tractatus contra passagium ad partes ultramarinas.*[127]

My first control for Arnau, the physician Galvano da Levanto, was a representative of the lively cultural scene in Genoa at the turn of the thirteenth and fourteenth centuries.[128] He dedicated to Philip IV of France

---

[123] For a description of MS Vat. lat. 3824 see J. Perarnau, 'L'*Allocutio christini* . . . d'Arnau de Vilanova', *ATCA* 11 (1992), 10–24. There at 47–65 Perarnau describes the internal development in Arnau's spiritual works as running from cabbalistic via scholastic to more practical texts which stressed the art necessary for acquiring true wisdom and spiritual salvation. On an ealier redaction of these texts in MS Vat. Borgh. 205 from *c.*1302 see A. Maier, 'Handschriftliches zu Arnald de Villanova und Petrus Johannis Olivi', in *Ausgehendes Mittelalter*, ii (Rome, 1967), 215–37 at 215–29.

[124] On the manuscript and the debate over Arnau's authorship see M. Batllori, 'Dos nous escrits espirituals d'Arnau de Vilanova', *AST* 28 (1955), 45–70; K.-V. Selge, 'Un codice quattrocentesco dell'archivio generale dei carmelitani contente opere di Arnaldo da Villanova, Gioacchino da Fiore e Guglielmo da Parigi', *Carmelus*, 36 (1989), 166–76, and 37 (1990), 170–2; Perarnau, 'Problemes i criteris', 70–8; Lerner, 'Ecstatic Dissent', 42, n. 37; G. L. Potestà, 'Dall'annuncio dell'Anticristo all'attesa del pastore angelico. Gli scritti di Arnaldo di Villanova nel codice dell'Archivio Generale dei Carmelitani', *ATIEAV*, i. 287–344.

[125] On the 'medical' allusions in *Expositio see* J. Mensa i Valls, 'Sobre la suposada paternitat arnaldiana de l'*Expositio super Apocalypsi*', in *ATIEAV*, i. 194 n. 281 (also in *ATCA* 13, 1994) and my remarks there at p. 406. The allusions do not necessarily reflect a medical background of the author, but are not incompatible with Arnau's authentic texts; hence they are not helpful in determining Arnau's authorship of the text.

[126] On the Greek versions of Arnau's work, see J. Carreras i Artau, 'Una versió grega de nou escrits d'Arnau de Vilanova, *AST* 7 (1932), 127–34; M. Batllori, 'Els textos espirituals d'Arnau de Vilanova en lengua grega', *Quaderni Ibero-Americani*, 14 (1953), 358–61.

[127] MS Genoa, Biblioteca Universitària, Manoscritti G. Gaslini, A. IX.27, fols. 101^V–110^V, 131^V–132^V; Perarnau, 'Problemes i criteris', 78–94.

[128] On Galvano see J. Leclercq, 'Textes contemporains de Dante, sur des sujets qu'il a traités', *Studi Medievali*, ser. 3, 6/2 (1965), 531–5, and 'Galvano da Levanto e l'Oriente', in *Venezia e l'Oriente fra tardo medioevo e rinascimento*, ed. A. Petrusi (Venice, 1966), 403–16 (at 404–5 biographical details); Paravicini Bagliani, *Medicina e scienze*, 43–5; G. Petti Balbi,

the *Liber sancti passagii*,[129] which was presumably written shortly after the fall of Acre in 1291 and not later than 1295. *Liber sancti passagii* contains no indication of the medical background of its author. Galvano does mention the efficacy of disease and the fear of death accompanying it in arousing religious fervour. He employs commonplace metaphors like 'antidote', but people with no medical background used similar expressions.

Galvano had special relationships with various primates at the curia, including the Pope himself and two of the Cardinals, Pietro Valeriano Duranguerra (d. 1304) and Luca dei Fieschi (d. 1331), to each of whom he dedicated a treatise. There is no evidence that he practised medicine in Genoa, and he may have devoted most of his time to meditation and studies. He was probably married and father of at least two children. After his death his name was inscribed in the anniversary book at the Franciscan convent in Genoa; together with the frequent dedication of his treatises to members of the Franciscan Order, this highlights his special relationship with the Franciscans.[130] He also profoundly admired the Dominicans, and may have led a pious life on the fringe of a monastic community. Of the two fifteenth-century Italian manuscripts which include Galvano's medical works, I have used MS Vat. lat. 2463 for four medical works and MS Berlin, Staatsbibliothek Preussischer Kulturbesitz, lat. quart.773 for three.[131]

'Arte di governo e crociata: Il *Liber sancti passagii* di Galvano da Levanto', *Studi e Ricerche. Istituto di Civiltà Classica Cristiana Medievale (Genoa)*, 7 (1986), 131–68 at 131–41. In 'Società e cultura a Genoa tra due e trecento', *Atti dela Società Ligure di Storia Patria*, n.s., 24/2 (1984), 123–49 and esp. 128–35, Petti Balbi discusses the cultural and social context and the thriving medical community in Genoa at the turn of the century. E. Wickersheimer, *Dictionnaire biographique des médecins en France au Moyen Âge* (Geneva, 1936), 164–5; D. Jacquart, *Supplément* to Ernest Wickersheimer, *Dictionnaire biographique des médecins en France au Moyen Âge* (Geneva, 1979), 79.

[129] MS Paris BN, nouv. acq. lat. 669. It was partly published by Ch. Kohler, in 'Traité de recouvrement de la Terre Sainte adressé vers l'an 1295 à Philippe le Bel par Galvano de Levanto, médicin génois', *Revue de l'Orient Latin*, 6/3 (1898), 343–69, text at 358–69; Petti Balbi, 'Arte di governo'.

[130] Ibid. 135 and n. 16.

[131] MS Vat. lat. 2463 is a well-made fifteenth-century manuscript which includes four treatises: fols. 1ʳ–68ʳ, *Thesaurus corporalis prelatorum ecclesie Dei et magnatum fidelium contra nocumentum digestionis stomachi*; 69ʳ–78ʳ, *Remedium salutare contra catarrum*; 78ᵛ–110ʳ, *Liber paleofilon curatius langoris articulorum multiplicis dolorosi Galuani*; 110ʳ–114ᵛ, *Salutare carisma ex sacra scriptura* (P. Micheloni, *La medicina nel primi tremita codici del fondo vaticano latino* (Rome, 1950), 40, no. 149). *Iter Italicum* III, 479ᵃ made me aware of MS Berlin SPK lat. quart. 773. It contains three treatises by Galvano da Levanto: fols. 3ʳ–21ʳ, *Chrisma sanatiuum tremoris cordis*; 21ʳ–69ʳ, *Liber saluatoris contra morbum caducum*; and 69ᵛ–100ʳ, *Liber doctrine curatiue langoris leprosi*.

Another collection—MS Paris, BN, lat. 3181—includes the spiritual writings Galvano submitted in 1303 to the scrutiny of Pope Boniface VIII, apparently without causing an acrimonious row over the right of a layman to engage in theological discourse.[132] This is not surprising since, unlike Arnau, Galvano did not express controversial ideas. He was loyal to the papal cause in this crucial period of growing strife and competition between the papacy and the French court. This has led Jean Leclercq to the conclusion that Galvano is of little doctrinal interest or importance, and that his spiritual texts do not deserve to be edited.[133] I do not intend to refute Leclercq's harsh indictment that, compared with Dante, Galvano's *Doctrina de inferno, purgatorio et paradiso*[134] is nothing but an unoriginal compilation of scriptural and patristic texts, or that the *Liber fabrice corporis mistici*[135] is of no particular doctrinal interest and lacks the precision typical of professional theologians. But Galvano's theological writings do contain much medical knowledge and language which allow his works to be evaluated in the same way as Arnau's spiritual writings, and will enable me to compare two contemporaneous cases of 'theologizing physicians'.

Galvano's three manuscripts are explicitly linked to each other. The author identifies himself in each treatise as 'Galvano genuensis de levanto umbre medici'. The Berlin manuscript refers to a treatise which appears in the Paris manuscript, the *Liber contemplationis neophyte de gratia dei gradiens super corpus humanum*. The Vatican manuscript refers to *Liber doctrine curatiue langoris leprosi*, which is in the Berlin manuscript.[136]

The second control is Giovanni da San Gimignano and his sermon literature, in particular the *Summa de exemplis et rerum similitudinibus locuplentissima* (*Sde* hereafter).[137] Not much is known about Giovanni. He was a *lector* at various Dominican houses and then Prior of the Dominican

[132] *Catalogue General des MSS Lat.* iv. 303–4. The manuscript appears in the 1311 Perugia inventory of the papal library. F. Ehrle, *Historia bibliothecae Romanorum pontificum*, i (Rome, 1890), 31, no. 53.

[133] Leclercq, 'Galvano da Levanto'.

[134] MS Paris, Vat. lat. 3181, fols. 45–56.

[135] Ibid. fols. 1–9.

[136] MS Berlin, SPK, lat. quart.773, fol.63^V. Cf. MS Paris, BN, lat. 3181, fols. 12^r–20^V. MS Vat. lat. 2463, fol. 5ra; cf. MS Berlin, SPK, lat. quart. 773, fols. 69^V–100^r.

[137] All the citations are from the 1583 Antwerp edition, which was the first of seven Antwerp editions (1597, 1609, 1611, 1615, 1629, 1630). I have checked the printed version against MS Basel, Univ. Bibliothek, B VIII 30, fols. 101^r–156^r and MS Berlin, SPK, Theol. lat. fol. 219, fols. 208^r–262^r. Printing in this case did not prove to be an agent of change, since the printed edition is loyal to the MS versions.

house at Siena between 1310 and 1313,[138] and thereafter played an important role in establishing a Dominican convent in San Gimignano. He is believed to have written the *Sde* during the first decade of the fourteenth century before he embarked on his administrative career in the Order. He may have been sent to a *studium generale* outside his province; it has been suggested that Barcelona was the most likely place in which he could have gained some of the wide knowledge he displays in the *Sde*, especially his insights into the Saracens and their culture. However, I have found no evidence that the Dominican house in Barcelona was a *studium generale* before 1303.[139]

The *Sde* was preserved in at least fifty manuscripts from the fourteenth and fifteenth centuries, many of which have survived only in fragmentary form.[140] By 1499 it had been printed seven times (Deventer, 1477; Venice, 1484, 1497, 1499; Cologne, 1485; Basel, 1499; and a seventh incunable *sine loco* from 1490), and its popularity did not diminish in the sixteenth century (Venice alone offers five more editions from 1576, 1577, 1582, 1583, and 1584); all this indicates its importance. I shall concentrate on one aspect of this work, the absorption by Giovanni of medical knowledge into religious discourse, which may explain the continuous interest the book aroused.

This encyclopaedic, yet widely neglected work is composed of ten books, each dedicated to a different scientific field, from which Giovanni draws lessons of theological or religious import for preachers' sermons.[141] I use the sixth book, dedicated to the human body. I also cite

---

[138] J. Longère, *La Prédication médiévale* (Paris, 1983), 113–14; Kaeppeli, *Scriptores* ii. 539–43; A. Dondaine, 'La vie et les oeuvres de Jean de San Gimignano', *AFP* 9 (1939), 128–83 at 157–64 on *Sde*; *DTC*, viii. 721–2; J.-Th. Welter, *L'exemplum dans la littérature religieuse et didactique du Moyen Âge* (Paris, 1927), 340–1; M. Oldoni, *Giovanni da San Gimignano. Un enciclopedico dell'anima* (San Gimignano, 1993), 7–33, and 'Giovanni da San Gimignano' in *L'enciclopedismo medievale*, ed. M. Picone (Ravenna, 1994), 213–28.

[139] Dondaine, 131. Prior to that date Barcelona had a lively cathedral school and the Dominican convent was also active. See W. A. Hinnebusch, *The History of the Dominican Order*, ii (New York, 1973), 12–13; A. Walz, *Compendium Historiae Ordinis Praedicatorum* (Rome, 1948), 127–30, 223.

[140] Thirty-two of the MSS are in German, Austrian, and Swiss libraries; seven are in Italian libraries; the rest are dispersed mainly in East European libraries. None is either in an English or French library. The obvious popularity of the text in the German cultural area is exemplified by the fact that in the 1340s the Dominican Konrad von Halberstadt compiled an abridged version of Giovanni's book.

[141] Bk. i. *De celo et elementis*; ii. *De metallis et lapidis*; iii. *De vegetabilibus et plantis*; iv. *De natalibus et volatibus*; v. *De animalibus terrestribus*; vi. *De homine et membris suis*; vii. *De visionibus et somniis*; viii. *De canonibus et legibus*; ix. *De artificibus et rebus artificialibus*; x. *De actibus et moribus humanis*.

a manuscript and two printed collections of his sermons in order to show that material from the manual did find its way into his sermons.[142] I have chosen the *Sde* as the main control for Arnau because Giovanni fits the chronological and perhaps also the geographical context in which Arnau worked. His text was so popular that any conclusion we draw from it can be a basis for a broader generalization. The *Sde* opens a window on to the genre of preachers' manuals and sermon literature which processed learned culture for the consumption of the *vulgus*.[143] Thus it is an excellent yardstick for measuring widespread notions and beliefs. As a manual, it was a working tool intended to be used rather than simply read.[144] Hence it should be regarded not merely as a storage place for abstract ideas concerning physicians and medicine, but as an insight into what was actually being disseminated.

In describing Giovanni's ideas I shall also refer to other preaching material that mirrors his line of thought in order to show that, despite his idiosyncrasies, he cannot and should not be regarded as an isolated representative of this genre. For this purpose I have examined a sample of sermons and preachers' manuals, mostly in print and mainly from the period between 1250 and 1350, from a variety of places in the Latin West, from northern and southern Europe (though with a strong bias to the south), whose authors belong to various Orders. Although each of the authors is doubtless unique and merits an independent study, since I am interested in the broad question of how they make use of medical subject matter in their manuals and sermons, I shall treat them largely as a group characterized by similar features. Despite the personal foibles of each preacher and the regional variations, it seems to be possible to speak of a 'European panorama of sermons'[145] of the period.

[142] MS London, BL Addit. 24998—a fourteenth-century manuscript which contains 151 Sunday sermons; Giovanni da San Gimignano, *Conciones funebres* (Paris, 1611), and *Convivium quadragesimale hoc est conciones et sermones . . .* (Cologne, 1612). Hundreds of sermons have been attributed to Giovanni, yet there is no systematic study of them.

[143] According to the prologue, *Sde* was edited 'Predicantium igitur commodo, curioso desiderio simplicium auditorum profectui desiderans inservire'. *Sde prol.* 3³.

[144] R. H. Rouse and M. A. Rouse, *Preachers Florilegia and Sermons: Studies on the Manipulus Florum of Thomas of Ireland* (Toronto, 1979), 3–90. On more examples from the same genre of moralized *exempla* see Welter, *L'exemplum*, 335–54.

[145] C. Delcorno, 'La predicazione volgare in Italia (sec. XIII–XIV). Teoria, produzione, ricezione', *Revue Mabillon*, 65 (1993), 83–107, at 83.

The Language of the Physicians who Produce Spiritual Texts

Language is neither a transparent medium for an accurate representation of a reality nor does it derive its meaning from some purified extralinguistic object or subject. Uncovering the hidden linguistic codes unique to every writer can yield important insights into his cultural background, motives, and personality. Does the language Arnau employs in his spiritual writings suggest possible links with his medical background? Does he introduce into his spiritual language anything which is specifically 'medical'? This we may learn from juxtaposing his medical and spiritual writings, seeking religious features in the medical texts and medical features in the spiritual texts, and locating points of convergence between the two worlds.

Marie-Christine Pouchelle has already reconstructed a physician's subconsciousness, imagination, and motivations by analysing the analogies in Henri de Mondeville's surgery book.[1] Henri, the third important medical figure of the period at Montpellier in addition to Arnau and Bernard de Gordon, was a surgeon to Philip the Fair and composed his treatise on surgery (*Chirurgia*) between 1306 and 1320. Pouchelle has compiled detailed lists of the metaphors Henri used and has produced some illuminating insights into his use of specific kinds of metaphors. In Henri's surgery book both priest and physician prescribe controlling the orifices for maintaining physical or spiritual health.[2] Disease emerges as a bestial thing; it is closely connected with sin and animality. Together with minerals and plants, animals are the most commonly used metaphors for pathologies, reflecting the notion that the intrusion of nature into the body is the essence of pathology. When discussing the healthy body and the medical

---

[1] M.-C. Pouchelle, *The Body and Surgery in the Middle Ages* (Cambridge, 1990). See also C. R. Backman, *The Decline and Fall of Medieval Sicily: Politics, Religion, and Economy in the Reign of Frederick III, 1296–1337* (Cambridge, 1995), 201–2, and 'The Reception of Arnau de Vilanova's Religious Ideas', in S. L. Waugh and P. D. Diehl (ed.), *Christendom and its Discontents: Exclusion, Persecution and Rebellion, 1000–1500* (Cambridge, 1996), 125–6.

[2] Pouchelle, *The Body and Surgery*, 150–1.

practitioners, Henri uses analogies relating to the organization of space, architecture, and the world of food and cooking. His medical writing also manifests the extensive social imagery associated with the body. However, it is difficult to grasp the significance of the use of such analogies, and it is not at all clear, as Pouchelle suggests, that this imagery actually influenced Henri's medical practice. What is the meaning of Pouchelle's finding that Henri is more interested in the human body as a whole than in its component parts?[3] Metaphors in medical texts may have been used as substitutes for dissections and pictorial illustrations. But does the writer's imagination as exposed through the metaphors he employs teach us anything significant about him and the cultural or social context in which he was acting?

Like Pouchelle, who stresses the need for further research similar to hers into the medical writings of other physicians,[4] I shall start to decipher a physician's imagination by looking at his medical texts. But the main way I have chosen to uncover the hidden linguistic codes unique to him is by examining his non-medical writings.

Religious Language in Medical Texts

Arnau employs the terms *sanitas* and *salus* interchangeably. In his medical texts these terms mean physical health or well-being, while in the spiritual texts they mean spiritual health. His spiritual texts are saturated with concepts such as *sana doctrina* (sound teaching) or *sanitas doctrine*,[5] *sanus intellectus* (sound understanding),[6] *sana mens* (sound mind),[7] and *sanitas* as spiritual health.[8] This shows that, at least linguistically

---

[3] Ibid. 191. [4] Ibid. 190, 204 .

[5] Correct teaching through which knowledge of the truth is transmitted is *sana doctrina*; it is useful and necessary for salvation (*salus*); *sanitas doctrine* is one of the expressions of the image of Christ. *De prudentia catholicorum scolarium* in Graziano di Santa Teresa, 'Il *Tractatus de prudentia catholicorum scolarium* di Arnaldo da Villanova', in *Miscellanea André Combes*, ii (Rome and Paris, 1967), 438; *Confessio Ylerdensis*, MS Vat. lat. 3824 fol. 175ra; J. Carreras i Artau, 'Del epistolario espiritual de Arnaldo de Vilanova', *Estudios Franciscanos*, 49 (1948), 393.

[6] The purpose of knowledge, understanding, and learning is *salus eterna* and this can be acquired only by *sanus intellectus*. *Allocutio super tetragrammaton*, in J. Carreras i Artau, 'La *Allocutio super Tetragrammaton* de Arnaldo de Vilanova', *Sefarad*, 9 (1949), 80, 82.

[7] *Sana mens* describes the state of one who knows and understands the truth as well as believes in it, while those who refuse to acknowledge manifest truth have *vellum ante oculos mentis*. Ibid. 97.

[8] In *Apologia de versutiis et perversitatibus pseudotheologorum et religiosorum*, MS Vat. lat. 3824, fol. 160[ra], Arnau determines that those who gnash their teeth at his writings are doubtless to be counted among depraved men afflicted by malignant spirits. All that is left to them is to pray that the merciful God will restore them to health ('ut deus ipsos pro sui misericordia restituat sanitati').

Arnau the physician and Arnau the spiritual mystic perceive the object of their activity as one and the same thing: health.[9] The overlap between physical and spiritual health, for which physicians are responsible, is also revealed in more practical texts. In 1310, after giving political advice to James II, Arnau offers a medical prescription, and openly proclaims that he has been occupied with the King's body and soul.[10] Similarly, James II alternates between *salus* and *sanitas* when he describes the venerable and prudent master Arnau as a necessary agent responsible for the conservation of his health and the well-being of his body.[11] *Peccatum* as a physical defect which causes a disease,[12] *lapsus* as a physical failure which can be corrected by the physician,[13] *purgatio* as a curing technique,[14] and even *passio*[15] were all key medical words which had acquired strong religious connotations.

Luke Demaitre has already cautioned against charging medical texts with moral meaning in translation into modern languages.[16] *Malus morbus* should not be translated as 'evil disease' but as 'nasty disease'; *peccatum humoris* is not 'sin of humour' but 'humoral defect' which is caused not by 'complexional malice' (*malitia complexionis*) but by 'imbalance of the complexion'. The result is 'breakdown of a faculty' (*corruptio virtutis*) and not a 'corruption of virtue'. Nevertheless, it is plausible to assume that the Christian connotations of these words helped, at least subconsciously, to dismantle the boundaries between the physician and the cleric in

[9] On the probable scriptural origin of this confusion of words, see Arnau's commentary on the term 'verbum sanum' or sound speech (Tit. 2: 8): ('Sanum, hoc est, ad salutem eternam edificans auditores' in J. Carreras i Artau, 'La polémica gerundense sobre el Anticristo entre Arnau de Vilanova y los dominicos', *Anales del Instituto de Estudios Gerundenses*, 5/6 (1950/51), 37.

[10] 'Unde quia multa percepi per passionibus cordis et corporis vestri, consulo . . .', in H. Finke, *Acta Aragonensia*, ii (Leipzig, 1908), 701.

[11] See letters from 1305 and 1308, ibid. 872/550, 877-78/554-55.

[12] On the concept of *peccatum humoris* or *humor peccans* see *Speculum medicine*, in Arnau de Vilanova, *Opera* (Lyons, 1520), fol.31vb; *Repetitio super can. Vita brevis*, ibid. fol. 276va; and *De parte operativa*, ibid. fol. 124ra. See also the following apocryphal treatises: *De conceptione*, ibid. fol. 213va; *De coitu*, ibid. fol. 273va; *Breviarium practice*, ibid. fol. 172ra. In polemical medical texts the noun *peccatum* often denotes the theoretical error which the writer purports to refute.

[13] *Speculum medicine*, fol. 23ra.

[14] *De simplicibus*, in de Vilanova, *Opera*, fol. 242vb; *De regimine sanitatis*, ibid. fol. 78ra (apocryphal).

[15] *De simplicibus*, fol. 242rb; *Speculum medicine*, fol. 31vb which explains the use of the term *passio* as one kind of the accidents of disease or their causes; *De parte operativa*, fol. 123ra.

[16] L. E. Demaitre, 'The Description and Diagnosis of Leprosy by Fourteenth-Century Physicians', *Bulletin of the History of Medicine*, 59 (1985), 339.

the eyes of the medical practitioner and his clients. This was hardly an intentional choice by medieval physicians, since the use of such terms in a medical context predates the Christian period and was part of the language of classical medicine. However, once these terms had acquired a strong Christian connotation, a possible link between the cleric and the physician was created. By using the term *peccatum* in a medical context, the physician put himself, at least linguistically, on the same level as a priest, in that each could be seen as offering a way to heal *peccata*.

Perhaps the clearest example of similarity in the language of physicians and clerics appears in *De consideracionibus operis medicine sive de flebotomia*, one of Arnau's earlier medical works.[17] The treatise includes a general discussion of the ways to produce the right therapeutic decision and also deals with the effect of air on the humours, pain and its treatment, and the quantities of blood to be evacuated by phlebotomy. The prologue to the treatise reveals the existence of factions among the physicians. The struggle between them is described in religious terms. Arnau and his followers pursue the way of truth (*via veritatis*), and are burning with desire for truth (*flagrantes desiderio veritatis*). They have duly read Galen and Hippocrates and therefore they monopolize medical truth. Their opponents, who are motivated not by equity and justice but by envy, cause infection of scandals (*pestilentia scandalorum*) and bodily destruction (*pernicies corporis*); they do not read the medical authorities themselves but only booklets and *summe*.[18] The language of the debate is significant. The contested texts are *scripture*; it is through them that the medical truth has been revealed as if by divine concession. The *empirici*, who do not properly read or master the authoritative texts, are not only ignorant but also heretical.[19] Unaware of the medical context of the argument, one might easily mistake this language for that of a theological debate. Medical texts appear here like spiritual texts in a religious polemic. This reflects the growing assimilation of medical science into

---

[17] *AVOMO*, iv. 131–7. On the polemical context of the treatise, see ibid. 51–2, 69–83; L. García-Ballester, 'Arnau de Vilanova (*c.*1240–1311) y la reforma de los estudios médicos en Montpellier (1309): el Hipócrates latino y la introducción del nuevo Galeno', *Dynamis*, 2 (1982), 109; M. R. McVaugh, 'The Nature and Limits of Medical Certitude at Early Fourteenth-Century Montpellier', *Osiris* (2nd ser.), 6 (1990), 68.

[18] L. E. Demaitre, *Doctor Bernard de Gordon: Professor and Practitioner* (Toronto, 1980), 34, raises the possibility that the target of Arnau's attack was Bernard de Gordon, with whom he may have had a running disagreement on the subject of practical compendia like Bernard's *Lilium medicine*.

[19] Arnau dedicates the book to Gusinus Coloniensis, saying, 'Sed compatimur tue sinceritati propterea quia lapsum quasi te videmus in heresim.' *AVOMO*, iv. 133.

the scholastic world, but it also clearly shows that medical practitioners perceived their role in religious terms. Thus in the *proemium* to *Antidotarium* (probably compiled by Arnau and then edited by his disciple, Pedro Cellerer), Arnau declares that he is about to unravel the secrets of medicine used often by the sons of the 'incarnate truth' (*incarnata veritas*), so that those who are engaged in the practice of healing will be 'orthodoxly illuminated' (*orthodoxe lucidati*).[20] If there existed a concept of medical orthodoxy, it is not surprising that Arnau labels 'profane' any medical theory which contravenes the medical scripture of Galen.[21]

Another example of this trend appears in Arnau's discussion of what he calls *medicus fidelis*.[22] The term *fidelis* also appears in his spiritual treatises, where it has a purely religious meaning. *Dyalogus de elementis catholice fidei*, a catechetical text from *c.*1296 dedicated to the king of Aragon for the education of his children, starts in this manner: 'Are you a faithful Christian (*fidelis*)? Indeed I am, Sir. Why do you say you are faithful? Because I have the right faith (*recta fides*). What is the right faith? The Catholic faith (*fides catholica*)'.[23] *Fidelis* in the medical context has a religious flavour which is slightly different from the usual meaning of the word when used in a purely religious context. It denotes a trustworthy, loyal (towards the patient), and honest practitioner. As well as swiftly attending the patient,[24] the *fidelis medicus* must be competent (*peritus*) so as to avoid inflicting harm through his treatment. That adjective, Arnau stresses, derives from the word *fides*, which itself originates from God who commands that we help each other according to our capacity. Arnau, however, preserves his instrumental approach to medicine by stressing that *fidelitas* must rest only on the firm foundation of competence (*peritia*) and the virtue of *caritas* which is common to medicine and the Christian faith. Medical ethics are thus enshrined in a religious structure, and Arnau sees a fusion between religion and medicine on an ethical

---

[20] *Antidotarium* in Arnau de Vilanova, *Opera*, fol. 243[vb]; M. R. McVaugh, *Medicine before the Plague: Practitioners and their Patients in the Crown of Aragon 1285–1345* (Cambridge, 1993), 120, and 'Two Texts One Problem'. The vocabulary of medicine was pervaded by religious terminology also in the writings of Henri de Mondeville; see Pouchelle, *The Body and Surgery*, 52–6.

[21] *Repetitio super can. vita brevis*, fol. 276rb.

[22] *Contra calculum* in de Vilanova, *Opera*, fol. 305vb–306ra.

[23] W. Burger, 'Beiträge zur Geschichte der Katechese im Mittelalter', *Römische Quartalschrift* (Geschichte), 21/4 (1907), 173.

[24] 'Medicus fidelis et sapiens cognitis agnoscendis, quanto celerius potest subvenit egrotanti.' *Medicationis parabole*, in *AVOMO*, vi. 1, 35/4. In the anonymous commentary which accompanies the printed editions of *Medicationis parabole*, in de Vilanova, *Opera*, fol. 103[ra]: 'Fidelitas est ut unusquisque faciat alteri quod facere tenetur secundum fidem.'

rather than on a practical level of the causes and the cures of diseases. Since the faithful Christian adheres to the correct faith, it is logical to regard the faithful physician as the adherent of the correct medical code of behaviour, which implicitly plays the role of the faith. The precept to be *fidelis* is grounded on the maxims of the faith (Christian and medical) and the well-attested, physically invigorating effect of the patient's trust (*fiducia*).[25]

In his commentary on *Medicationis parabole*, Arnau links the efficient performance of the faithful physician to his moral and religious disposition. The physician who wishes to cure usefully (*utiliter medicari*) should acquire a noble desire (*nobilis appetitus*) which is expressed by religious devotion and through readiness to help his neighbour. Only a continuous, unrelenting attachment to God, which creates a correctness of purpose (*rectitudo intentionis*), can ensure useful medical practice.[26] Arnau does not explain how this usefulness is manifested, if at all, with regard to the treatment itself. However, he states that the faithful physician who persists in that desirable pattern of behaviour will feel its impact on his reputation amongst the living and on his position with regard to divine grace. Guided by charity, he secures eternal salvation and earns good money from his work.[27] Nowhere in the medical texts is it suggested that the moral/religious behaviour of the patient was deemed to have any repercussion on his physical health.

As Michael McVaugh has shown,[28] the analytical language used by physicians was sometimes influenced by the philosophical discourse in the faculties of arts or theology. The medical masters of the thirteenth and fourteenth centuries treated natural-philosophical questions as wholly analogous to those raised in the arts or theological faculties, though they arose from very different contexts. McVaugh shows that Arnau wrote *Aphorismi de gradibus* (the first Western attempt to assemble all the earlier works on pharmaceutical theory into a single unified interpretation of the

---

[25] For more about the clinical importance of *fiducia*, see *Repetitio super can. Vita brevis*, fol. 279[rb]. For a similar use of religious concepts in a medical context by a Renaissance physician, see R. French, 'The Medical Ethics of Gabriele de Zerbi', in *Doctors and Ethics: The Earlier Historical Setting of Professional Ethics*, ed. A. Wear, J. Geyer-Kordesch, and R. French (Amsterdam and Atlanta, 1993), 72–97 at 84–6.

[26] *Commentum super quasdam parabolas*, in *AVOMO*, vi. 2, 155.

[27] 'tunc splendebit peritia medici et erunt omnia opera interiora eius postquam ex charitate fiant; nam apud deum merebitur gratiam, et ab hominibus etiam emolumentum.' *Repetitio super can. Vita brevis*, fol. 279[va].

[28] Introduction to *Aphorismi de gradibus*, in *AVOMO*, ii. 3.

subject) mindful of the thirteenth-century philosophical discussion over the question of qualitative change and its theological significance.[29] Arnau was concerned about whether his conclusions would accord well with the judgements of contemporary philosophy, and made a special effort to demonstrate the philosophical soundness of his work. Like the Franciscan Richard of Middleton (d. *c.*1305) in his commentary on Lombard's *Sentences*, Arnau used the concept of *quantitas virtutis*,[30] applying it not to the usual theological question of increasing charity but to changing primary qualities. Like Middleton, Arnau was able to talk quantitatively about qualitative intensification. Middleton's views were the source for Peter of John Olivi's explanations of the manner in which qualities intensify. This suggests the possibility that Olivi, who was lecturing on theology in Montpellier when Arnau was there, is the source for the latter's philosophical foundation for his mathematical theory of compound medicine. A direct link between the two remains uncertain.[31] Be that as it may, this affinity in language enabled the physician to feel at home in the field of metaphysical speculation and it reduced the natural inhibitions of an outsider entering a foreign intellectual field; when you master the analytical language of the other discipline, the leap into it is always less terrifying.

The Metaphoric Level of Medicine

So far I have attempted to show that in Arnau's medical texts and on the linguistic level the ground had been prepared for a fusion between religious and medical discourse. Before examining the other side of the equation, namely Arnau's use of medicine in his spiritual writings, we should ask ourselves whether he was aware of the possible links between medicine and spirituality. It is evident from his commentary on the first aphorism of *Medicationis parabole* that Arnau had in mind a possible spiritual interpretation of his aphorisms (and perhaps of medicine in general). He explains why he entitled the treatise 'The Parables of Cure' rather then 'The Canons of Cure' by saying that, since the visible can describe the invisible, all the canons concerning the cure of bodily failures in this treatise can be aptly adapted to spiritual failures. A parable

[29] *AVOMO*, ii. 89, 91–2.

[30] *Quantitas virtutis* expressed the notion that charity as a force (*virtus*) has a quantity too. This counter-Aristotelian approach viewed the increase of charity 'as taking place by the addition of real qualitative parts to a number of pre-existing qualitative parts' (ibid. 91). It deviated from the Aristotelian distinction between the categories of quality and quantity.

[31] Ibid. 96.

is an exemplary model (*similitudo*); hence each of the canons is an exemplary model for a spiritual cure.[32] Arnau formulates the principle without offering a specific spiritual interpretation of any of the medical aphorisms he discusses.

The same notion appears (albeit more vaguely) in the four concluding aphorisms of the treatise, where Arnau calls the wise reader to draw a lesson from Christ the *parabolanus* (a talker of parables) and to reshape (*reducere*) the aphorisms as parables. This is reinforced by two further examples for the usefulness of parables. The parables in the Book of Proverbs show that the results of reflections on natural things can be adapted to moral issues through a suitable figure (*metaphora*). Efficient teachers use parables based in tangible things to make hidden things plain.[33] This part of *Medicationis parabole* has no commentary; hence we do not know how such a recommended conversion of the aphorisms can be achieved in order to unfold their moral meaning. But this passage, together with the previously discussed commentary, clearly reveal Arnau's belief that medical principles can deliver a spiritual message.

As early as his first spiritual treatise, *Introductio in librum Ioachim De semine scripturarum*, Arnau expresses the conviction that all knowledge is figural and hence prophetic. Every art and every science expresses a *mysterium* which hides diverse layers of knowledge concerning the Creator. Cognition is thus causally linked to prophecy: increased cognition will inevitably lead to increased prophecy. The rules of rhetoric and grammar, the terms of logic and geometry, the laws of mathematics, all produce parts of the *ymago misterii*. The astrologer, the physician, and the lawyer can reveal prophetic knowledge by exercising their professions. The physician, whom Arnau calls the lover of well-being (*salutis amator*) who confers health (*sanitas*), extends the inquiry of the intellect into things natural, non-natural, and counter-natural only as much as is necessary for the

---

[32] 'omnes canones hic expressi de medicatione corporalis lapsus, convenienter possunt spiritualibus lapsibus adaptari: nam invisibilia per visibilia designantur. Et ab ista consideratione vocavit supra in titulo canones hic descriptos parabolas. Parabola enim similitudo interpretatur; et unusquisque istorum canonum medicationis corporalis est similitudo vel quedam exemplar canonis particularis ad medicationem spiritualem.' *AVOMO*, vi. 2, 153.

[33] '1. Parabole Salomonis ostendunt quod que sapientes in considerationibus naturalibus protulerunt, convenienti metaphora moralibus adaptantur. 2. Doctor gratiosus et efficax parabolis utitur ad occulta per sensibilia declaranda. 3. Eterni doctoris evangelica lectio testatur eundem fuisse parabolanum. 4. Sapiens igitur ad exemplum illius premissa reducet in parabolas oportunas.' *Medicationis parabole*, in *AVOMO*, vi. 1, 127, 129.

acquisition of health mysteriously.[34] The medical way and the mysterious way for achieving good health are complementary; the first serves the second and is limited in its power to cure. Medical knowledge is thus tightly connected to the *mysterium* which is responsible for health. Arnau's spiritual writings do not demonstrate direct, explicit borrowing of material from medical sources. However, they do indicate a general awareness of medicine's spiritual dimension, which provides an infrastructure for a more meaningful exchange of ideas between the medical and spiritual worlds and hence offers a further explanation for Arnau's spiritual inclinations. Item 67 in the inventory of Arnau's minor possessions prepared in December 1311 by the executors of his will is 'a book concerning spiritual life and corporeal life' (*unum volumen de vita spirituali et de corporea*).[35] Whilst it is impossible to identify the book, it does provide further evidence that Arnau was interested in the mutual relationship between body and soul.

A juxtaposition of Arnau's notion of medicine's metaphoric dimension with Ramon Llull's perception of the metaphors of medicine in his *Liber principiorum medicine* (henceforward *LPM*)[36] leads to the conclusion that the two shared here a common notion of medicine's spiritual dimension. Arnau only implied a spiritual content in medicine; Llull (*c.*1234–*c.*1316) went far beyond him and explicitly allotted the content of his medical theory a metaphoric meaning. Llull and Arnau frequently appear together in contemporary accounts and modern essays.[37] In *Tractatus quidam*, an anonymous theological treatise from the early

[34] 'Hic salutis amator accedit ut conferat sanitatem, videlicet, medicus, qui, rerum naturalium, non naturalium et contra naturam diversitatem enumerans, tantum in ipsis profundat indaginem intellectus quantum adquisitioni salutis misterialiter est necesse iuxta illud Apostoli "Non plus sapere quam oportet".' *Introductio in librum Ioachim De semine scripturarum*, in R. Manselli, 'La religiosità d'Arnaldo da Villanova', *Bullettino dell'Istituto Storico Italiano per il Medio Evo e Archivio Muratoriano*, 63 (1951), 48, 57–9 at 58; H. Lee, 'Scrutamini Scripturas: Joachimist Themes and *Figurae* in the Early Religious Writing of Arnold of Vilanova', *Journal of the Warburg and Courtauld Institutes*, 37 (1974), 42–8. The distinction between natural, non-natural and counter-natural things was a starting-point of medieval medical instruction.

[35] R. Chabás, 'Inventario de los libros, ropas y demás efectos de Arnaldo de Villanueva', *Revista de Archivos, Bibliotecas y Museos*, 9 (1903), 192.

[36] In *Quattuor libri principiorum*, with an introduction by R. D. F. Pring-Mill (Paris, 1969: reprint from the *Opera Omnia*, i (Mainz, 1721). On the book, see *Selected Works of Ramon Llull (1232–1316)* ii, ed. and tr. A. Bonner (Princeton, 1985), 1009–116 (with an English translation); R. Lulle, *Principes de médecine*, tr. A. Llinarès (Paris, 1992), at 221–30 a selection of his key medical allusions; A. Llinarès, 'Les *Principes de médecine* de Raymond Lulle', in *Le Corps et ses énigmes au Moyen Âge*, ed. B. Ribémont (Caen, 1993), 121–31.

[37] M. de Montoliu, *Ramon Llull i Arnau de Vilanova* (Barcelona, 1958); J. N. Hillgarth, *Ramon Lull and Lullism in Fourteenth-Century France* (Oxford, 1971), 97, 261.

fourteenth century whose attribution to Arnau has been contested, Arnau, Joachim, Peter of John Olivi, and Ramon Llull appear to belong to the same group of *moderni nuntii* who possessed true, divine knowledge and were persecuted by the cunning dragon.[38] Arnau and Llull were Catalan, shared the claim to have received divine revelation, and were considered equally 'fantastic' by their contemporaries, who often reacted violently to their religious teaching. The only historically verifiable encounter between them (1308) was in a religious/political context. There is no evidence for an encounter between the two on the medical level.[39] Thus, it may not be possible to determine who influenced whom (if at all), but the fact that Arnau is not alone in this attitude to medicine is of significance.

It is beyond the scope of this book to analyse Llull's contribution to medieval science or even to expound his medical theory in full. This, as has been shown, could only be done by a full analysis of Llull's *Art*, which was conceived as a system for a perfect and universal language with which to convert the infidels.[40] I shall elaborate on Llull's medicine only as far as it serves as a source of religious truths.

LPM was composed between *c.*1273 and 1275, at a period which coincides with the earliest phase of the development of the Llullian Art. In it Llull attempts to supply a logical method through which the knowledge of degrees might be attained. The concept of degree (*gradus*) was fundamental for the pharmaceutical discussions in the thirteenth century. *Gradus* was the degree of the intensity of the effect of a particular substance used as an ingredient in a medicine. But Llull is not interested in medicine for its own sake, as the final *distinctio* (no. X), entitled *Metaphora*, reveals. According to Llull, metaphor is anything which signifies one thing through another (*significat unam rem pro alia*).[41] For him

---

[38] *Tractatus quidam*, MS Rome, Archivio Generale dei Carmelitani III, Varia 1, fol. 65rb (also in M. Batllori, 'Dos nous escrits espirituals d'Arnau de Vilanova', *AST* 28 (1955), 68.

[39] M. Pereira, 'Le opere mediche di Lullo in rapporto con la sua filosofia naturale e con la medicina del xiii secolo', *Estudios Lulianos*, 23 (1979), 29–30, and *The Alchemical Corpus Attributed to Raymond Lull* (Warburg Institute Surveys and Texts, 18; London, 1989), 38.

[40] For a comprehensive analysis of Llull's medical works see Pereira, 'Le opere mediche di Lullo', 5–35. F. A. Yates, 'The Art of Ramon Lull', *Journal of the Warburg and Courtauld Institutes*, 17 (1954), 115–73 dealt particularly with Llull's attitudes to astronomy and his explanation of heaven (*celum*), yet gave some important insight into his medical thought at 129–31, 151–5.

[41] In the following discussion I shall adhere to this definition when using the term 'metaphor', which could be translated in modern English as 'analogy' or 'example'. For Llull's concept of metaphor, see M. D. Johnston, *The Evangelical Rhetoric of Ramon Llull: Lay Learning and Piety in the Christian West around 1300* (New York and Oxford, 1996), 101–2.

urine, pulse, appetite, and the rest of what he calls 'metaphors' are accidents, examples, and signs by which causes of disease (fever, in his exemplary discussion) are diagnosed and accidents of health are revealed. The metaphoric or exemplary dimension of medicine is thus an integral part of the medical occupation. In this way understanding (*intellectus*) is enhanced both vertically, in the specific art itself, and horizontally into other arts, because it simultaneously allows a deeper understanding of various forms of meaning (*species*). Grasping the metaphorical dimension of medicine is initially necessary for the immediate concern of the physician who diagnoses diseases, finds their causes, and finally prescribes a fitting therapy. Yet the metaphorical art, which links the three faculties of the soul (memory, reason, and will) permits a better and deeper insight into fields of knowledge other than the one of immediate concern, and adds other meanings to a given phenomenon. Llull explicitly states that theology (together with law and natural philosophy) can be illuminated through the metaphorical aspects of medicine,[42] and that it is permitted to descend to other sciences such as philosophy, law, and medicine when expounding Scripture and theological authorities.[43]

Medical metaphors which lead, according to Llull, to a better insight into medical, ethical, and theological truths are interspersed throughout *LPM* and especially in *distinctio* X of the book. Thus, the purgative power of turpeth (*pomoea turpethum*), which dissolves phlegmatic humours, 'may be understood metaphorically to denote the fact that while virtues assemble in the middle point between two extremes, vices are at the extremes themselves'.[44] The thirteenth metaphor discusses springtime, when phlebotomy, frequent baths, and reduction in the quantity of food and drink are recommended by physicians for the preservation of good health, thus securing full and efficient revival and restoration of the complexional and elemental foundation of the body. This medical regimen for the spring follows the natural example of nurturing a tree in

---

[42] 'De Metaphora autem in hac Arte tractamus ad hoc, ut sit ars ad exaltandum intellectum in ista Arte et in aliis Artibus; per Metaphoram enim corroboratur intellectus ad intelligendum; nam per istam uno eodemque tempore super diversas species gyratur . . . ideo est in hac Arte Metaphora, ut per hoc . . . possint etiam intelligi ea, que de aliis scientiis existunt, sicut de Theologia, Jure et Philosophia naturali et aliis, per quas intellectus exaltatur in intelligendo'. Llull, *LPM*, dist. I, v, 5$^{1-2}$. See also dist. X. c. 36, Metaphora 7, ibid. 40².

[43] Llull, *Ars compendiosa Deil* 30 ii, in *Opera Latina* 134, ed. M. Bauzà Ochogavía (*CCCM* 39; Turnhout, 1985), 329: 1362–67.

[44] 'potest metaphorice intelligi, quod virtutes in medio duorum extremorum conveniunt, vitia autem in ipsis extremis'. Llull, *LPM*, dist. I, v, 6^{1}.

springtime if we wish it to blossom properly, metaphorically signifying that in Lent we are expected to fast and decrease the quantities of food we consume. Divine providence enjoins us to fast at exactly that time of the year when nature orders us to avoid food harmful to our health.[45]

We shall look more closely at two pharmaceutical examples which deal with the Trinity, but before doing so a short explanatory note is necessary. Llull, who is sometimes depicted as the forerunner of modern symbolic logic and computer science, bases the combinatory nature of his art on the symbolic notation of its alphabet, relating everything to the exemplification of God's dignities. His explanation relies on hierarchical rings which are in analogical relationship with each other. The lowest—that of the elements, which included the medical doctrines of his time—constituted a valid scientific basis for arguments projected to a higher level. The peculiarity of his thought also lies in the use of letters of the alphabet combined on geometrical figures to work out philosophical problems. In the application of his art to medicine, the letters A, B, C, and D represent respectively the four elemental qualities (hot, dry, humid, and cold). It is possible to describe every simple matter by virtue of the specific combination of these four qualities, which characterize it in different degrees. Thus the simple matter Llull labels with the letter *E* is hot (A) in the fourth degree, dry (B) in the third, humid (C) in the second, and cold (D) in the first. The simple matter *S* is hot (A) in the first degree, dry (B) in the second degree, humid (C) in the third, and cold (D) in the fourth. The simple matter *K* is dry (B) in the fourth degree, cold (D) in the third, hot (A) in the second, and humid (C) in the first. Another key term in Llull's medical theory is the *punctum*, a basic unit of measurement for calculating the degrees. Of all the *puncta*, the seventh is the most important one, for it is incorruptible and without opposition (*contrarietas*). It desires in every elemental body a simple body. Searching for this body, it attracts all the lower *puncta*, for which it is the form. Thus simple water, which is the original matter in the formation of compound water, retains its seventh point in order to control and conserve its simple form in the new compound.[46] The following two examples from *LPM* discuss doctrinal topics by using these terms and combinations.

---

[45] 'Unde cum hoc ita sit, idcirco per dispositionem et ordinationem divinam et naturalem tibi metaphorice revelatur, quod in Quadragesima debeas jejunare et parum comedere, et etiam quod Quadragesima est in maxime conve[ni]enti tempore anni, excipiendo tamen cibos sanitati contrarios'. Ibid. metaphora 13, 42[1].

[46] Llull, *Ars demonstrativa* II.8.3, in *Selected Works of Ramon Llull (1232–1316)*, ed. and tr. A. Bonner (Princeton, 1985), i. 350.

Llull says that if you wish medically (*medice*) to understand the most holy revelation of the Trinity, you should know that if the combination of *E* and *S*, which involves greater contrast than *E* and *K*, produced a harmonious compound (*concordantia*), then there would be a greater difference, agreement, and equality or uniformity (*differentia, concordia, equalitas*) in the compound *ES* than in *EK*, since originally there was a greater contrast between *E* and *S*. This reflects the Trinitarian doctrine of a unified deity composed of sharply different elements. Because it is agreed that there is a greater harmony and uniformity or equality (*concordantia, equalitas*) in God than in created things, it should also be acknowledged that this uniformity originates in a greater difference (*differentia*, though without any opposition or *contrarietas*) between the divine persons.[47] Thus the medico–pharmaceutical theory exactly fits the theological truth and can be used to illuminate and explain it.

In the simple matter *E*, which I discussed above, there are thirteen *puncta*. Seven *puncta* come from the hot quality (A) which is in the fourth degree, three *puncta* come from the dry quality (B) which is in the third degree, two *puncta* come from the humid quality (C) which is in the second degree, and one *punctum* comes from the cold quality which is in the first degree. These thirteen *puncta* represent Christ and the twelve apostles. Christ is represented by the seventh point (*septimum punctum*), which is the form of all the other twelve points and hence determines the compound's dominant quality. The seventh point also signifies the Sabbath, which is the form of all other days.[48] The simplicity of the number seven and the fact that it is the form of all the remaining elements in the body are metaphorically used for portraying the incarnation, which was the ultimate completion of God's creation.[49]

Llull's complex theory, which attempted to unite all knowledge into one comprehensive explanation, automatically subordinated each branch of knowledge to that ultimate end. In his spiritual approach to medicine and the thirty metaphors in *distinctio* X, Llull apparently must have believed that in the elemental process, particularly as worked out in the science of medicine, he had found a pattern that could be used metaphorically—as an *exemplum*—in ethics and theology with such precision as to provide a way of mathematically calculating exemplarism. This could be dismissed as a mere idiosyncratic characteristic of Llull's peculiar mysticism; but it can also serve as an example of the possibilities of extending the scope of medicine far beyond the technical aspects of therapy. His belief in the certainty that medicine provides, both within and beyond the narrow boundaries of the discipline, parallels Arnau's absolute conviction that he possesses the keys to certain knowledge. Llull provides us with a vivid example of a thinker, contemporary with Arnau and from the same geographical area, who regards medicine as more than a therapeutic art; medicine provides its initiates with keys to higher knowledge.

Language barriers play a key role in demarcating fields of knowledge; and the above discussion shows how permeable they were in the case of medical and religious or moral discourses. Arnau's medical texts employed language and conceptual terms which were loaded with religious meanings. Within the medical treatises these terms had a purely medical meaning, but by using them he implicitly presented the medical practitioners as holding a clerical function, implying that medical knowledge hid a spiritual dimension. Llull went even further, and believed that medicine's metaphorical dimension fashioned it into an important instrument for deciphering divine truths. To establish whether this has any explanatory force in Arnau's movement between medicine and spiritual speculation, it is necessary to provide more explicit textual evidence. At this stage we may be content with describing the phenomenon and suggesting that it paved the way for a more substantial exchange of ideas and practices between physicians and clerics.

Medical Language in Religious Context

How does Arnau employ his medical knowledge in his spiritual writing, and is his pattern of using medicine different from that of other contemporary thinkers—physicians and theologians alike? Here I introduce a concept which I shall be using from now on, a 'level of medical language', differentiated between 'high' and 'low'.[50] A religious text which I describe as 'high-level medical language' includes medical terms and concepts which originate specifically in academic medical discourse, and displays knowledge that is particularly expressive of a medical background. References in such a text to specific medical authorities should automatically classify it as using high-level medical language. A text that uses low-level medical language will contain banal medical terms such as references

---

[50] The term 'level of medical language' is Michael McVaugh's; the following discussion is my development of his initial idea and the outcome of a fruitful discussion between us on this question.

to organs of the body, the senses, and diseases, or allusions to the humoral theory, terms which do not signify any specific medical knowledge and training and which could have originated in biblical, philosophical, or theological sources. The overall level of medical language in a text should be determined both by the quality and quantity of the terms employed.

Thus, there may be texts which qualitatively use low-level medical language, yet these terms saturate the text to such an extent that the quantity acquires a qualitative value. By quantity I mean not only the simple density of the use of medical language (per page or per treatise) but also the proportional density, namely the density in comparison with other metaphors used. Furthermore, the context in which the medical language appears should not be ignored. There is, for example, a difference between Thomas Aquinas talking about the ensoulment of the foetus, where the use of medical language would be expected because embryology is essential to his argument, and his use of medical language in a debate over a strictly metaphysical question. The latter case would be more striking and could serve as evidence for the 'medicinalization of religious language', which involves the adoption of medical knowledge and language for simplifying religious messages. Can level of medical language serve as a litmus test for the author's medical background? In other words, is the medical language employed by theologizing physicians usually of a higher level than that of theologians who have no particular medical background?

What, then, is the level of the medical language employed by Arnau in his spiritual writings? Let us first look at four exemplary sections, chosen because of their centrality in the religious discourse of the period in general and not because they are interrelated in any form.

The Use of Medical Knowledge for the Description and Explanation of Abstract Religious Messages: The Case of Generation

In one of his earlier treatises written in *c.*1292 Arnau tries to give a Christological interpretation for the Hebrew Tetragrammaton.[51] He asserts that the Hebrew characters of the Tetragrammaton signify the mystery of the Trinity, and attempts to prove it by an analysis of the letters according to three categories: shape (*figura*), meaning (*potestas*), and order (*ordo*) within the word. After having explained that the divinity is

---

[51] Carreras i Artau, 'La *Allocutio super Tetragrammaton*', 75–105. See also 'Arnaldo de Vilanova, Apologista Antijudaica', *Sefarad*, 7 (1947), 49–61. Lee, 'Scrutamini Scripturas', 48–53.

a whole, simple, and indivisible essence, he claims that the intellect can grasp this notion as easily as it can comprehend that the whole soul is found in every bodily organ.[52] The philosophy of language, semiotics, and attitude to the Hebrew language displayed here are of no concern to us. What matters is Arnau's use of medical knowledge in a religious or philosophical context.

Comparing the meaning of the letter 'h' in Hebrew and in Latin, Arnau argues that the shape of the Latin 'h' signifies the Holy Spirit which descends perpendicularly from heaven to touch the upper part of the human curve (*curvitas humana*), that is, the spiritual human nature. Spiritual human nature is bent as a result of Adam's sin, and is likened to a circle in two ways. The first is as a contagious disease: the crooked or corrupt elements of the spiritual nature are endlessly transferred from generation to generation through the biological process of generation of bodies. Once Adam's body was corrupted by an infected soul, all its offspring were also corrupted.

The second reason for the circular characteristic of human nature also relates to the generation process.[53] For Arnau, physical human nature revealed to him in his work on the human body discloses the mysteries of spiritual human nature as well. The process of generation begins and ends with the sperm. The sperm unites with blood to form the body, an idea originating from Aristotle's notion of generation. From the body dung is produced, creating moisture which is appropriate for the growth of vegetation. Plants and then fruits are the results of this moisture. The fruit is used as food which then is turned into chyle. Chyle, which originally was the extracted juice of a plant, had acquired by the fourteenth century the medical meaning of a white milky fluid formed by the action of pancreatic juice and bile on chyme.[54] Blood is formed of chyle, and then through the phases of moisture and transformable matter sperm is produced. These terms used by Arnau echo quite distinctly the academic language of natural philosophers who dealt with the issue of generation. The cyclical development of the body is manifest not only in the microscopic

[52] Carreras i Artau, 'La *Allocutio*', 90.

[53] 'Secundo vero circulum imitatur in generatione quantum ad naturam corpoream. Nam ex spermate et sanguine fit humanum corpus, et ex humano corpore fit fimus, et ex fimo fit humiditas apta vegetationi, et ex tali humiditate fit planta, et ex ea fit fructus, et ex fructu fit cibus, et ex cibo fit chylus, et ex chylo sanguis, et ex sanguine ros, et ex rore cambium et ex cambio fit sperma. Et sic redit secundum speciem ad id quo inchoavit. Similiter ab impotentia membrorum incipit infantia, et ad eandem redit in senio.' Ibid. 93. Cf. *Speculum medicine*, fol. 2[rb].

[54] Chyme is food converted by gastric secretion into acid pulp.

level of the sperm, but in the whole stature of the body which starts and ends its existence in a phase of physical impotence. This cyclical development is detected in the spiritual level of discretion, since humans start and end their life in a state of spiritual impotence. They progress from sensible to intellectual understanding before the onset of the inevitable intellectual decline which accompanies old age and leads them to a stage of idiocy. This decline can be halted only through the contact of the believer's soul with the Holy Spirit. The physical rules thus decide everything—except for the rare cases in which divine agents intervene.

The biological concept of generation is useful to Arnau when he discourses further on the letter *vav* (equivalent to the Latin 'v'). This letter signifies the Son, and Arnau attempts to prove the perfection of the begotten. He who is conceived retains the essence of the conceiver, and this is a general phenomenon in the world of animated forms. God produces a perfect entity resembling Himself, and it draws its essence directly from Him. However, Arnau is aware that the *modum generationis* which is at the basis of his discussion may create some logical difficulties; for in a human-like mode of generation the offspring will contain the essence of both parents and not only of the father, an unacceptable conclusion for believers in Christ as the son of God alone. Here Arnau borrows from the current approach to the question of conception. The premise for his argument is that God is perfection and thus can produce only perfectly. But in human generation, the mother is an imperfectly reproducing agent, because she does not actively generate in herself: she reproduces not by herself but through someone else. Since no imperfect manner of generation can be attributed to Christ, the offspring of the perfect being, he derives his means solely from the Father whose male mode of conception (unlike all male animals) is perfect and who generates actively and concomitantly *in se* and *ex se*.[55] The divine mode of generation is different from that of the male animal; for male animals reproduce by themselves (*ex se*) but still have to achieve this in someone else (*in alio*). Here Arnau still echoes the Aristotelian view which postulated a radical distinction between the male and female contributions to the generation process. It asserted that the woman provides only the passive material (menstrual blood), which the male semen, the sole carrier of the soul, forms into the foetus. The argument about the passive role of women in the generation process could not have been effective had the Galenic theories of embryology been used in this context, for Galen, to whom the

---

[55] Carreras i Artau, 'La *Allocutio*', 94–5.

discovery of the ovaries is attributed, asserted that male and female semina operated according to the same principles and contributed in an
active manner to the form as well as to the matter of the foetus.[56] Arnau,
the vehicle of Galenism, was surely aware of this facet of Galenic medicine, so he seems to have deliberately chosen to use the traditional
Aristotelian theories to promote his argument. He ignores the potential
contradiction between Galenic medical theory and the rival Aristotelian
theory, which retained its role in theological debate.[57]

How do Galvano da Levanto and Giovanni da San Gimignano employ
generation in a spiritual context? In the third treatise of MS Paris, BN,
lat. 3181,[58] Galvano asserts that understanding the structure of the physical body and the regimen it requires should enable the author to make
his modest contribution to theological discourse. He divides the treatise
into three chapters, each dealing with an aspect of the human body which
then receives a moral interpretation. The first chapter, entitled 'On the
Generation and Nature of the Structure of the Human Body and the
Optimally Healthy Body and its Moral Significance' (*De generatione et
constitutione fabrice corporis humani et optime sani ad iusticiam et eius moralitate*), mainly deals with the generation of the exterior body, and attempts
to create parallels between its characteristics and that of the interior body.
Galvano elaborates on the philosophical aspects of generation rather than
on its physical or embryological ones. The exterior body is created with
temperateness of principal causes (*formales, agentes, moventes*) and elements.[59] The result of the process is 'due consistency of complexion,
orderly arrangement and unity' (*complexionis, compositionis et unitatis debita consistentia*) which is Galvano's definition of optimal health (*optima
sanitas*).

The introduction of the term *complexio* creates a further opportunity
for Galvano to reveal his professional medical background. Avicenna is

[56] J. Cadden, *Meanings of Sex Difference in the Middle Ages: Medicine, Science and Culture*
(Cambridge, 1993), 30–7.

[57] For the use of Galen's and Aristotle's embryology and physiology by the Franciscan
School (Bonaventura and Scotus) and by Thomas and Albertus Magnus respectively, in the
context of the debate on Marian anthropology see K. E. Børresen, *Anthropologie médiévale
et théologie Mariale* (Oslo, 1971), 70–90. See J. W. Baldwin, *The Language of Sex: Five
Voices from Northern France around 1200* (London and Chicago, 1994), 294 n. 23, 318 n. 9
for the use of Galenic embryology in biblical commentaries of Peter the Chantor (d. 1197).

[58] 'Contemplacio de gracia dei neophyta gradiens super corpus humanum et eius regimen conseruatiuum et curatiuum'. MS Paris, BN lat. 3181, fol. 12[rb]–20[v].

[59] 'temperantia suarum causarum principiorum et elementorum'. Ibid. fol. 12[vb]. He
mentions a *Liber medicine anime* and a *Liber sanitatis obsequiose* which he has written, yet neither is part of the present compilation and they seem to have been lost.

his source for the definition he offers of God-given complexion, which paves the way for the introduction of the soul into the body.[60] *Compositio* is the uniformity of the organs (*equalitas membrorum orcanicorum*), and *unitas* is the nature in which the organs relate to each other (*natura in qua utraque communicant membra*). A long philosophical analysis follows in which the vegetative soul (*anima vegetativa*) is discussed, citing Aristotle's *Metaphysics* when proving God's role as first principle and Avicenna on the fourfold properties of nature as the originator of motion (*principium movendi*).[61]

The generative power as the supreme of the three powers of the vegetative soul is the focus of Galvano's discussion, and it has one purpose—to serve as a foundation for the argument concerning the likeness between the generation of man's physique and his soul. God is responsible for creating the soundness of the exterior body by giving it a temperate complexion, uniformity, and unity, and its aptitude for self-preservation and self-improvement. In this divinely ordained biology, medicine was also created by God as a fulfilment (*complementum*) of his creation and a help (*adiutorium*) in securing the proper management of the body. The outcome of this divine intervention is optimal health (*optima sanitas ad iustitiam*).[62] Galvano cites Galen's *De diffinitiva doctrina*[63] as the authority for the common notion of the divine origin of medicine and avoids in this context Ecclesiasticus 38. In exactly the same manner God

---

[60] 'Complexio quidem est eucrasia membrorum consimilium quam secundum avicennam libro primo capitulo secundo deus donauit homini temperationem quam in hoc mondo esset possibile cum suarum uirtutum conuenientia quibus agit et patitur secundum exigentiam forme ultime introducende in eo que est anima rationalis.' MS Paris, BN lat. 3181, fol. 12vb. Cf. *Avicenna Liber canonis*, i. fen 1, 3.2 (Venice, 1507), 3^1 (literal citation).

[61] Ibid. fol. 13^{ra-b}. All the Galenic texts that he employs deal with the ethics and philosophy of medicine; Avicenna is his main source for the more practical aspects of medicine.

[62] 'Jam igitur patet quod sicut deus dedit homini exteriori nobiliorem complexionem ex generatione et sanitatem optimam ad iusticiam que consurgit ex temperata complexione membrorum consimilium et equali compositione orcanicorum et debita unitate que est natura communis in qua utraque communicant membra ex quibus consurgit immediate optima ipsius hominis exterioris consistentia habens a natura aptitudinem quod preserueret et duret et aptitudinem quod proficiat in melius, secundum Galenum de diffinitiua doctrina, complementum tamen recipit ab adiutorio medicine a deo create ... sic et deus post spiritus celestes et spiritum humanum assumptum homini interiori id est anime dedit nobiliorem naturam et iusticiam originalem.' Ibid. fol. 13vb.

[63] See n. 78, Ch.3. The content of the argument attributed here to Galen's *De diffinitiua doctrina* bears some resemblance to Galen's discussion in *De foetuum formatione libellus* in Galen, *Opera omnia*, iv. ed. C. G. Kühn (Leipzig, 1822), 652–701. I could not, however, find a direct relationship with this Galenic text. I am grateful to Vivian Nutton, who suggested such possible secondary use of *De foetuum formatione*.

has given man a noble nature, that is, the soul, and a basic virtue of original justice which creates moral uprightness (*rectitudo anime hominis*, equivalent to physical health) and the means of its preservation. This may be supplemented by divinely installed correctness of will (*rectitudo voluntatis*) which nourishes the soul as food nourishes the body.[64]

This discussion demonstrates how Galvano uses his professional knowledge concerning the body to examine the soul, which he regards as within his medical jurisdiction. Galvano is far more philosophical and 'academic' in his approach to generation than Arnau, and he also explicitly cites various medical and philosophical sources. Though both he and Arnau use physical generation as an exemplary aid to a logical argument, Galvano regards his knowledge as a well of hidden spiritual information, which he is competent to decipher. On this particular occasion Galvano's body has a spiritual dimension, which is missing in Arnau's discussion.

Doubtless Arnau's or Galvano's medical experience was what brought the particular allusion to the fore, but the application of scientific knowledge on reproduction to a theological context was not unique to them. Medical terminology was also used by natural philosophers and theologians like Thomas Aquinas and Albertus Magnus, who probably acquired it by studying Avicenna's *Canon* as carefully as any medical master.[65] Examining Giovanni da San Gimignano's use of his knowledge of generation will help us to grapple with the question raised.

Giovanni compares physical conception to the spiritual conception of the penitent through God.[66] It is one of a number of medical similes he offers for penance, which can be signified by the lungs, the eyelids, bile, the spleen, and even the four kinds of stomach ache, according to Avicenna. For conception a suitable matter (*materia conveniens*) is required. This is the menstrual humour or the female seminal humour (*humor menstrualis sive seminalis femine*). Spiritually, this humour represents the remembrance of sin (*recordatio peccati*) since the penitent should

---

[64] 'Rectitudo ergo uoluntatis anime habet ipsam nutrire per dei patris potentiam, augmentare per filii sapientiam et generare per spiritus sancti bonitatem.' MS Paris, BN lat. 3181, fol. 13[va]. Anselm, Augustine, and a certain Galfridus are his sources for this discussion.

[65] M. R. McVaugh, 'The *Humidum Radicale* in Thirteenth-Century Medicine', *Traditio*, 30 (1974), 270–1.

[66] *Sde*, vi. 54, 338[4]–9[1]. Cf. Bartholomaeus Anglicus, *Venerandi patris Bartholomei Anglici . . . opus de rerum proprietatibus* (Nuremberg, 1519), vi. 4 (*de creatione infantis*). For the overwhelming dominance of medical analogies in the 13th-century theological and pastoral discussion of penance, see N. Bériou, 'La confession dans les écrits théologiques et pastoraux du XIIIe siècle: Médication de l'âme ou démarche judiciaire', in *L'Aveu: Antiquité et Moyen Âge* (Rome, 1986), 261–82, at 269–73 and 278–82.

regard himself as conceived spiritually by God (*quasi spiritualiter Deo concipitur*). The second requirement for conception is a suitable place (*locus expediens*), which is the womb (*matrix*); spiritual conception happens in the mind, which fulfils the role of the womb. Third, an efficient cause is required which is the male seed (*semen viri*) 'according to the Philosopher'; Giovanni thus introduces to a hitherto Galenic explanation of conception (which started with the female seminal humour) the Aristotelian notion of the primacy of the male sperm. Spiritually this male seed is the fear of God (*timor Dei*). Fourth, an instrumental cause (*causa instrumentalis*) is required; this is provided physically by the natural heat which influences the powers of the body and sets them in order (*calor nature, virtutem corporis influens et disponens*). As for the formation of the child's body, this does not happen at once but gradually and in a specific order. First the principal organs—the heart, brain, and liver—which are the foundation for all the others, are formed. Giovanni gives a detailed description of the embryo from the stage when all these principal organs are united by the same sanguine matter, through their separation into independent members, and the growth of the other organs from them (from the head the nerves and the spinal cord, from the heart the arteries, and from the liver the veins). He ascribes all this to Galen, but also mentions that Aristotle thought that the heart was the origin of the veins. Giovanni does not seem to be disturbed by blending two such different medical sources in one example; he selects the one most convenient for his religious message. The bones are then formed in order to defend the interior organs (the skull, the pectoral bones, and the ribs). Subsequently, the secondary bones are gradually formed (hands, legs, and arms). It is this gradual development of the emerging body that links it to penance. The penitent does not immediately become perfect; the three principal organs correspond to the three theological virtues, faith, hope, and Christian love (*caritas*); the secondary and defensive organs correspond to the intellectual virtues; the functional organs of the body correspond to the moral virtues. All can reach the state of perfection only gradually. From Galen, Giovanni borrows the term stages of creation (*gradus formationis*) which analyses the four stages of foetal formation and compares them to the phases of penance.[67] The first one resembles milk (*lacti vicinus*, the reference here being to the seminal fluid itself), which is equivalent to the acknowledgement of sin (*recognitio peccati*), since in both stages the material involved can easily become either good or corrupt. The

---

[67] *Sde*, vi. 54, 339²⁻⁴.

second stage is the mixing of semen and blood, and it corresponds to exe-
cration of sin (*detestatio peccati*); admitting sin and recalling it to mind
(*agnitio et recordatio peccati*) is mixed with pain and feelings of abomination (signified by the blood) towards sin. The third stage occurs when the
three principal organs have been formed, but the other organs have not
yet separated into autonomous units. Confession of sin (*peccati confessio*)
is the equivalent moral stage; the three distinct organs are the three kinds
of mortal sin (against God, one's neighbour, and oneself—*in Deum, prox-
imum et in seipsum,* or in the heart, speech, and action—*in corde, ore,
opere*). These sins must be privately confessed whilst all the others will be
confessed later in the communal confession. The fourth stage is satisfaction, in which the body is completed and ordered (*organizatum*) to receive
the soul.

The similarity between penance and the formation of the foetus is
also patent in relation to the minimal duration of each phase;[68] the milky
stage (*gradus lactis*) lasts 6 days, the sanguine stage (*gradus sanguinis*) 9
days, the stage of lump of flesh (*gradus masse carnis*) 12 days, and the
fourth stage, at the end of which corporeal perfection is achieved, lasts
18 days. These 46 days *in toto* (counting the first and the last days) correspond to the four grades of the elect. The successful birth depends on
the gradual formation within the chronological framework of time
described above. Thus the sooner the foetus is formed the earlier the
birth will take place, and the child's chances of survival will decline.
When the formation of the body reaches completion within 30 days, the
child will be born in the sixth month and will definitely not be able to
survive; completion of formation in 35 days often involves a seventh-
month birth, and children are known to be able to survive such an early
birth. Those whose formation is completed in 40 days are born in the
eighth month and cannot survive the premature delivery. The reason
for this peculiar behaviour of the foetus is given by Galen and
Constantinus Africanus. They claimed that, should the child have
strong enough impulse (*motus*) in the seventh month, and he is not
born prematurely in that month, his powers will be debilitated. If born
in the eighth month his chances of surviving (*convalescere ad vitam*) are

---

[68] Ibid. 339⁴–340². See the use of this information in Giovanni da San Gimignano,
*Convivium quadragesimale hoc est conciones et sermones tam sacri quam suaves singuli totius
quadragesimae feriis et dominicis* (Paris, 1611), 479, when he discusses the long duration
which is necessary for the production of good things, and the ease with which they can be
ruined. The 40 days which are necessary to form a human being are contrasted with the
immediacy of death.

non-existent. If he stays in the womb and gains more powers until the ninth or even the tenth month, he could be born a healthy child. Similarly those who reconvert to God may do so fast or slowly. The birth itself is an agonizing process which causes sadness (*tristitia*) though soon sheer happiness is to follow; an identical change of mood is detected among penitents.

Giovanni thus shows that physicians were not alone in finding in the generation process a useful source for moral, spiritual, or theological speculation. He is interested in the embryological aspects of generation and his text communicates a high level of practical knowledge. Yet he uses the medical knowledge as a basis for an imaginary simile rather than for a logical argument. Unlike Giovanni, Arnau does not mention the sources for the theories he expounds, and the medical subject matter is interpolated in the spiritual debate in a natural and unforced manner. Arnau employs generation theories as exemplary models for abstract religious truth. For him the generation process, like all other physical aspects of the body, has no autonomous moral/spiritual meaning or existence. Unlike him, Galvano and Giovanni hold as a premise that the body as such has a spiritual/moral meaning. This distinction gives more credence to Arnau's 'rational', 'scientific' image among the scholars.

For the moment let us content ourselves with the insight that two patterns of using medical knowledge in religious debate can be distinguished. First there is the informative pattern, manifest in the discussion of generation by Arnau and Galvano. Medicine creates exemplary logical aids which support a well established theological truth and are used as informative analogies. In this case the medical example relies on the natural properties (*proprietas rei*) of the exemplary object or phenomenon which do not contain hidden layers of meaning. Second, there is the mystical pattern (Galvano's and Giovanni's approach), in which medicine is a source of knowledge which reveals a deeper moral and spiritual level of meaning. In this case the medical matter maintains by definition a moral/spiritual existence.

Both patterns give physicians ample space to exercise their knowledge in religious contexts. Galvano's behaviour, which fits both patterns, suggests that they are not mutually exclusive. Both patterns take it for granted that the human body is a storehouse for information that transcends its obvious physical dimension. However, both patterns were also used by non-physicians; hence neither of them is specifically medical.

A Medical Approach to Apostolic Poverty?

Any attempt to establish an inherent connection between physicians and apostolic poverty must entail some study of the social and professional composition of the followers of this idea. It has been suggested that Arnau's ideas of medical perfection, of open knowledge which enables the common people (*vulgus*) to know more than the learned sage (*sapiens*), and of *caritas* as the infrastructure of the physician's practice were directly connected to his ideas about evangelical life.[69] But this philosophy of medicine was not unique to Arnau, so why do we not detect an unusually strong presence of physicians among the radical spirituals? Since the idea of poverty is so central to Arnau's spiritual writings, I shall present the few examples which seem to reflect Arnau's medical background and which appear in his discussion of the topic. It is to the style rather than to the content that I would like to draw attention.

Arnau frequently employs categories of body and soul in defining poverty, and the body provides him with numerous analogies. It is essential, he claims, that those who aspire to apostolic status not only raise the dead, heal lepers, and drive away demons, but also cure the sick (*ut infirmos curent*).[70] Thus, for him, there is a direct relationship between the occupation of a physician and practising apostolic poverty. He describes the importance of apostolic poverty for the status of perfection through a comparison with the importance of the leg and hand to the body because 'even though man could live without limbs—albeit not wholly or perfectly, in the same way the condition of evangelical perfection is not whole without poverty which directs the practitioner of evangelical life constantly to avoid expensive and grand things'.[71] He also compares the lack of apostolic poverty with the unbecomingness that results from the lack of a beard in a person who is otherwise physically perfect. Each of these metaphors represents very low-level medical language and betray no evidence of the author's medical background. However, they are part of Arnau's figurative world which, I shall claim, relied almost solely on bodily and other medically related imagery.

---

[69] C. Crisciani, '*Exemplum Christi* e sapere. Sull'epistemologia di Arnaldo da Villanova', *Archives Internationales d'Histoire des Sciences*, 28 (1978), 284–7.

[70] *Gladius iugulans Thomatistas*, MS Vat. lat. 3824, fol. 185rb. Arnau concludes at 185vb: 'Sicut impossibile est hominem esse sine anima et corpore sic impossibile est quod euangelica seu apostolica perfectione quis pauper existat, si proprietarie quicquam possederit.'

[71] 'licet homo possit esse sine ipsis non tantum integre uel perfecte, sic nec status euangelice perfectionis est integer sine usu paupere per quem preciosa et pomposa regulariter euitantur.' Ibid. fol. 185vb–186ra.

Arnau calls for strict observance of the behavioural rules that are
derived from the idea of poverty. For him, the idea is just the basis for
practice. Even the consumption of the basest of things, such as beans and
olives (an allusion to the diet of such spiritual groups), should be performed with due temperance if people really aspire to evangelical perfection. Yet despite his call for the strict observance of the code of behaviour appropriate to evangelical poverty, he rejects the notion that this
code is identical for all. In doing so, Arnau uses the idea of range (*latitudo*), which was a subject of medical interest in 1300 when applied to
health, complexion, and pharmaceutical theory. We encounter here again
the medical or scientific side of his personality; lifestyle, even of those
imitating apostolic poverty, should be adapted to natural circumstances.
Geography, climate, age, and health will determine its unique character
for every person.[72] As in previous instances, Arnau does not sound like a
delirious mystic; he is a physician who has crossed the boundary between
his profession and the clerical domain by applying his medical experience
to the description of spiritual matters, but he has not abandoned his original intellectual preoccupation.

Senses, Organs, and Corporeal Spirituality

Wisdom, if not the direct gift of God, is acquired by the correct use of
man's intellectual powers (*vires facultatis*). Arnau interprets these as the
various senses, especially sight and hearing, which thus link intellectual
achievements with physical attributes. Every sense and every bodily
organ functions both physically and spiritually, and the perfect employment of the sense must involve both levels. Therefore 'those who solely
perceive things by the corporeal sense of hearing have ears to hear and
hear not, for though they may have corporeal ears, they nevertheless do
not hear through the ears of their heart'.[73] Arnau uses the sense of taste to
convey a spiritual message. Salt, in accordance with Matthew 5: 13 ('ye are
the salt of the earth') creates taste; the role of the monastic communities

---

[72] 'usus pauper in temporalibus non est determinatus siue restrictus ad indiuisibile, ymo
latitudinem magnam habet secundum diuersitatem locorum et temporum ac etiam personarum; proinde medium seu mensura debita parcitatis non est eadem in septemtrionalibus et
meridionalibus et in yeme et estate et in iuuene et in sene et flegmatico et colerico.' Ibid.
fol. 186[rb]. On *latitudo*, see McVaugh's introduction to *AVOMO*, ii. 21–2.

[73] 'Nam, qui solum auditu corporis percipiunt, aures habent et non audiunt, quia, licet
aures habeant corporis, non tamen audiunt auribus cordis.' *Tractatus de tempore adventus
Antichristi*, in J. Perarnau, 'El text primitiu del *De mysterio cymbalorum ecclesiae* d'Arnau de
Vilanova', *ATCA* 7/8 (1988/9), 134–69 at 134–5; Ezek. 12: 2; *De prudentia catholicorum scolarium*, 437.

is to preserve the faithful by the sanctity of their speech and way of life, and to render the people 'tasteful' (*sapidum*) to the creator. However, excess salt ruins the whole dish. Arnau therefore criticizes the excessive numbers of monasteries and monks whose sole preoccupation is the incessant quest for alms. The result is a failing of morality and duty, since even salt may lose its power to generate tastefulness amongst the people.[74]

Arnau treats the soul itself like physical matter which needs the quality of heat in order to function properly, namely to love God. Consequently he can proceed to discuss the extent (*mensura*) of the love due to God and the utility and advantage that one can draw from it.[75] He also frequently uses bodily organs (especially the heart, the ear, and the eye) in describing intellectual and spiritual phenomena. Those who do not correctly understand Scripture are characterized by veiled eyes, blindness, a blinded or coagulated heart, and obdurate or deaf ears. Like the physical eye, the spiritual one can also be irritated by dust, closed by a growth of flesh or by blood, turn white owing to white spot (*albugo*), or be overshadowed by tumours.[76] A bent back (*dorsum incurvatum*) is the hallmark of those who indulge in worldly pleasures and always desire terrestrial things.[77] Arnau presents the understanding of Scripture as a physical process in which stiffness and heaviness are removed from the mind and the coagulated heart.[78] The state of belief, epitomized by praise, meditation, and prayer is also described physically. Prayer is defined as 'requesting God with an upright heart and a prostrate body'.[79] Indeed, because the essence of prayer is spiritual, Arnau determines that man

---

[74] *De morte Bonifatii*, MS Vat. lat. 3824, fol. 211[ra]; cf. C. Iannella, 'Malattia e salute nella predicazione di Giordano da Pisa', *Rivista di storia e letteratura religiosa*, 31 (1995), 177–216, at 189 for Giordano da Pisa's use of the metaphor of taste.

[75] *Allocutio Christini* in J. Perarnau, 'L'*Allocutio Christini* . . . d'Arnau de Vilanova', *ATCA* 11 (1992), 83–4.

[76] '[M]ale vident quorum oculi vel turbati sunt pulvere, vel oppressi carnositate aut sanguine, vel candentes albugine, vel panniculis obumbrati.' J. Carreras i Artau, 'Del epistolario espiritual de Arnaldo de Vilanova', *Estudios Franciscanos*, 49 (1948), 394, 399; *Allocutio super Tetragrammaton*, 83–4: 'obscurati sunt oculi eorum . . . quia excecatum est cor eorum, et aures etiam obturate ut audientes verba sacre scripture non intelligant' (cf. Isa. 6: 10); *Apologia de versutiis*, MS Vat. lat. 3824, fol. 152[ra].

[77] *Tractatus de tempore adventus Antichristi*, 137; cf. Ps. 68: 24 and Rom. 11: 10. *Sde* vi. 36, 321[4] uses the simile of back pain to denote the inability or the unwillingness of the slothful to bear heavy loads (moral and spiritual).

[78] *Allocutio super Tetragrammaton*, 85; on coagulated hearts, see *Tractatus de mysterio Cymbalorum*, in Perarnau, 'El text primitiu', 88.

[79] 'Deum rogare cum erectione puri cordis et inclinatione corporis', in *Dyalogus de elementis catholice fidei*, in Burger, 'Beiträge zur Geschichte der Katechese im Mittelalter', 176.

should always pray first for the spiritual objects and only later for the physical ones, for the soul is nobler than the body. Here he adheres loyally to the conventional clerical attitude to the body–soul relationship.[80]

Throughout all his treatises the heart plays an important role as a metaphor for the origin and focus of all religious thoughts, desires, and actions. It is also the centre and core of any spiritual disorder, and the shelter for all the diseased, bestial thoughts which produce wrongful actions. As the heart is the origin of corporeal impulse, so the desire which rises from it is the prime spiritual impulse. By alluding to the heart as the source of all the powers which control animal life, Arnau, the Galenic physician, again echoes a medical notion which is of Aristotelian origin.[81] As with the theory of generation, here too Arnau does not hesitate to use a rival theory as long as it serves his religious argument.[82] It could be an indication that at least in this case the term is not 'medical' at all, but is borrowed from scholastic philosophy or from preachers who used it in similar contexts.[83]

Certain members of the body always have positive association. Thus the womb is the place from which the sinners are rejected, as in biblical language like that of Psalms 57: 4 (58: 3)—'the wicked are estranged from the womb'. Arnau introduces two terms *vulva* and *uterus*, which are usually used synonymously in religious texts. He distinguishes the two, as behoves a physician who is well familiar with their subtle differences (the function of the first is to mix the two seeds, the second is the uterus

---

[80] Burger, *Beiträge zur Geschichte der Katechese im Mittelalter*, 182.

[81] 'Nam sicut cor est principium motus corporalis sic desiderium est principium motus spiritualis'. Ibid. 186. Similar example is given in the Catalan version of *Confessió de Barcelona*, from July 1305, in Arnau de Vilanova, *Obres Catalanes*, i. ed. M. Batllori (Barcelona, 1947) 115. Within the context of providing Scriptural proof for the approaching reign of Antichrist, and after having cited II Thess. 2: 1–9, Arnau produces this example: 'As from the heart all the powers of corporeal life are issued to all the organs, similarly from it are issued or should be issued all the powers of spiritual life, first of all by example and afterwards by teaching.' See also *Raonament d'Avinyó*, in Arnau de Vilanova, *Obres Catalanes*, i. 174, 178, 193; Pouchelle, *The Body and Surgery*, 120–2.

[82] On Arnau's attempt to harmonize the two approaches, see *De diuersis intentionibus*, in Arnau de Vilanova, *Opera*, fol. 36vb–37ra, and García-Ballester, 'Arnau de Vilanova', 148–50.

[83] J. Le Goff, 'Head or Heart: The Political Use of Bodily Metaphors in the Middle Ages', in *Fragments for a History of the Human Body*, iii, ed. M. Feher, R. Naddaff, and N. Tazi (New York, 1990), 12–27; *Sde* vi. 64, 352^2–3^3 (as a simile for the perfection of holy men—*perfectio sanctorum virorum*); N. Bériou, 'La prédication synodal au xiiie siècle d'après l'exemple Cambrésien', in *Le Clerc séculier au Moyen Âge* (Paris, 1993), 242–3 (for Guiard de Laon, bishop of Cambrai, 1238–48).

itself), so that one denotes the Scripture and the other the Church.[84] Pope Benedict XI is hailed as one 'whom Christ nourished from infancy and cherished in his bosom'.[85] Other organs alternately receive positive or negative associations. The motherly bowels of compassion (*viscera matris*) refer to the great care of Jesus for the faithful people.[86] In a later treatise against the Thomists, Arnau says he is motivated to write the treatise by the desire to reveal the dung in their bowels (*stercora viscerarum*).[87]

This is only a selection of individual organs and senses employed by Arnau as analogies and metaphors. But are they specifically medical? Spiritual interpretation of the senses appears also in Giovanni's *Sde*, where the sense of hearing and the structure of the ear reveal truths about the interior sense of hearing, the sense of touch denotes *caritas*, physical vision explains contemplation, and taste and its organs (tongue, lips, and saliva) are similes for wisdom.[88] In a culture which stressed sense perception and gave sensory experience priority over intellectual judgement, sensual religious language was not uniquely medical.[89] However, the density of such metaphors and analogies in Arnau's spiritual treatises, their spontaneous intercalation within the text, and the fact that they constitute the overwhelming source of figurative vocabulary, clearly create a link to his professional preoccupation with the body.

The Body as a Category and Foundation of Corporeal Spirituality

Does the body as a product of divine creation further spiritual speculation? In *Allocutio Christini* Arnau reveals some of the philosophical presuppositions which seem to be linked to his profession. There are two ways to know God (*Deum cognoscere*) in this world. The first is through created things (*per creaturas*) or nature, the second through divine scripture (*per scripturas divinas*) or the Bible. When discussing the world of the created things Arnau mentions fitness of organs (*membrorum decentia*) and bodily strength *(robur corporis)* together with various intellectual faculties

---

[84] 'Uulua quidem est uteri janua. Nec ignoratis quin sacra scriptura sit janua per quam ad uterum superne matris, scilicet ecclesie triumphantis ingrediuntur electi, que gignit eos in utero karitatis dei que diffusa est in cordibus eorumdem.' *Apologia de versutiis*, MS Vat. lat. 3824, fol. 136[rb]; 'alienati a uulua et errantes ab utero.' *Tractatus de mysterio cymbalorum*, 70: 277.

[85] 'quem Christus ab infantia nutriuit et fouit in gremio suo', in *De morte Bonifatii*, MS Vat. lat. 3824, fol. 212[ra].

[86] *Tractatus de tempore adventus Antichristi*, 134.

[87] *Carpinatio poetrie theologi deviantis*, in MS Vat. lat. 3824, fol. 193[vb]. *Sde* vi. 53, 337[1] uses the *viscera* as a simile for particular sinners.

[88] *Sde*, vi. 11, 301[4]–303[2]; vi. 13, 304[3]–306[2]; vi. 16, 309[4]–310[4]; vi. 65, 354[1–4].

[89] J. Huizinga, *The Waning of the Middle Ages* (London, 1955), 192–201.

like discretion, subtlety, wisdom, and prudence, as intrinsic characteristics of the human being which epitomize the benefits and love bestowed by God on man, and so should evoke similar love toward God on the part of man.[90] Thus scrutinizing the body and its organs can lead to loving God and ultimately to knowing him; it provides man with the necessary data which will enable him eventually to reach the desirable religious conclusion.

In one of his last treatises Arnau takes a negative attitude to the body, which confuses the issue but does not undermine the above reading of his texts. In an *exemplum* in the treatise, which is devoted to the idea and practice of *caritas*, he deems excessive care by an abbess of her body to be a sign of sinfulness, based on desire for vainglory and total addiction to temporal or corporeal life. Her attitude, like that of secular women, is the hallmark of her failure to lead a proper, exemplary evangelical life.[91] In his later treatises he regards excessive preoccupation with physical health, which leads even the regular clergy to seek medical advice from non-Christian physicians, as illustrative of their blasphemous behaviour. This attitude of ambivalence towards the care of the body would appear odd in the case of a practising physician, and it seems to be a development of Arnau's very last years. This may be due to his increasing distance from the medical setting (the faculty at Montpellier, where we cannot show that he taught after 1300) and its discourse, an attempt at self-justification by speaking unlike a physician, or the influence of the spiritual or Beguin circles he was affiliated with—a hypothesis I tend to favour. Ambivalence towards and, in extreme cases, disparagement of excessive medical treatment was a not uncommon form of religious piety among the laity. Nevertheless, even at this stage he did not abandon the overwhelming use of metaphors and analogies associated with the body.

Discussion of specific organs inevitably leads to discussion of the body as a whole, which Arnau frequently uses as a descriptive category for every collective unit he writes about. Depiction of the Christian faith, Scripture, and knowledge, and of Christ or Antichrist as bodies, was again not Arnau's invention. As before, each of these metaphors on its own could be employed, and indeed had been so, by non-medical religious thinkers. It is their concentration in Arnau's work which makes it plausible to suggest

---

[90] *Allocutio Christini*, 85: 62–4.

[91] *Epistola ad priorissam de caritate*, in Manselli, 'La religiosità', 73–4; in *Lliçó de Narbona* (written between August 1305 and December 1308) Arnau preaches the rejection of life in this world and total devotion to the needs of the soul. Arnau de Vilanova, *Obres Catalanes*, i. 149.

that his corporeal spirituality is connected to his preoccupation with the human body. Faith is a body of knowledge, and is literally so treated by Arnau. There are fourteen articles of faith, like the fourteen separate joints in the hand necessary for sensation.[92] Christ and Antichrist are described as the heads of antithetic, competing bodies composed of organs such as the believers on one side and the followers of Antichrist on the other. Here this bodily metaphor corresponds with the Galenic notion of the brain's role in controlling the movement of the organs through the nerves. 'For in a body which is properly formed the head precedes the organs, but the contrary happens in a monstruous body.'[93] The clergy is described as a body afflicted from head to toe (soles to vortex, in the medieval construct) by love of temporal things. The effect of this love is compared to the effect of a leech which sucks the body until all moisture is drained from the organs.[94] Since the Christian community is a body, fluid flows through it. In the case of corrupt bodies it is pestiferous venom; conversely, the heads of salubrious Christian bodies are filled with marrow (*medulla*) which in the theological language of the period usually denotes grace.[95] The mystery of the saviour hidden in Scripture is like a body buried in a tomb.[96] Arnau's visionary allegorical description of the end of time is saturated with anatomical language. Germany, for example, will be overwhelmed by the pain of the viscera, and her neck will be broken; the lungs of its people will contract; their blood will be polluted.[97]

The perception of the Christian community as a body allows Arnau to use the imagery of amputation for corrupt organs. Speaking of the corrupt rich and the necessity for capital punishment under certain circumstances, he compares the rich to a gangrenous organ that should be severed from the body. The removal of the corrupt part should be total, so that it will no longer be able to corrupt the body by action, by bad advice, or even by memory. Under no circumstances should the corrupt rich be allowed to remain organs of the body, even if they guarantee to do no evil, because their very presence is detrimental to the whole

---

[92] *Dyalogus de elementis catholice fidei*, 173.

[93] 'Nam in corpore, quod recte formatur, caput precedit membra, e contrario vero in corpore monstruoso.' *Ars catholicae philosophiae*, in J. Perarnau, 'L'*Ars catholicae philosophiae:* primera redacció de la *Philosophia catholica et divina*', *ATCA* 10 (1991), 72: 235–6.

[94] Ibid. 92: 522–5.

[95] Carreras i Artau, 'Del epistolario', 398. Cf. *Sde* vi. 30, 319⁴–320¹, where bone-marrow is the simile for grace.

[96] *Allocutio super Tetragrammaton*, 85.

[97] *Tractatus de mysterio cymbalorum*, 102–3.

body.[98] Arnau also uses the concepts of evacuation and repletion—one of the pairs of non-natural things—to denote his ambitious enemies who are replete with impiety and 'evacuated' of compassion.[99]

The body of the rich is the focus of an *exemplum* which Arnau introduces in *Raonament d'Avinyó*. An attempted murder of a certain surgeon is foiled, the conspiracy is revealed, and the rich man who was behind it stands trial. The story focuses on the attempts by the rich man's powerful friends to persuade the king to be lenient with him. It gives Arnau an opportunity to attack the *falsarii*, who in this case are the rich, but also signify the false pious—the prime target of his criticism. The main argument against them is that they lack the natural traits which should signify their humanity, and so behave contrary to nature. They think that they are of a better, purer nature than other humans. But they live a lie. To demonstrate this Arnau resorts to other examples which seem to stem from his occupation as a physician. The rich neither have a different origin nor are made of different matter. They neither reproduce in a different manner nor enjoy any privileges when dying. From their souls flows the stench of bad reputation. Since they have been excessively nourished on a delicate and moist diet, such as chicken, geese, and other food pounded in a mortar (hence refined), they tend to decompose more quickly. Consequently their bodies stink worse than the poor, who did not indulge in excessive eating and drinking, and consumed only dry food such as bread, *carnsalada* (a greasy piece of salted pork), cheese, garlic, and biscuits. The varying modes of human putrefaction are likened to the difference between a decomposing goose and a decomposing crane.

Not satisfied with this example from the world of animals, Arnau then substantiates his argument by human examples. When people from Urgell or Penedes want to carry the corpse of a rich man to Poblet or Sentes Creus in summertime, they have to whitewash it and smear it with pitch to prevent the smell.[100] If the corpse is that of a sailor or a farmer such precautions are not necessary. He adds the contemporary case of a

---

[98] *Raonament d'Avinyó*, 193–4. Job-like tribulation is one of the seven means to cure a diseased soul; it is compared in *Sde* v. 53, 476³–479⁴ to the removal of putrid organs (*putridorum resecatio*).

[99] 'Nam presumptuosus et ambitiosus impietate repletur et evacuatur omni compassione.' *Apologia de versutiis*, MS Vat. lat. 3824, fol. 154vb.

[100] Poblet and Sentes [Santes] Creus are two major monasteries in Catalonia, situated north-west and north-east of Tarragona respectively. Urgell is a cathedral town and the name of a diocese in north Catalonia. Penedes lies to the west of Tarragona. Roughly the distance as the crow flies from Urgell to the monasteries is about 120 km.; from Penedes it is about 40 km.

rich man in Provence who, while staying in a monastery, was stricken by a disease and suddenly died. To honour him, as was the custom in that hypocritical community, his hosts buried him on the same day in the middle of the choir. Within days such a stench filled the church that even these monks could not bear it, and they could hardly find porters who would exhume the body and bury it outside in the common cemetery.[101] These stories are indeed anecdotal, but they join Arnau's other tropes to reflect his medical occupation.

The analogy of the body is the pivot on which Arnau develops a more substantial argument. For example, he grounds the universal right of every Christian to pronounce on theological matters on the image of Christ's body. If each baptized person becomes an organ of Christ's body, and if through baptism the door is open for the Holy Spirit to distribute at its own discretion the powers of knowledge, science, and health, then no-one can deny physicians the right to reveal what has been given to them by virtue of divine gift, whether or not it has been sanctioned by the authority of recognized masters.[102]

Both physicians and those who had no medical training frequently saw the body as a reflection of the social order.[103] Arnau's political thought does not contain such commonplace use of metaphors of the body. In his writings, health in general acquired political significance, and health care became a moral obligation of the political authority. In 1301 (in the context of the deteriorating relationship between the papacy and Frederick III of Sicily) Arnau gives Boniface VIII political advice explicitly as a physician. He says that physicians believe high winds harm both body and soul, and then equates them with accidents and external dangers. Consequently, he recommends that Boniface resume his former policy, which aimed at convincing Frederick to choose the way of *caritas* in international relations.[104] In a letter to Frederick III (*c.*1310) Arnau reveals the norms and ideals of the Christian ruler. He advises promoting public utility and preferring it over his own private utility, implementing justice equally among all subjects, and imitating Christ. Imitation of Christ requires the Christian king to visit the major hospital

---

[101] *Raonament d'Avinyó*, 191–2.

[102] 'Si ergo magistralis inflatio sibi appropriat id quod apostolus dicit spiritum sanctum distribuere membris christi sicut uult, nonne per tales inflatos doctrina irritatur, apostoli et medici negantur esse de corpore christi et esse fratres eorum in christo? Nam si medici baptisati de corpore christi sunt, constat quod uiuunt per spiritum christi.' *Apologia de versutiis*, MS Vat. lat. 3824, fol. 148ra. See Ch. 3, n. 103 for the whole argument.

[103] For Henri de Mondeville's example, see Pouchelle, *The Body and Surgery*, 101–24.

[104] Finke, *Acta Aragonensia*, i. 102.

which is situated in his domain three times a year (at the octaves of Christmas, Easter, and Pentecost); during these visits he should give alms to the needy. Similarly, the queen should imitate Mary by performing acts of charity and humility. Among other things, four times a year she should visit a hospital and console its patients (usually the destitute rather than the sick). Furthermore, Arnau advises the ruler to abstain from sexual intercourse with his pregnant wife, but wait until she has given birth and has been purged. Physical contact during pregnancy is religiously unacceptable because it causes mutual pollution and because it may be detrimental to the complexion and composition of the foetus. The king is therefore expected to maintain continence by revering God. Arnau also advises the rejection of superfluities of food, drink, and clothing, and establishing a hospital for the poor.[105]

Arnau's political radicalism was influenced by a broader perception of man's place in nature as an animal of a special species. Every man with political authority should refrain from injustice for the well-being (*salus*) of his soul as well as for his dignity. His vigilance to preserve justice should involve mind (*mens*) and body. He should constantly meditate on how to avoid stifling and injuring justice, as if it were a body.[106] He should also visit and be physically present wherever it is necessary to control his officials and ensure that justice is upheld. A prince who neglects justice, says Arnau, is senseless in body and numb in soul.[107]

Arnau's attitude towards nature derives from his medical observation of the human body and its generation, and leads him to preach a political message of equality. Respect for the poor is an essential characteristic of the just prince, since 'although God made him in his reign more honorable and more honoured than the poor, nevertheless by nature he is no better than they are for they were born from the same matter and in the same way just as he was, and they are not less loved by God than he is'.[108] In every political system, therefore, there should be an absolute

---

[105] *Informació espiritual*, in Arnau de Vilanova, *Obres Catalanes*, i. 227–31, 238; *De helemosina et sacrificio*, 615: 208–9. On the process by which health acquired political and moral characteristics and became a moral obligation of the public authority, see L. García-Ballester, 'Medical Ethics in Transition in the Latin Medicine of the Thirteenth and Fourteenth Centuries: New Perspectives on the Physician–Patient Relationship and the Doctor's Fee', in *Doctors and Ethics*, 38–61, at 47–59.

[106] 'vulnerari et suffocari iusticia'. *Allocutio Christini*, 106: 343.

[107] 'in mente sopitur et in corpore torpet'. Ibid. 108: 366.

[108] 'licet Deus fecerit eum in suo principatu magis honorabilem et magis honoratum pauperibus, tamen non est per naturam melior ipsis cum ex eadem materia et eodem modo sint geniti, prout ipse, nec minus etiam dilecti sint a Deo quam ipse.' Ibid. 109: 391–5.

preference for the public good over the private good of the prince. It is the prince's duty to honour and reward the deserving, to direct or suppress as necessary, and to remove those who are incorrigible from the community 'like rotten organs which corrupt the rest of the body'.[109]

Arnau neither systematically discusses the body nor treats it as a mystical object. In this respect he is different from lay mystics (many of whom were women), whose visions of Christ were overwhelmingly physical and sensual, and for whom the use of bodily metaphors and the essential metaphor of illness for the union with Christ were central. Arnau spontaneously uses the body as a physical entity to describe moral and spiritual phenomena. This, along with his frequent use of metaphors of specific organs, may reflect his medical background and the physician's preoccupation with the physical human body.

Let us look at the way Giovanni and Galvano regard the body and employ its images in their texts. In *Sde*, which discusses three main categories of bodily similes, every organ also communicates a higher, religious message. The first category is anatomic similes which describe and explain various aspects of orthodox Christian life. C*aritas* is equated with the nerves, the innate heat of the soul (*calor anime*), the legs, the back, and the heart. Grace is described as bone marrow, and the reception of the divine word as physical digestion, the sense of hearing or the ears themselves, and the formation of voice. Prayer is described within the context of breathing, and pastoral care is compared with breast-feeding. Each simile includes a detailed anatomical or physiological description which is then moralized.[110] The second category consists of similes describing the anatomy of the Christian body, whereby each of the main groups within the Christian community is likened to a certain organ.[111] The third category consists of similes which depict the anatomy of the human mind and intellect. Memory is depicted as the stomach, thoughts as hair, mind as the chest, wisdom as taste, tongue, and saliva, knowledge as the nose, and contemplation as sleep, blood, and eyes.[112]

There is no need to speculate about Giovanni's perception of the human body; the penultimate chapter of book vi of *Sde* explicitly reveals it.[113] According to Giovanni, the body is not a mere corporeal structure but a complex combination of abstract principles which conceal moral,

---

[109] 'tamquam membra putrida ceterorumque corruptiva'. Ibid. 114: 454–5.
[110] See Appendix Ic.   [111] See Appendix Id.
[112] See Appendix Ie.   [113] *Sde* vi. 78, 362²–363¹.

ethical, and religious truths. As such, a person who possesses scientific knowledge of the body can more easily obtain this extra-scientific knowledge. The organs exist in the body in harmonious unity, and reflect similar unity among the faithful of the Church. Organs are attached to each other in some harmonious proportion; the faithful should be similarly connected by *caritas*. The organs share their powers (*virtutes*) and actions (*operationes*), and the faithful should behave in this manner towards one another; those who have received grace should administer it to others, and as the superior, principal organs help, direct, and control the inferior ones, the *maiores* should similarly direct the *simplices*. The *inferiores* also should obey and support the whole structure just as the legs support the body. As long as the organs are governed by the soul, they will remain healthy and able to fulfil and complete their function. When deprived of the *regimen* of the soul, they are harmed. Similarly, as long as the faithful are within the unity of the Church and governed by *caritas*, they remain spiritually healthy; the schism of mortal sin will render them pestiferous and noxious. The unity of the organs is such that, when an organ is harmed, humours from other organs flow to cure it; and a similar pattern of relationship should exist among the faithful, who should rush to the aid of a member in need. The organs are also mutually comforting; pain in one organ might mitigate pain in another (as is the case of phrenesis, when pain in the arms or shanks counteracts a headache). Similarly, the passion of Christ and the suffering of the saints alleviate human pain and toil. In the body, the more noble the organ, the more quickly it is likely to experience harm: this is why the eye suffers more from a small grain of dust than the arm by a major bruise. Similarly, the joints are highly sensitive and, when harmed, shatter the harmony of the whole body: this is why the sins of the *maiores* who display a bad example are more harmful and constitute a cause for scandal. Finally, the seventh and last reason for the simile is that the love among the organs is so great that sometimes when one of them is damaged another is liberated, as happens in cautery, phlebotomy, and surgery, and as is revealed in parallel manner by Christ's passion.

The body is a form of communication which enables religious and ethical truths to be uncovered through the prism of scientific medical knowledge combined with knowledge of Scripture. Giovanni's body is not the product of fear. It is used to express social relations, but it derives its power from a combination of scientific observation and religious beliefs. Thus, while the social experience tends towards setting a low value on the physical functions of ingestion and excretion,[114] Giovanni's scientific observation tends to set a high value on sweat, vomit, intestinal worms, proper evacuation, and any excrement connected with efficient digestion. At the basis of all this remains the belief that body and soul mutually affect each other; the soul follows the complexion of the body, bodily sense organs serve intellectual perception and, by other bodily organs, the soul performs exterior actions.[115] Therefore the knowledge of the one will contribute to knowledge about the other. However, he also stresses that the human body is only one of the organic bodies in nature which, when properly understood, reveal divine truths.

Giovanni's exploration of the human body should encourage a re-examination of the notion that horror of the body was a hallmark of the medieval period.[116] Some people certainly did abominate the body, yet this was not universal: there were also those who were so fascinated by it as to incorporate it into their religious language. Thus, when discussing the existence of sharing and participation (*participatio* and *communio*) in the Church, the Dominican Aldobrandino da Tuscanella employed around 1280 the analogy of the body. The brain which communicates the senses to all the organs, the stomach which is the vessel of digested food for the whole body, the heart which is the source of all the spirits and of life, and the liver which is the source of natural heat, function harmoniously. Aldobrandino described how, despite this harmony, independent organs may be afflicted by paralysis caused by a block in the normal flow of nutritive and vital spirits, and he compared such an organ to the sinner who does not share the goods of the Church.[117] Positive attitudes to the body also appear in thirteenth-century Franciscan sources, suggesting that we are dealing with a more general mood which is not uniquely Dominican.[118]

Giovanni's thinking that there was a tight relationship between body and soul was shared by theologians, who from the second half of the thirteenth century came to treat the body as integral to the person and regarded it as being the focus of personal specificity. These theologians held

[114] M. Douglas, *Natural Symbols: Explorations in Cosmology* (London, 1970).

[115] 'Sed quoniam complexio corporis quam anima in pluribus sequitur et organa corporea sensuum qui intellectuali cognitioni deserviunt ceteraque corporis membra per que interior anima actus exteriores exequitur.' *Sde*, Prol., 4².

[116] J. Le Goff, 'Body and Ideology in the Medieval West', in *The Medieval Imagination* (Chicago and London, 1985), 83–5.

[117] Aldobrandino da Tuscanella, *De scala fidei*, in MS Oxford, Bod. Lib., Laud. Misc. 41, fol. 21^(ra–b); see also Pouchelle, *The Body and Surgery*, 109.

[118] D. D'Avray, 'Some Franciscan Ideas about the Body', *AFH* 75 (1991), 343–63.

that body and soul were inseparable, that the human person was a bodily animal, and that the body was an essential element in human life.[119]
Under such circumstances it may not be so surprising that some
Christian physicians at the turn of the thirteenth century were reluctant
to confine their interests solely to the body.

Galvano entitles one of his spiritual treatises 'The Book of the Structure of the Mystical Body and the Regimen Related to the Head which
is Christ the Lord from whom the Whole Mystical Body which is the
Church Receives its Motion and Senses' (*Liber fabrice corporis mistici et
regiminis eius relati ad caput quod est Christus dominus a quo totum corpus
misticum quod est ecclesia recipit motum et sensum*). It describes and
explains the role of Christ and his successors, the Popes, who lead and
direct the Church as the head rules the body. It discusses the hierarchical order of the mystical body, from the Trinity through the angels
to Peter and the bishops, in a fashion favourable to papal claims of
absolute sovereignty over the Christian community. Galvano introduces many conventional medical metaphors in this treatise, as he does
in his other spiritual treatises. He is particularly fond of the term 'antidote' (*antidotum*), which is supplied by Christ, the new physician who
cured mankind, and which denotes a specific religious text or practice
such as indulgences. The antidote offered by the celestial physician to
fight the various sorts of sensual paralysis purges the filth of disbelief
and cures blindness, bleary eyes, and white spots on the eyes. When the
antidote of Scripture, blended by God from matter of the most simple
complexion like milk, honey, and balsam oil, trickles through the ears,
it affects the soul.[120] Galvano describes the pathologies of sin, speaks of
the divine word as a medicine and nourishing milk,[121] and repeatedly
employs the metaphor of Christ the good, new physician who offers a

---

[119] B. Davies, *The Thought of Thomas Aquinas* (Oxford, 1992), ch. 2 and esp. 207–15; C.
Walker Bynum, 'The Female Body and Religious Practice in the Later Middle Ages', in
Fragmentation and Redemption: Esssays on Gender and the Human Body in Medieval Religion
(New York, 1991), 222–35.

[120] *Liber neophytus spiritualis thesauri indulgentiarum*, MS Paris, BN lat. 3181, fol. 9[vb];
Liber de amando deum, fol. 21[va]: 'quibus fideliter et deuote susceptis ab auribus sordes
incredulitatis abstringitur; cecitas, lippus et albula occulorum curatur . . . sic et antidotum
sacre scripture ex lacte, melle et oleo balsami compositum, si distilletur in aures hominum
operatur in animas eorum scilicet ex gratia unionis nature diuine et nature humane
assumpte.'

[121] Ibid. fol. 27[r] deals with the poison (*pernicies*) invading the body and causing corrod-
ed kidneys and darkened eyes. On the Catholic faith as medicine and the divine word as
milk, see fol. 61[ra–b]; at fol. 66[rb] Ecclus. 38 is paraphrased to present the 'new physician'
who offers a 'new medicine'.

new medicine and who is opposed to the evil physician who is sterile.[122] The act of incarnation is perceived by him as a pharmaceutical process. 'I have come as physician not as judge. Hence I am made the companion of those who languish, I am subjected to stench and dung so that I may provide the remedies', his Christ exclaims.[123] Yet Galvano's medical background is particularly reflected by the manner in which he employs the physical structure of the body as a convenient starting-point for elaborating on complex Christian ideas. Unlike Arnau, he introduces medical and natural philosophical sources to substantiate his ideas.

The sacraments are described as nourishing milk which is given to children and which helps them to develop to the stage of adolescence and youth. The skull allegorically represents the maxim of divine law (*allegorice omne divine legis significatur preceptum*). These precepts are also described by a comparison with the bones, which are the foundation of the human body. Avicenna's claim that there are 248 bones leads Galvano to declare that there is an equal number of affirmative precepts in the divine law. The 365 days of the year signify an identical number of negative precepts.[124]

The formation of the body and the relationship among its organs fascinate him. From eternity the Maker and Creator decreed that the heart should be the first organ to be formed and the last to die, asserts Galvano, confusing the pagan idea of eternity and the Christian notion of creation. Naming Aristotle and Averroes as his scientific authorities, he contemplates with amazement the diversity of the organs of the body and their functions. The brain, the liver, and the testicles grow from the heart, and assume with it the status of principal organs. The rest of the organs emerging from these four principal ones are called inferior organs, even though they are absolutely necessary for the perfection of the body's structure. Nature, by divine will, created this diversity in bodily functions and arrangements neither solely as an ornament nor to induce praise of God's wisdom. Through diversity of bodily organs ('officers', *ministri*),

---

[122] *Liber neophytus spiritualis thesauri indulgentiarum*, MS Paris, BN lat. 3181, fol. 26ʳ, 66ʳᵇ.

[123] 'Nam medicus ueni et non iudex. Ideoque conuiua fio languentium, patiorque fetorem ut prestem remedia.' *Tyriaca mortis spiritualis gradiens super tyriacam medicorum*, MS Paris, BN lat. 3181, fol. 42ʳᵇ.

[124] 'Sunt enim precepta legis diuine in corpore mistico. Sicut ossa in corpore fundamenta humano. Ut sicut in uniuerso ossa corporis humani sunt ccxlviii, secundum Auicennam, ita precepta affirmatiua in lege diuina sunt tot idem.' MS Paris, BN lat. 3181, fol. 2ʳᵇ. Cf. Avicenna, *Liber canonis*, i. fen 1, 5. 30, 18ᵛᵇ.

their services and functions (*ministeria*) are performed more diligently and executed more promptly.[125]

Consequently, he leaps smoothly from the discussion of the physical body to the mystical one. Relying heavily on Aristotle's approach (without mentioning him by name), Galvano describes the various officers of the Church. Allowing the heart as the source of the spirit, an overriding influence over the entire body, while simultaneously subscribing to the Galenic doctrine of four principal members and other inferior organs, Galvano is able to discuss the supreme jurisdiction of the Pope within the Church, and the principal position of the bishops, archbishops, and patriarchs who create the inferior members of the Church (parish priests, abbots, and deans).[126] The seven sacraments unite all these organs into one harmonious system. Baptism and Confirmation give the spiritual and vital essence (*esse*) to the mystical body, as the heart gives the vital spirit to the physical body. The Eucharist performs the role of the liver in infusing the mystical body with spiritual heat (*spiritus caloris spiritualis*). The spirit produced in the course of the sacrament of penitence is likened to the animal spirit which is produced in the brain. Ordination, which creates spiritual offspring, is likened to the testicles which are responsible for the formative spirit (*spiritus formativus*). The absolute supremacy of the heart over all the other anatomical systems of the body leads

[125] 'Constat inquit opificem genitoremque deum sic statuisse ab eterno quod in fabrica corporis naturalis humani primum membrum quod formatum sit cor et primo uiuit et ultimo moritur secundum phylosophum 15 de animalibus. Reliqua uero membra eius sue generationis a corde principium sumunt secundum avert. (sic) in suo coliget inter que cerebrum, cor, epar et testiculi simul cum corde principalitatis sortiuntur et nomen. Reliqua uero omnia membra hiis comparata inferiora dicimus licet ad perfectam organizationem fabrice corporis humani necessaria sint. Non solum enim ad decorem nutu dei uariauit natura corporis officinas nec ut sua sapientia diuersis institutionibus lauderetur. Sed ut fideliora seruitia prouenirent ex diuersitatibus ministrorum forent diligenciora ministeria et executiones occurrerent promptiores hoc autem non uacat a ratione misterii.' MS Paris, BN lat. 3181, fol. 6vb–7ra. Cf. Aristotle, *De Gen. Anim.* ii. 5, 741b .

[126] 'Sane sicut in corpore humano quadam membra principalia sunt sicut cor, cerebrum, epar et testiculi reliqua uero omnia hiis comparata inferiora dicuntur et sicut omnia membra corporis humani relationem passiuam habunt ad cor quia omnia recipiunt ab ipso influenciam mediante spiritu uitali, naturali, animali et formatiuo que secundum diuersitatem operationum diuersi dicuntur et tamen unus spiritus per respectum ad cor uitalis dicitur, per respectum ad epar naturalis, per respectum ad cerebrum dicitur animalis, et per respectum ad testiculos dicitur formatiuus, ut plane lacius dictum est per me in libro medicine anime, sic in toto corpore universali ecclesie militantis Christus deus et homo instituit unum principalem antistitem a quo executionem iurisdictionis maiorem et minorem membra corporis ecclesie militantis recipiunt. Membra autem principalia huiusmodi episcopi, archiepiscopi, primates et patriarche et maiorem iurisdictionis extensionem accipiunt. Inferiora uero membra corporis ecclesie militantis sunt creati, scilicet presbiteri parochiales, prebani, archipresbiteri, abbates, decani et huiusmodi.' MS Paris, BN lat. 3181, fol. 7ra.

Galvano initially to abandon the conventional metaphor which depicts Christ or the Pope as the head of the Church. Both should be described as the heart, while the metaphor of the head should be used in describing the Roman Church as the head of all the other Churches in the world.[127]

Yet the general predominant influence of the heart over all the other organs is according to truth (*secundum veritatem*); according to appearance (*secundum manifestationem*) the head takes the supremacy. Through a meticulous description of the head as the source of senses and thought of all kinds, Galvano vindicates the usefulness of the metaphor of the head when describing Christ or the Pope, who, as we have seen above, can be signified by the heart. He cites medical authorities to describe the three ventricles of the head, the first of which is hot, dry, full of animal spirit and little marrow, and is the organ of common sense (*sensus communis*, the clearing house for all sensation), fantasy (*fantasia*), and *imaginatio*, which receives and retains the sensible forms. The second is the organ of cognition, is hot and humid, full of spirit and marrow, and is called by Johannitius of Alexandria *cerebrum*. It contains two powers: the imaginative power (*vis imaginativa*), which works on the material stored up in the *imaginatio*, joining and dividing forms to make new ones; and the estimative or judging power (*virtus extimativa*), which perceives meanings in the sensations brought to it by the common sense, fantasy, and *imaginatio*. The third is the organ of memory, which is cold and dry, and according to Avicenna contains little spirit and marrow.[128] Seven pairs of nerves are responsible for translating feelings and thoughts into action. Galvano describes what he is doing as transumption or transfer from the natural human body to the mystical body in order to manifest its hidden properties.[129]

---

[127] 'cum caput non influat in cor sed potius econtra, ergo Christus dici debet magis cor corporis mistici quam caput.' Ibid. fol. 7[ra–rb].

[128] 'In capite etenim omnes sensus apparent. Ibique sensus eminenciorem situm habent. Et in capite sunt uentriculi siue cellule tres ad senciendum ita quod prima scilicet, anterior est organum sensus communis, fantasie et ymaginationis, que forte calida et sicca est multum habens de spiritu animali et parum de medulla. Secunda autem est organum uirtutis ymaginatiue humane rationis decorate nec non et extimatiue que forte calida et humida est tam in spiritu quam in medulla multum habundans ex quo anthomasice [sic] a johannitio alexandri cerebrum appelatur. Tertia autem est organum uirtutis memorie que forte frigida et sicca est cui parum de spiritu et medulla attribuitur ab ipso ergo capite secundum Auicennam.' Ibid. fol. 7[rb]. Cf. Avicenna Latinus, *Liber de anima*, I. v. 87–92; E. R. Harvey, *The Inward Wit: Psychological Theory in the Middle Ages and the Renaissance* (London, 1975), 39–46.

[129] 'transumptio corporis naturalis humani ad corpus misticum . . . ad manifestare eas proprietates spirituales latentes'. MS Paris, BN lat. 3181, fol. 7[rb].

Galvano performs the transumption on various occasions in his other treatises. The properties of the teeth, for example (they are white on all sides, they are strong and fleshless, they cannot bear anything to intrude between them; there is no worse ache in the body than toothache, they chew the food for the whole body, they are defended by the lips), provide him a useful comparison with the monastic orders (*viri religiosi*).[130] The unity (*unio*), the provision (*subministratio*), and the exchange (*communicationis vicissitudo*) which characterize the organs of the physical body merely portray the features of the spiritual one.[131] The ensuing description of God as *medicus optimus spiritualis*, who pours wine and oil over wounds and restores spiritual health, is thus a natural development of that worldview. Christ should be called the head of the mystical body, since from him originate the seven sacraments through which the believer receives the spirit of divine knowledge and the inclination to charit-able conduct.

A similar pattern appears in Galvano's medical collection in MS Vat. lat. 2463. The third treatise in the manuscript is dedicated to Albertus de Flisco, and deals with diseases of the joints (such as gout, podagra, and sciatica). At the end of the prologue Galvano writes: 'And since we find hiding dormant in them the spiritual medicine for the sick mind, we therefore add a second treatise concerning the wholesome interior person.'[132] That second treatise starts with a declaration linking Galvano's professional interest in the body with his interest in spiritual health. He has transformed past intellectual engagement with the human body and other disgraceful (*turpis*) things into a new interest in spiritual health, improvement of ecclesiastical devotion (*cultus*), and contribution to the spiritual well-being of humans. The link to the previous treatise about the joints is Isaiah 48: 17, which Galvano partially cites and fuses with his own original interpretation: 'I am the Lord thy God which teacheth thee to profit' is immediately followed by 'from the organs'. Galvano thus creates a link between the body and divine secrets.[133]

This is followed by thirteen chapters which give a moral interpretation to all the organs described in the previous section on arthritic diseases (the

---

[130] MS Paris, BN lat. 3181, fol. 63ra, 67vb. This congruence is based on simple observation rather than on deep medical knowledge, and it is found in preachers' manuals. Cf. *Sde* vi. 63, 351^1–4.

[131] *Liber spiritualis thesauri indulgentiarum*, MS Paris, BN lat. 3181, fol. 10ra.

[132] 'Et quia in illis et membris eorum inuenimus mentis languentis medicinam spiritualem iacere, ideo adiungitur tractatus secundus interioris hominis salutaris.' MS Vat. lat. 2463, fol. 79^v.

[133] 'Ego dominus deus tuus docens te utilia ex membris.' Ibid. fol. 110rb.

arms, hands, fingers, knees, shins, shoulders, back, and neck). Here there are few medical allusions; Galvano describes the function (*ministerium*) of the organs, and introduces moral associations which are linked to the specific function. In chapter 10, for example, the back, which is defined as *conexura spondilium* (knot of vertebrae), is said to give the body its erect stature; Galvano elaborates on the need to direct one's thought and desires to heaven. Although the content of the treatise does not reflect specific medical knowledge, its context reveals a theologizing physician for whom the body, as the object of his profession, communicates moral and spiritual messages to be assimilated and explained to the wider public exactly like physical information. He performs this transformation under the umbrella of *caritas,* which obliges him to supply medical care. Galvano stresses in the prologue to the treatise that, driven by divine grace, he is supplying mankind with useful information concerning its health; in the case of physicians, this information is usually specifically medical, but this time it is of a spiritual character.

Hitherto I have dealt with the broad issue of contemplation and observation of the physical body leading to similar observations on the mystical body. Let us now look at two specific examples of the smooth leap from medical to spiritual contemplation through the medium of the body, examples which also reveal Galvano's level of medical language.

In his devotional treatise 'The Book of the Spiritual Treasure of Indulgences' (*Liber spiritualis thesauri indulgentiarum*), Galvano discusses the virtue of humility which is the medicine for man's tumour of pride and is one of Christ's key virtues. The metaphor of man as a worm (*vermis hominis*) (Job 25: 5–6), used so often by Galvano and other pious writers of the period (including Arnau), together with Micah 6: 14 which says 'and thy casting down shall be in the midst of thee' (*humiliatio tua in medio tui*), provides him with an opportunity to interpret the digestive system morally by fusing the scriptural verses and medical knowledge. Interpreting Micah, Galvano holds that the verse speaks about the stomach, which is not simply an organ but a divine vehicle for spiritual messages. The stomach forces the human being constantly to observe, to feel, to contemplate, and to be aware of his humble origin (*materia sue humilitatis*). The general condition of the viscera, which are sometimes silent and passive and sometimes move violently and produce murmuring noises, sometimes rest and sometimes emit violent gases, determines the disposition of the whole body and makes us aware of our vulnerability. The intestines are a hothouse for various kinds of parasitic worms and serpents, which, according to Avicenna, are useful for the digestion. Thus even worms may be of value when looked at through the eyes of the physician.[134]

Elsewhere Galvano moralizes on the eye. For this purpose he employs more than banal metaphors which depict the blood of Christ as medicine of the eyes (*medicina oculorum*),[135] or white-spot in the eye of the faith (*albugo in oculo fidei*) as the disease afflicting the arrogant, who follow human reason (represented by Aristotle and his disciples) rather than Christ and his disciples (represented by Saint Bernard).[136] Complete blindness is the state of those who utterly ignore the light of divine contemplation. Bleary eyes, in which the pupils are healthy yet the sight is spoiled by the uncontrolled flow of humours into the eye, are found in those whose minds are obscured by carnal actions despite their inclination towards knowing the truth.[137]

In the treatise 'Treasure of Monastic Poverty' (*Thesaurus religiose paupertatis*) Galvano praises the mendicant orders, in particular their founders. He devotes to the eyes a major part of his discussion of St Francis, whom he calls 'the organic eye of Christ' (*oculus officialis organicus Christi*).[138] Galvano starts with a scientific description (explicitly attributed to Avicenna and Johannitius of Alexandria) of the structure of the eye resembling Johannitius's analysis of the physiology of the eye in *Ten Treatises on the Eyes* translated into Latin by Constantinus Africanus.[139] This includes a detailed description of the three humours: vitreus, crystalline, and albuminoid (*humor vitreus, cristalinus, albugineus*) and the seven membranes: sclera, choroid, retina, arachnoid, uvea, cornea, and conjunctiva (*tunice—sclirotica, secundina, rethina, tela aranea, uvea, cornea, coniunctiva*). These membranes perform the role of separating the humours (*sequestratio humorum*), and each of them contributes to the proper functioning of the eye and the transformation of the visible image to the brain. The eye thus introduces light to the body, and creates perception and cognition of the shape (*species*) and colour of all things. Galvano then describes how Francis, as the eye of Christ, supplies the

---

[134] MS Paris, BN lat. 3181, fol. 25^{rb-va}; cf. Avicenna, *Liber canonis* iii. fen 16, 5. 1, 331^{ra-b}. [135] MS Paris, BN lat. 3181, fol. 35rb.

[136] *Liber neophytus spiritualis thesauri indulgentiarum*, MS Paris, BN lat. 3181, fol. 10rb; *Liber de amando deum*, ibid. fol. 22ra.

[137] 'Nam in lippis oculis pupille sane sunt sed humore defluente languente palpebre grosescunt quorum quia infusione crebra conteruntur, acies uitiatur, pupillatio queritur.' MS Paris, BN lat. 3181, fol. 22rb.

[138] Ibid. fol. 64vb–65va.

[139] D. C. Lindberg, *Theories of Vision from Al-Kindi to Kepler* (Chicago, 1976), 34–42, and *Pecham and the Science of Optics* (Madison, Milwaukee, and London, 1970), 249–50, n. 93.

world with light and knowledge.[140] He is endowed with three spiritual humours, faith, hope (mentioned implicitly), and *caritas*, and seven spiritual membranes, which provide him and his followers with protecting shields. One of these shields is obedience, which is also called the membrane of contemplative life (*tunica vite contemplative*); it corresponds to the membrane called *tunica sclirotica* because of the hardness (*durities*) which characterizes both. *Pietas* is another shield, and it corresponds to *tunica secundina*, which originates from the interior cerebral membrane called 'pious mother' (*pia mater*, the inner coat of the optic nerve). The love of poverty (*amor paupertatis*) corresponds to the *rethina*, and a preference for chastity (*prelibatio castitatis*) corresponds to the membrane called *tela aranea*.

Moralization on the eye supported by significant knowledge of its physiology was not a mode of expression limited to physicians at the turn of the thirteenth and fourteenth centuries. Giovanni described the seven *tunice* which represent the seven divine gifts that should decorate the mind of the preacher, and the three humours of the eye which designate the three theological virtues. He mentioned Haly as the source for this optical knowledge, which he interpolated into a sermon on the theme of Luke 10: 23 ('Blessed are the eyes which see the things which ye see').[141] By discussing the three humours of the eyes and their role in the transmission of the sight, the nerves which transmit the image to the brain and the pupil which is the instrument of vision, he explained to his audience the concept of beatific vision and ways for attaining it.[142]

Pierre de Limoges wrote his highly popular treatise 'On the Moral Eye' (*De oculo morali*), which also mixed *exempla*, moralism, biblical exegesis, and current scientific knowledge.[143] According to Pierre, acquaintance

---

[140] 'Sic beatus Franciscus dei seruus ex tribus humoribus et 7 tunicis spiritualibus a deo dotatus factus est oculus Christi, officialis organicus prestans mundo lucem.' MS Paris, BN lat. 3181, fol. 65[ra].

[141] *Sde* vi. 59, 344[I]–345[I].

[142] 'Item in medio occuli posita est pupilla que est principium instrumentum uisiue uirtutis . . . habet autem pupilla magnam dignitatem quia, ut dicit aly, omnia que in occulo sunt aut sunt pupillam iuuantiua aut pupille seruientia.' MS London, BL Addit. 24998, fols. 182[vb]–85[va] at 183[rb–vb].

[143] On the treatise see D. L. Clark, 'Optics for Preachers: The *De oculo morali* by Peter of Limoges', *Michigan Academician*, 9/3 (1977), 329–44. It is not clear whether this Pierre is the same one who was Dean of the faculty of medicine in Paris in 1267 and 1270 or a different Pierre de Limoges—a bachelor of theology who died in 1306 as a canon at Évreux. (The second was a Fellow of the Sorbonne and, together with Thomas le Myésier, constituted the party supporting Llull at the University of Paris. Hillgarth, *Ramon Lull and Lullism*, 158). E. Wickersheimer, *Dictionnaire biographique des médecins en France au Moyen Âge* (Geneva, 1936), 645; Jacquart, *Supplément* to Wickersheimer, *Dictionnaire*, 237. I have consulted MS Oxford, Bod. Lib., Bodley 315, fols. 28rb–59vb.

with the physiology of the eye is 'useful for acquiring a fuller knowledge of divine wisdom'.[144] Alhazen ('alahacen') and Constantinus are the source for the scientific knowledge he employs. The seven parts of the eye needed to protect the pupils which are the source of vision are equivalent to the seven principal virtues that defend the soul called 'the spiritual eye' (*pupila spiritualis*). The three fashions of seeing—by reflected, broken, or direct lines—depict the three modes of beatific vision in the state of glory (*status glorie*) which culminate in perfect, direct vision. Like physical vision, spiritual vision also demands an external existence of the shape and quality of the seen object. Pierre extensively quotes Ptolomaeus's *Sciencia perspectiva* when the interior process of transferring the image via the visual nerves to the brain is discussed. Spiritual vision follows similar patterns; one should not judge anything *prima facie*, but only after sincere inner deliberation.[145] The twelve properties of the eyes also hide religious truths, and turn the eye into the judge of the soul (*iudex animi*). In addition to physiognomic ideas about the colour and shape of the eyes and their moral meaning, Pierre also mentions the principle according to which one eye compensates for the other, which gives him some insight into the idea of community.[146] Specific eye conditions like white-spot (*albugo*) and an overflow of the crystalline humour correspond to specific sins, which acquire medical names like *albugo spiritualis*.[147]

The human body was therefore a powerful source for spiritual speculation and expression, and it was universally employed as such by physicians as well as thinkers with no specific medical background. As the example of Giovanni shows, in the early fourteenth century even citing specific medical authorities is not automatic proof of the writer's medical background. The way Arnau, Galvano, and Giovanni used medical knowledge in their spiritual writings suggests that these metaphors may have their origin in Scripture rather than in any medical experience. Galvano and Giovanni employed a much higher level of medical language than Arnau. Only a few of Arnau's medical figures reflect any knowledge which can be described as a product of academic medicine. It seems clear, then, that, as previously concluded, Arnau uses the body and its organs as a storehouse of examples and generally retains their simple physical characteristics. Galvano and Giovanni start from the distinction

---

[144] 'utilis ad habendum diuine sapiencie notitiam pleniorem'. MS Oxford, Bod. Lib., Bodley 315, fol. 28[va].   [145] Ibid. fol. 29[rb–vb].

[146] Ibid. fol. 34[ra] and *passim* to 39[ra].   [147] Ibid. fol. 39[vb]–40[ra].

between the exterior and the interior body, and proceed to moralize about it on the basis of intensive use of medical authorities. Yet the quantity and the relative density of the terms employed suggest that Arnau linked his spiritual activity to his medical background. One further example will illuminate this observation before a final appraisal of this section.

The Vocabulary of Disease

Arnau frequently alludes to diseases—from tumours and moles to malignant cancer, from sterility to madness, from catarrh to lethargy—when he writes of his critics. These diseases are characterized by malignancy, contagion, and incurability. They are employed as metaphoric types, and I have found no detailed clinical description of them by Arnau. The intensifying use of the vocabulary of disease, poisons, and antidotes may reflect his growing interest as a physician in practical pharmacology, poisons, and antidotes in the latter part of his life.[148] Yet, if my reading of his subtext is correct, Arnau's references to disease, plague, infection, and pestilence, matters on which he is expert, elucidate the medical path which led him to the spiritual domain.

As I have concluded in previous sections, the level of medical language Arnau employs is quite low if taken trope by trope. It is also quite conventional; twelfth-century thinkers had frequently equated erroneous religious ideas with disease.[149] But analysing Arnau's use of the language of disease as a whole, a picture emerges of a physician diagnosing spiritual diseases and claiming to be able to cure them. Arnau regards the vocabulary of disease, pestilence, inflammation, poisoning, and bodily corruption as especially useful in attacking those he condemns as pseudo-Christians and his opponents in general. Thus the theologians of the University of Paris and the Bishop of Paris who supported them in their campaign against Arnau in 1300 suffer from sterility of the mind (*sterilitas mentis*), probably as incurable as the physical state. The bishop's misbehaviour in this case is for Arnau so outrageous that even madness, or weak or utmost insensitivity and stupidity, would not excuse it.[150] Also sterile is the Pope, who does not fulfil his duty to fight every deviation from evangelical truth. This danger to the body of the Christian community

---

[148] M. R. McVaugh, 'Two Texts, One Problem: the Authorship of the *Antidotarium* and *De venenis* Attributed to Arnau de Vilanova', in *ATIEAV* ii. 75–94.'

[149] R. I. Moore, 'Heresy as Disease', in W. Lourdaux and D. Verhelst (ed.), *The Concept of Heresy in the Middle Ages (11th–13th c.)* (Leuven and The Hague, 1976), 1–11.

[150] *Protestatio facta coram domino rege Francorum*, in M. Menéndez y Pelayo, *Historia de los heterodoxos españoles*, iii (Buenos Aires, 1951), p. lxxxiii.

affecting it from head to toe is much graver than the 'pestilence of the Templars'.[151] In Arnau's interpretation of the dreams of the Aragonese kings towards the end of his career, he describes the clergy as utterly sterile (*omnino steriles*). This whole treatise conveys a picture of the Church as corrupt and sick, suffering from debilitating ills (*languores*), moles (*macule*), corruption of doctrine *(corruptio doctrine*), and pest (*pestis*).[152]

Arnau opens *Ars catholicae philosophiae* (*c.*1302) with a quotation from Proverbs 29: 8, 'scornful men bring a city into a snare' (*homines pestilentes dissipant civitatem*), and defines the pestilential people 'as if inflicting pestilence which is the corrupt disease that generally overwhelms the inhabitants or ravages the crops necessary for life'.[153] The root of their evil is an immoderate appetite (*appetitus immoderatus*) for vainglory, and they are afflicted by seven malignant spirits.[154] During the heated debate on Arnau's eschatology initiated by the Dominicans of Girona and led by Fr. Bernardus de Podio Cercoso at the end of 1302 or the beginning of 1303, Arnau calls those who misinterpreted him and Scripture 'either heretics or insane' (*vel heretici vel insani*). Throughout his polemic at Girona the motif of insanity together with impurity and corruption of the mind occupies a major place, and was to become a common trait of all his future treatises.[155] The 'theologizing philosophers' or the 'philosophizing theologians', as Arnau derisively calls the scholastic theologians who oppose him, are intellectually wounded. They suffer from injury to the capacity for natural reason (*vulnus naturalis discretionis*), for they are unable to understand that man's wisdom is limited to what he has learnt and hence is always partial if not occasionally erroneous.[156] Those presumptuous

---

[151] H. Finke, *Papsttum und Untergang des Templerordens*, ii (Münster, 1907), 82, 94–8 (in a letter to James II in 1308).

[152] *Interpretatio de visionibus in somniis*, in Menéndez y Pelayo, *Historia de los heterodoxos*, iii, pp. liv–lv.

[153] 'quasi pestilentiam ingerentes, que est corruptio morbi generaliter opprimens incolas aut fructus necessarios vite communiter vastans.' *Ars catholicae philosophiae*, 57. Leprosy appears as characterizing Arnau's critics in 1304 in his anti-Thomist treatises. *Denunciatio tertia facta Massilie cum carpinatio*, MS Vat. lat. 3824, fol. 204ra.

[154] *Presumptio, ambitio, cupiditas uel auaritia, ypocrisis, inuidia, obstinatio, perfidia. Apologia de versutiis*, MS Vat. lat. 3824, fol. 151va.

[155] *Eulogium de notitia verorum et pseudo-apostolorum*, in Carreras i Artau, 'La polémica gerundense', 33, 37.

[156] *Apologia de versutiis*, MS Vat. lat. 3824, fol. 140[r]; F. Ehrle, 'Arnaldo de Villanova e i "Thomatiste". Contributo alla storia della scuola Tomistica', *Gregorianum*, 1 (1920), 496–7; F. J. Fortuny, 'Arnau de Vilanova: els límits de la raó teològica. Arnau en oposició a Averrois, Maimònides i Tomàs d'Aquino', in *El debat intercultural als segles XIII i XIV*, ed. M. Salleras (Barcelona, 1989), 31–59 and esp. 43–56.

teachers who claim that God, by his ordained power, could not make known the end of time show such a lack of understanding of Scripture that they can be proclaimed mad.[157]

Speaking about his Dominican opponent Martinus de Atheca in 1304, Arnau determines that 'unless he can be excused due to insanity or lethargy, he certainly argues unjustly'.[158] Arnau seems to be implying that insanity and health reasons could explain irrational behaviour; but it is evident from his bitter attack on them that he regarded his opponents as fully responsible.

In the scathing attack he unleashes against the Thomists in 1304 Arnau speaks of the ignorant mockers who have become diseased animals, and whom 'we know to have diseased eyes inflicted with the disease of envy or some other malice for they cannot tolerate the benefit of light'.[159] Held up by excessive folly, they abhor the sound (*sana*) and catholic interpretation of divine scripture. In *Antidotum*—the treatise which is perhaps the most thoroughly saturated with images of sickness—Arnau determines that while disease (*morbus*) and drunkenness (*ebrietas*) are possible causes for the outrageous opinions of his opponents, sickness rather than distilled wine explains their behaviour. Thus he holds them fully responsible for it, since spiritual like physical disease is caused by deviation from the correct regimen. Because disease is the prime cause for their behaviour, he can also diagnose it accurately and concentrate his criticism on the behavioural flaws which cause it.[160] Sickness of the mind (*egritudo mentis*) disables their mental capacity from reaching or accepting the truth, and is therefore the cause of their pathological behaviour.[161]

However, the corrupt false religious who maliciously avoid or even fight divine truth are not the only ill people. Malignant, infectious diseases are only one kind of infirmity; there is a less virulent disease which nevertheless needs treatment. This is lethargic sleep (*sompnum litargicum*), from which sufferers can only be wakened by the sharp sound of

[157] Carreras i Artau, 'La polémica gerundense', 45.

[158] 'nisi per insaniam aut litargiam excusaretur . . . certum est quod inique arguit et non iuste' in *Antidotum contra venenum*, MS Vat. lat. 3824, fol. 244ra; *Prima denunciatio gerundensis*, in Carreras i Artau, 'La polémica gerundense', 51; *Tertia denunciatio gerundensis*, ibid. 56.

[159] 'cognoscemus eorum occulos esse morbidos uel in morbo inuidie uel cuiusquam malicie quia non possunt lucis beneficium tolerare.' *Gladius iugulans Thomatistas*, MS Vat. lat. 3824, fol. 183vb–184ra, 191vb.

[160] *Antidotum*, MS Vat. lat. 3824, fol. 253[ra], 254[rb].

[161] Ibid. fol. 241[vb], 254[ra].

the trumpet.[162] Arnau equates the mental state described as *intelligendi gravedo* (slowness in understanding) with heaviness of the limbs or catarrh, thus transforming a spiritual state into a physical one.[163] He describes the reform of the Church, for which he has campaigned since 1304, as the removal of a stain or a mole from the face of the bride of Christ.[164]

Arnau regards the desire for vainglory as one of the main causes of human corruption. In later treatises he accuses not only theologians but also natural philosophers, physicians, and lawyers of being infected by that disease. All these academically trained intellectuals who lay down the truth to laymen and the ill-informed through their disputations subvert their listeners. Quoting 2 Timothy 2: 17 ('And their word will eat as doth a canker'), he continues: 'namely, it corrupts the faithful like the disease of cancer which gnaws the organs'.[165] The belief that words and ideas may affect the soul spiritually like a cancer was not peculiar to Arnau,[166] who may have drawn that metaphor from the *Glossa Ordinaria*, which he frequently used, or from contemporary use of the metaphor by clerical authors. In fact, it seems that Arnau has in mind a disease similar to that described by Nicholas of Lyra (*c.*1270–1340) who repeats in his commentary on II Timothy 2: 17 the notion of the slow, corrupting effect of the illness already expressed in the interlinear gloss, and says: 'that is, it gradually spreads and aims at the corruption of truth'.[167] However, the choice of the metaphor highlights my argument that the goals of Arnau the physician and Arnau the spiritual man are one—to fight disease on both the spiritual and the physical plane.

The malignancy of disease should not be confused with the inherent

---

[162] Carreras i Artau, 'Del epistolario', 396; *Tractatus de mysterio cymbalorum*, 56.

[163] *Allocutio super Tetragrammaton*, 85. On *catharrus* (a process in which the brain, preternaturally affected by cold, produced a qualitatively unbalanced humour in excessive quantity that passed down through the pores in the palate and by way of the trachea to the lungs) see *The Cambridge World History of Human Disease*, ed. K. F. Kiple (Cambridge, 1993), 635–6.

[164] *De morte Bonifatii*, MS Vat. lat. 3824, fol. 213rb.

[165] 'Lo loro parlare si spignie innanzi come il cancro'; cioè coronpe li fedeli comme la infermità del cancro rode le membra.' *Per ciò che molti*, in Manselli, 'La religiosità', 98.

[166] The fourth canon in the Council of Tours (1163) described the Albigensian heresy spreading *more cancri*. J. M. Mansi, *Sacrorum conciliorum nova et amplissima collectio* (Florence and Venice), xxi. 1177; P. Thompson, 'The Disease that We Call Cancer', in *Health, Disease and Healing in Medieval Culture*, ed. S. D. Campbell, B. B. Hall, and D. N. Klausner (Toronto, 1992), 1–11.

[167] 'Id est paulatim tendit ad corruptionem veritatis.' *Glossa Ordinaria* on II Tim. 2: 17, in *Biblia sacra, cum glossa ordinaria . . . et postilla Nicolai Lyrani*, vi. (Lyons, 1589), 741; the gloss cites there Jerome and John Chrysostom for other explanations to the disease.

weakness (*infirmitas*) which characterizes human existence owing to original sin. Arnau compares the effect of sin on the soul with the effect of poison on the body. The spiritual nature of humans has been bent or corrupted by original sin. The fall of Adam's soul infected his body and poisoned it, and this infection was then transferred to his offspring by contagion.[168] The poisonous character of his opponents' words is a favourite image in his latter writings. In February 1304 Arnau makes two declarations to Durandus, Bishop of Marseilles, in which he urges him to fulfil his duty and resist the venomous doctrine of the false prophets.[169]

Arnau describes pride as a tumour (*tumor superbie*) when discussing the obstacles that hinder the learned members of the faculty of arts from searching for the truth.[170] Being aware of one's origin, and of the miseries and defects of one's nature, is the first stage in removing that tumour, which will disappear only when the present phase of pilgrimage ends. Is this the origin of Arnau's obsession with eschatological thoughts? If there is no cure for infirmity in this world, one should look for it elsewhere, and this he does.[171]

For all these diseases Arnau comes up with a therapy which will restore health (*sanitas* or *salus*). His language implies that the salvation of souls is like a physical process of cleansing (*mundatio*) which is attained in two phases: first, the cleansing of the corrupt spirit, and second, the cleansing of corrupt flesh. The salubrious and useful knowledge contained in his treatises offers an assured route to salvation. Arnau the physician can diagnose sickness, detect its causes, and also provide the means to overcome it. The *Antidotum*, written in 1304/5 possibly in Barcelona, and directed to the Bishop of Mallorca, is an antidote not only against the venom emitted by the Dominican Martinus (Martí) de Atheca, but against all his opponents who are struck by malignant spirits and pour out poison everywhere, and whose rabid bites he counteracts

---

[168] 'Et primo quantum ad infectionem peccati, nam ex lapsu anime primi parentis incidit corpus in infectionem. Et ex infectione corporis orta ab anima generantis contagiata est postmodum anima generati cuiuslibet more humano.' *Allocutio super Tetragrammaton*, 93.

[169] MS Vat. lat. 3824, fol. 180vb, 192^v. *Carpinatio poetrie theologi deviantis*, MS Vat. lat. 3824, fol. 193vb.

[170] *Introductio in librum Ioachim De semine scripturarum*, 58. Carreras i Artau, 'Del epistolario', 402.

[171] 'peccatum veniale, quod in presenti vita non potest omnino vitari propter infirmitatem nostram, et ideo per ipsum retardatur hic fervor karitatis. Sed in patria ubi tota nostra infirmitas erit absorbta, fervebit ad plenam karitas et continuo, quia neque peccato veniali neque aliqua infirmitate vel defectu nostro fervor eius poterit impediri.' *Dyalogus de elementis catholice fidei*, 188.

with medicine.[172] Humanity should be purged of all diseases, and Arnau expresses his desire to do it.[173] Just as in the physical world, discipline of souls (*regimen animarum*) is essential to gain eternal salvation; if it is not preserved (Arnau especially mentions piety in this context) the inevitable results are verbal infections diffused by preaching sermons and spread through libidinous insanity.[174]

It is not surprising, therefore, that the bishop's duties are defined in terms of those of a physician. In *Confessio Ylerdensis* from 1303, which sums up his criticism concerning the regular clergy, Arnau tries to recruit the Archbishop of Tarragona to fight his enemies. Calling the archbishop Christ's vicar in his diocese, Arnau asserts that he should 'give moral education to his herd in word and example and teach it the truth of faith and also cure it from disease or spiritual feebleness'.[175]

All this shows that Arnau uses short metaphors of disease in order to tarnish his enemies, to shock his readers and listeners, and to convince them that his cause is just. In so doing, he utterly ignores the sin–disease link that preachers were so fond of employing. The relative density of his vocabulary of disease together with the extensive use of general medical imagery hint at a medical frame of mind, which enables Arnau the physician who treats the physical body to perceive his spiritual role as an extension of his medical one. Typical for this frame of mind (which will be discussed in the next chapter) is the ending of a *consilium* Arnau gives in 1304/5 to Bremon, lord of Montferrer. He moves there from prescribing an eye-salve (*collyrium*) produced from sea-water and seeds of serapine for improving the sight, to prescribing the sapphire of Christ who should be incessantly applied to the spiritual eyes.[176] A glance at the way Galvano employed the language of disease in a spiritual context

---

[172] *Antidotum*, MS Vat. lat. 3824, fol. 248rb–va. On Martinus de Atheca, confessor to the king of Aragon who in 1304 wrote a book attacking Arnau's eschatological ideas and thus stimulated other Dominicans to preach against Arnau, see T. Kaeppeli, *Scriptores Ordinis Praedicatorum Medii Aevi*, iii (Rome, 1980), 106–7; F. Santi, *Arnau de Vilanova: L'obra espiritual* (Valencia, 1987), 126.

[173] In the Castilian version of *De helemosina et sacrificio*, 623: 490–3, Arnau explicitly asserts that he attempts to heal all human infirmities. '[E]sto todo dize por dar a entender las çircunstançias de la hunmanidat con la qual quiso sanar e guaresçer nuestras enfermedades todas hunmanales.'

[174] The term *libidinosa insania* describes the pseudo-religious and the pseudo-prophets who preach sexual promiscuity. *Interpretatio de visionibus in somniis*, pp. lxvi–lxvii. In *Raonament d'Avinyó*, 170, 174, Christianity in general is defined as *al regiment del hom*.

[175] 'gregem suum uerbo et exemplo de moribus informare ac de fidei ueritate instruere, necnon curare de morbo siue languore spirituali.' MS Vat. lat. 3824, fol. 178va.

[176] Carreras i Artau, 'L'epistolari', 26.

clearly shows that he too perceived his spiritiua interests as an extension of his medical activity.

Galvano maintains that every system, including the human body, relies on a sound foundation from which all other parts of the system directly or indirectly draw their stability. Thus the heart as a principal organ is first formed in the process of bodily generation. It is the foundation of all other organs, and if diseased the well-being of the whole body is jeopardized. Similarly, the sinner undermines the foundation of his soul (this is especially true for the sin of pride).[177] A small quantity of vinegar renders a much larger quantity of solvent totally sour. Similarly, even a small vice corrupts the whole soul.[178] The same categories of description and explanation may be applied to the human morals and the human body. *Discrasia* (complexional imbalance), which is the cause of all diseases, can also be used for describing decaying morals. Galvano describes immoderate ambition and uncontrollable desire for honour as irregularities in appetite caused by indigestion which wreaks havoc on the sense of perception, the intellect, and reason. The intake of undigested food causes nausea; similarly, the intake of undigested words, which do not translate into actual good deeds, leads the person to destruction. Avarice is metaphorically caused by corruption of the blood which spreads to all the organs of the body as a result of retention of matter that should have been digested. The stomach behaves like the mind; both should vomit when they come in contact with putrid matter.[179] However, like the preachers, Galvano does not adhere to a rigid scheme of specific diseases which signify precise sins. In the *summa phisica*, where Christ is

---

[177] MS Paris, BN lat. 3181, fol. 16vb; here he cites again his two lost treatises *Liber caritatis obsequose* and *Liber medicine anime*.

[178] Ibid. fol. 28ra. This is repeated in a later treatise *De neophyta doctrina de inferno purgatorio et paradiso*, fol. 51rb. More chemical information is provided in *Tractatus alphabeti christifere*, MS Paris, BN lat. 3181, fol. 59^{v}–60^{r}, where a list of metaphors is attributed to the Virgin Mary and is arranged in alphabetical order according to the letters which construct her name. Only three of the metaphors echo a medical background. Maple (*myra*) is said to be most useful in curbing putridity, and fighting wind and tumours. *Amigdala* (almond extract) is described as a useful food for the sick, and hyssop (*isopus*) is a purgative medicine for the chest and a cure for tumours of the lungs.

[179] 'Si uero diu retineas que iam digessisse debueras humores concorrumpis et saucias, sanguinem inficis ut impurus transeat, et ad membrorum alimenta cum corruptione perducis; sic totus languens nisi medicinaliter parsimonie studio conforeris. Non igitur erroganda retineas nec dispensanda conserues. Alioquin auaritie labe corrumperis et infamie ueneno necaris, uerba digeras ante quam fiant.' *Ars nauigatiua spiritualis*, MS Paris, BN lat. 3181, fol. 31rb. Cf. MS Paris, BN nouv. acq. lat. 669, fol. 47^{r-v} and 48^{r-v}; *Sde* vi. 14, 307^{1} (stomach as mind); *Sde* x. 74, 485^{3}–487^{4} (proper digestion and healthy appetite as similes of appetite for the word of God and of the proper digestion of spiritual food).

a physician and the sinner a sick patient, acute fever may denote lust, quartan fever is avarice, paralysis is gluttony, *phrenesis* is pride, medicines are penitence, and diet is fasting.[180]

The medical approach to vices helps Galvano to grade them according to their potential danger. The notion that diseases which originate from a hot cause are more dangerous than those which originate from a cold cause enables him to differentiate between sloth, which is of a cold origin, and careless zeal for the love of God (*indiscretus feruor dilectionis dei*, a common disease which afflicts the newly converted), which is of a hot origin and is therefore much more dangerous.[181]

Yet in MS Berlin, SPK, lat. quart. 773 he employs his medical knowledge for moral/religious purposes more elaborately and with greater sophistication. The three practical treatises in the manuscript provide a curative regimen for tremor of the heart (*tremor cordis*), epilepsy, and leprosy, and have nothing obvious to do with moral and religious questions. Indeed, the larger part of each treatise is purely medical; Galvano meticulously describes the disease and offers means to cure it using the usual medical authorities, especially Avicenna. However, each of the two later treatises has a second part tacked on dealing with the spiritual aspects of the disease. It is this leap from the physical to the spiritual that I would like to illustrate, concentrating in my description on the medical contents and omitting the supporting biblical references.

The prologue to the treatise on epilepsy is a short moralistic essay which hardly mentions the topic of the treatise. Like Arnau, Galvano declares himself compelled to write at the instigation of the Holy Spirit and in thrall to the passion of *caritas*. The diseases of the filthy body and the diseases of the soul have been part of the divine scheme since original sin; the former are caused by the latter, and he as a physician must pay attention to both. He describes diseases in general as the direct result of man's dedication to a life of sin and vice. Although his collected medical material is largely from non-Christian classical or Arabic sources, he justifies its use by the fact that medicine, like every art, originates from the grace of the Holy Spirit, and that the faithful are enriched by it. He himself does not use it indiscriminately, but chooses lawful and useful knowledge (*licita et utilia*) and rejects the vile material of the experts (*vilia expertorum*) which is incompatible with Christian orthodoxy. Loyal to Avicenna's definition of medicine, he determines that the power of the physician has been limited by the Creator to the prevention of an over-rapid

---

[180] MS Paris, BN lat. 3181, fol. 66ra.   [181] Ibid. fol. 32vb.

dissolution of the radical humour and the ensuing putrefaction of the body. Galvano ends the prologue in declaring that 'in this corporeal disease and its cure we have found lying dormant the disease of spiritual lunacy and its spiritual cure',[182] and prepares the ground for the second and much shorter part that will be dedicated to spiritual lunacy.

The first and longer of the two parts which compose the treatise (fols. 22^V–60^V) deals in twenty-nine chapters with various aspects of physical epilepsy, child epilepsy, analepsy (which rises from the stomach, the liver, or the spleen), and catalepsy. Though strictly medical in their content, the descriptions are saturated with frequent formulaic exclamations invoking divine aid. Galvano's piety thus influenced the style of his medical writing far more than Arnau's. A combined version of Matthew 17: 15 and Luke 9: 39 ('Lord, have mercy on my son for he is lunatic and sore vexed; for ofttimes he falleth into the fire and oft into water and he foameth') furnishes him the link between physical epilepsy and what he defines as spiritual lunacy (fols. 60^V–69^r). The first of the eight chapters of this second, shorter part defines the lunatic spiritual disease (*lunaticus morbus spiritualis*), reports its symptoms, and recounts its various types. It is written in a medical style, and is directly linked to the discussion of physical epilepsy in the first part of the treatise. Three elements—instability, folly, and loss of sense and motive powers—constitute the common symptoms of physical epilepsy in Galvano's earlier discussion, and they determine also the structure of his discussion of spiritual lunacy, the sole addition being that they are based in Scripture. Spiritual lunacy is inconstancy of the soul. It rises out of folly, and prevents human sense and reason from performing their due activities and motions and from holding the body fully erect.[183] Since the state of spiritual health is so far apart from the state of disease, medical cure (*curatio medicinalis*) will not lead to health unless it specifically and congruently targets the disease. Galvano therefore proceeds to give the names of the three types (*species*) of that spiritual disease (lust, proneness to anger, and greed) which, he stresses, correspond to the three types of physical epilepsy discussed in the first part.

The second chapter of the spiritual part of the treatise discusses the double name of falling disease (*caducus*) and lunatic disease, or the disease

---

[182] 'in hoc morbo corporali et in cura eiusdem inuenimus morbum spiritualem lunaticum et curam ipsius spiritualem iacere.' MS Berlin, SPK, lat. quart. 773, fol. 22^V.

[183] 'Inquam ergo spiritu sancto duce quod langor mentalis lunaticus est humane mentis inconstancia et stulticia prohibens sensus hominis ab operationibus sensus et motus et erectione non integra'. Ibid. fol. 62^V.

of the moon-struck (*morbus lunaticus*). Both fit the spiritual condition which involves falling away from (*cadi facere ab*) dignity, humility, and love, and also constant change and instability, which ties in with the changing size of the moon that affects people's mood.

The third chapter discusses the differences between and the shared characteristics of spiritual and physical infirmities. In both cases, when the cause is interior rather than exterior the cure is more difficult and doubtful. Galvano compares imbalance (*malitia*) with a sin against the Holy Spirit (such as living without penitence); both are fatal. A man who rejects grace, which was given to us as a cure, is like a patient who rejects the physician's advice. Furthermore, the same eight impediments which hamper physical cure hamper the spiritual healing process.

THE UNIVERSALITY (*generalitas*) of the disease is that which determines its degree of pestilence, infectiousness, and contagiousness. The more universal and widespread the disease is, the more dangerous it is and difficult to overcome. So how should one diagnose the spiritual disease with which we are all inflicted? Just as leprosy infects one person and then spreads everywhere without control, so the leprous sins of vanity and pride, cupidity and avarice, carnality and moral filth, anger, hatred, and discord, gluttony and intoxication, envy and spite, torpor and sloth infect and corrupt the congregation of the Christian Church. Hence we should speak of pestilence when we analyse the moral condition of people.[184]

THE DURATION (*diuturnitas*) of the disease. Galvano asserts that the spiritual pestilence by which we are inflicted has been with us since the days of Adam and Cain, and that it grows ever stronger. When diseases such as phthisis and hectic or quartan fevers turn chronic, the condition of the patient becomes more precarious. Similarly, the state in which sin becomes habitual is most dangerous.[185]

THE OPPOSITION OR CONTRARIETY TO THE AFFLICTION (*contrarietas morbi*). The more complex and compound the affliction is, the more difficult is the cure, since a cure for one of its elements (which usually is based on prescribing a counter-effective measure) may damage another organ or exacerbate other diseased elements. The various elements of the compound disease are interrelated, and the cure, if

---

[184] MS Berlin, SPK, lat. quart. 773, 64^V–65^r.

[185] 'periculosa est infirmitas diuturna cum in cronicam uertitur egritudinem ut pthisis ethica et quartana. Sed periculiosior est molita consuetudo peccandi a qua uix potest desistere.' Ibid. fol. 65^r.

possible at all, is most difficult. People who are both sinfully envious, avaricious, and lustful suffer from such a compound spiritual disease, which can hardly be cured. The first two sins affect a cold mind (and demand a warm medicine to counter them); the third excessively stimulates and heats up the flesh (and demands a cold medicine). Similarly, those who overflow by prodigality and are dried up by cupidity can only be cured with great difficulty, since one condition demands a dry medicine and the other a moist one.

THE INTENSITY AND FEROCIOUSNESS OF THE DISEASE (*acuitas, furiositas*). Does not Galen tell us, asks Galvano rhetorically, that an acute disease is that which approaches its end speedily, and is thus called great and dangerous? It ends quickly in destruction of the body, and is immune to almost any kind of medicine. In acute fever and phrenesis the disease penetrates the vital spirit and destroys it. Those who slander, disparage, and defame the people who have morally corrected them suffer from similar disease which penetrates their vital spirit. Spiritual vices like pride, vainglory, hate, envy, and pomposity penetrate the intestines of the heart like acute fever, and extinguish the vital spirit which is *caritas*.[186]

THE RESISTANCE OR INCOMPATIBILITY OF TIME (*temporis repugnantia*). Diligent physicians should direct their attention to the opportune time when prescribing cures. Thus, in times of great heat and dissolution of the humours, no medicine can be offered—unlike times of great cold, which lead to immoderate constriction of the elements of the disease and solidification of the humours.[187] Galvano cites Hippocrates's advice to adapt the cure by purgation to the opportune celestial constellation, and couples it with Ecclesiastes 3: 3 ('A time to kill and a time to heal'). This allows him to leap into the spiritual domain and apply the

---

[186] 'Nempe secundum Galenum morbus acutus dicitur qui cum uelocitate sui finis dicitur esse magnus, id est periculosus. Cito enim interimit et uix recipit medicinam sicut apostema quod dicitur noli me tangere. Qualis est hodie inquam pluribus qui si ab eo corrigantur de maliciis uel uiciis suis. Mox calumniant corrigentem, detrahunt uel infamant. Ex quo talis morbus de facili intrat et penetrat usque ad spiritum uitalem ut patet liquidius in febre acuta et frenesi. Sic hodie uitia spiritualia ut superbia uanagloria, odium, inuidia, pompa et huiusmodi tamquam febris acutissima usque ad intestina cordis transeunt et extingunt spiritum uitalem, i.e. caritatem.' Ibid. fol. 65^V.

[187] 'In forti enim calore propter nimiam dissolutionem humorum nec in forti frigore propter nimiam coacentrationem eorum ac immoderatam materie morbi compactionem nequaquam medicina porrigitur. Monito ypocratis dicentis sub cane et ante canem moleste sunt purgationes. Tempus enim curationis congruum medici periti attendunt.' Ibid. fol. 65^V.

same rule to the physicians of the soul, who are sometimes advised to desist from employing the word of God as a cure, since the environmental or climatic imbalance (*malitia temporum*) may render it ineffective, or rather, counter-productive. For it is hateful for the proud to be preached at about humility, or for the lustful to be lectured about continence.

THE INCOMPETENCE OF PHYSICIANS (*imperitia medicorum*). According to Galen, an inexperienced physician is an enemy rather than an aid to the sick person, and should be judged as the worst of all murderers. Similarly, an inexperienced spiritual physician does not cure but wounds when, despite pretending in his sermons to be experienced, he neglects the well-being of his patients.[188]

THE INSUFFICIENCY OF MEDICINES (*medicinarum insufficientia*). Penance, like physical medicine, must be proportional to the spiritual disease it is supposed to cure and to the disposition of the patient if it is to be effective at all.

THE DISOBEDIENCE OF THE PATIENT (*infirmorum inobedientia*). There is no hope of cure if the patient abhors the medicine and disparages the physician's advice. The same principle applies in the priest/believer context. He who despises the divine law and the word of God neglects the health of his soul.

This particular chapter could well have been written by a preacher or a theologian who was acquainted with these comparisons. As I shall show in Chapter 4, similar discussions of the priest/believer relationship frequently appear in various contemporary sermons, preacher's manuals, and moralistic treatises; however, they are much shorter and more schematic than Galvano's version. The more 'medical' character of Galvano's treatment of the topic is revealed through the medical authorities to whom he refers in the text, and of course from the context of the discussion.

The practical part of the discussion of spiritual epilepsy shows that Galvano thought he could provide the cure for the disease he has diagnosed. The fourth chapter lists the six things essential for a cure to spiritual epilepsy; these fit the six common modes for the cure of corporeal epilepsy discussed in the first part of the treatise. They include confession, compassion, discretion (the willingness to approach the true physician), faith, trust in the possibility of being cured on the part of the patient, and mercy on the part of the physician. In the fifth chapter

---

[188] 'Nam secundum Galenum imperitus medicus est inimicus et non adiutor infirmi. Quin ymo homicidiis speculatoribus deterior iudicatur. Sic medicus spiritualis imperitus non curat imo sauciat.' Ibid. fol. 66^{r}.

Galvano discusses the cure for lust—the first species of spiritual epilepsy or lunacy. On the basis of the rule that every cure is made through a suitable contrary (*omnis cura per congruum contrarium fiat*), he prescribes continence (*ieiunium libidinis*). This will maintain the purity of the kidneys (*renes pudicorum*), which are the seat of lust. Although temperance in the consumption of food and drink is advised, total abstinence is not required. The sixth chapter suggests maintaining the fear of God in the heart, kindness in responding and disputing, and gentleness in social intercourse as a triple chrism (*salutaris krisma*) for anger, which is the second type of spiritual epilepsy. The cure for cupidity which is the third type of spiritual epilepsy, discussed in the seventh chapter, consists of a fundamental change in attitude to life: rejecting the desire to possess temporal goods, and recognizing that only divine glory can bestow a feeling of fullness and satisfaction. The book ends with a short chapter which describes the signs of a patient fully restored to health. They include the revival of the sense of discretion (*recuperatio sensus discretionis*), the ability to confess (speaking) and to perform good deeds (motion), and renewed devotion.

The third treatise in the manuscript (on leprosy, at fols. 69^V–100^r) is similarly structured. Its first and main part consists of seventeen chapters which offer careful description and diagnosis of the four types of leprosy and prescribe specific therapies. It relies heavily on Johannitius, Avicenna, Isaac, and Galen. Yet, in the prologue, it formulates among its targets a non-medical aim: to understand what corporeal leprosy is and how it should be treated facilitates the understanding of spiritual leprosy and its cures.[189] The prologue to the second part, entitled 'The Second Treatise Concerning the Curative Doctrine of Spiritual Leprosy' (*Tractatus 2us de doctrina mundatiua lepre spiritualis*) explicitly presents Galvano as an imitator of Christ. He asks the readers to recognize him as a herald (*preco*) who has particular information regarding the interior man, and whose prophetic ability relies heavily on his medical background. After having discussed meticulously the exterior man, he deems himself fit to venture into the interior aspects of the disease. He beseeches the Christian readers to believe in his teaching as they believe in Christ, who was the true cleanser of leprosy.[190] This open comparison

---

[189] 'ut per eam ad doctrinam anime mondatiuam lepre spiritualis christi opitulamine facilius conscendatur.' Ibid. fol. 70^r.

[190] 'ergo uos obsecro o christicole ad quos peruenerit hec salubris doctrina lepre aures uestras mihi preconi credite tam Christo ihesu lepre uero utriusque hominis mundatori; qui enim audit dogmata eius secundum intellectum sanum reparatur secundum affectum dei caritate acensus non morietur'. Ibid. fol. 96^r.

between the theologizing physician and Christ is something Arnau did not dare to utter. However, Galvano's heralds (*precones*) and Arnau's watchmen (*speculatores*)[191] have an identical function. By virtue of the special knowledge and particular insights they possess, they divulge spiritual messages to the public. It may not be a coincidence that two physicians present themselves roughly at the same time as divine agents with access to divine messages which others cannot see and which they feel obliged to reveal to the world.

The spiritual part comprises three chapters which, Galvano claims, reflect the Trinity. In the first, Galvano defines spiritual leprosy and specifies its four types. He starts with Avicenna's definition (already quoted in chapter 1 of the treatise concerning corporeal leprosy), according to which leprosy is a malignant, destructive, destabilizing, fatal, and contagious illness (*mala infirmitas*) resulting from the spread of black choler throughout the body and the ensuing unnatural disposition (*dispositio contra naturam*) which is pathological. Galvano determines, referring to John of Damascus, that leprosy of the soul is similarly a mortal disease caused by the dispersion of the filth of sin throughout the body. It affects in the soul a *dispositio contra naturam* which is pathological and irrational. Physical leprosy involves the loss of many natural goods such as complexion, shape, and senses; similarly, spiritual leprosy causes the loss of goods of fortune and grace, and excludes sufferers from the ability to perceive punishment, to hear God's words, and to smell the stench of their sins. In physical leprosy, the harder one strives to suppress the disease the more violently it boils over. Similarly, in spiritual leprosy, the more hidden and untouched by confession the dung of sin is, the uglier it appears when finally it is revealed. The raucous, hardly audible voice typical of the corporeal leper characterizes the spiritual leper, who cannot be heard by God. The social isolation of lepers applies also to their spiritual counterparts. Galvano's sources for the description of the state of sin are Augustine, Gregory the Great, and John of Damascus, and they are smoothly fused with the medical definition. The four types of leprosy correspond to four mortal sins. *Alopicia* corresponds to avarice (the name, according to Galvano, is related to the browless wolf, whose notorious bad breath symbolizes the stench of money).[192] *Tyria* (from the serpent *Tyrus*, which loses its old skin) corresponds to lust, which causes a

---

[191] See Chapter 3 below, pp. 129–31.

[192] *Alopecia*, or baldness, denotes today absence of hair from areas where it normally grows.

triple loss of skin—temporal, corporeal, and honorial. *Leonina* corresponds to anger, and the gravest type, *elephantina*, to pride—the severest sin.

This chapter ends the long comparison between the two diseases with another medical paragraph. Corporeal leprosy falls under the jurisdiction of three kinds (*genera*) of diseases: first, imbalanced complexion (*mala complexio*), which dries out the organs of the body; second, functional diseases (*egritudo officialis*), which deform the body's shape; and third, chronic diseases (*egritudo communis*), which destroy the links between the organs. Similarly, spiritual leprosy introduces to the interior man three infirmities: ignorance of the law, aversion towards the good, and diffidence when facing difficult challenges (*diffidentia ardui*).

After the definition of the disease Galvano reverts to its diagnosis, and chapter 2 is entitled 'By which Signs is Spiritual Leprosy Recognized?' (*Quibus signis cognoscitur lepra spiritualis*). From the many signs of physical leprosy Galvano picks three—stained and swollen face and eyes, broken and hoarse voice, and discoloured skin—and parallels them to the blemish of concupiscence which turns the voice of confession hoarse. Excessive and superfluous ornaments are equivalent to the changing colour of the skin. The last chapter discusses the cure. The real therapy for leprosy involves surgery (*cyrugia* [sic], which probably here means phlebotomy), medical potions, and medicinal diet, administered in that order. He then fuses this medical programme with the description in Leviticus 14: 8–12 of how lepers could purge themselves. This description is interpreted as applying to the cure of spiritual leprosy. Washing the clothes corresponds to phlebotomy, and signifies the need to unravel all the hidden associations and to wash out evil mores with tears of contrition. Shaving the stricken part of the body corresponds to medicine that banishes and eradicates the diseased humours, and signifies eradicating vices and sin by the sword of confession. Finally, the leper is ordered in Leviticus to offer two immaculate lambs and purest wheat flour besprinkled with oil. This corresponds to diet, and signifies the two types of innocence expected from spiritually cured people—not to oppress anyone and to aid others, and thus lift themselves to moral heights. The wheat flour signifies the lack of the bran of vainglory.

Is Galvano writing here as a physician? What is particularly medical in these texts? Moralizing about diseases was common amongst preachers and theologians, as will be shortly revealed, but I would like to argue that Galvano speaks here as a physician and draws from his medical profession the authority and legitimacy to pronounce religious utterances.

Although the spiritual content of the texts is banal, it is based not only on scriptural references and patristic commentaries, but on a direct link with the medical text; the context in which the two spiritual annexes to the medical treatises appear clearly highlights this link. Galvano does not copy encyclopaedic descriptions of diseases and therapies, but fuses his medical knowledge with his religious beliefs in a way which suggests that he at least thought that a physician could cure the interior as well as the exterior man. Nowhere does he allude to the need to exclude and banish the leper (and hence the sinner) from society. He does mention that leprous patients are banned from human company, and that they often behave immorally; but in doing so he is in line with the diagnostic opinion of Avicenna, which he further elaborates when he discusses the explanation of the disease's origins.

It remains to examine the way in which preachers employed the language of disease. Like Arnau, preachers were aware of the rhetorical value of disease imagery. But unlike him, they identified specific diseases with specific vices and sins, and linked moral behaviour to health. King Hezekiah's disease (Isaiah 38) was thus diagnosed by the Franciscan Bertrand de la Tour (d. 1332) as an abscess or ulcer (*apostema scilicet ulcerus*) and as the 'affliction of kings' (*morbus regium*). For being ungrateful and proud, Hezekiah was justly struck by a mortal disease. Consequently, Bertrand specifically tied diseases with mortal sins: pride with madness, envy with epilepsy, anger with fury, avarice with dropsy, sloth with lethargy and paralysis, gluttony with apoplexy, and lust with leprosy.[193]

Other preachers were eager to display a deeper knowledge of medical terminology and theory when discussing diseases. Dropsy,[194] for example, was loaded with moral meaning. Bonaventura discusses avarice, lust, and pride through the three accidents of dropsy—swelling, bad breath, and extreme thirst. Just as abundance of corrupt and melancholic humours in the body generates a variety of skin diseases (from scabies and impetigo to leprosy) which pollute it, so an abundance of unclean thoughts generates corrupt humours in the heart and inordinate carnal desires.[195] Similarly, the Dominican Giordano da Pisa (1260–1311), when describing the corrupting

---

[193] 'Ista egritudo gravissima multiplex est. Est enim superbia sicut frenesis. Invidia sicut epylepsia. Ira sicut furia. Avaritia sicut ydropisis. Accidia sicut litargia et sicut paralisis. Gula sicut apoplexia. Luxuria sicut lepra. Pro his omnibus egritudinibus debet peccator egrotus orare celestem medicum.' Bertrand de la Tour, *Sermones quadragesimales epistolares* (Strasbourg, 1501/2), fol. xiiii^v–xix^va at xv^r. See also Giordano da Pisa, *Quaresimale Fiorentino 1305–1306*, ed. C. Delcorno (Florence, 1974), 221–2.

[194] Kiple (ed.), *The Cambridge World History of Human Disease*, 689–98.

[195] Bonaventura, *Sermones de tempore*, in *Opera Omnia*, ix (Quaracchi, 1901), 416^a.

effects of sin, juxtaposes the destructive characteristics of the putrid phlegmatic humours (*mali omore*) in the case of the dropsy-stricken person with destructive temporal love (*male amore*).[196] But the most accurate medical description of the disease is in Giovanni's *Sde*, where the three different species of dropsy—subcutaneous, abdominal, and tympanitic (*hyposarcha, alchites, tympanis*)—correspond to avarice, lust, and pride. He incorporates this medical description into a sermon, which introduces envy, self-love, and pride as the spiritual equivalents.[197]

In addition to dropsy, fever, paralysis, epilepsy,[198] lethargy, apoplexy, and leprosy[199] prominently appear in sermons and receive moralizing interpretations. These diseases played a role similar to that of cancer, TB, and AIDS, as Susan Sontag has portrayed them in modern society.[200] It was, of course, the Church Fathers who first identified them with sins. Hence it would be false to deduce that these were the commonest diseases at around 1300. Indeed, missing from the preachers' list were the three great killers of medieval children—smallpox, dysentery, and diarrhoea—and the major pre-Black-Death diseases which included, in addition to leprosy, St Anthony's fire, influenza, tuberculosis, malaria, and

---

[196] 'Così adviene del peccatore come dell' idropico, che la medicina sua si è l'abstinenzia. . . . L'idropico quanto più mangia e beie, quelli omori si corrompono tutti e convertonsi in mali omori flemmatici. E però quanto più beie e mangia, tanto più enfia e cresce il male, e più ha sete. Così è de' peccatori. I beni del mondo tutti si convertono in mali umori.' Giordano da Pisa, *Quaresimale*, 120: 128–38; Iannella, 'Malattia e salute', 202 n. 108, 216. See also Antonio da Padova, *Sermones dominicales et festivi ad fidem codicum recogniti*, II. ed. B. Costa, L. Frasson, and I. Luisetto (Padua, 1979), 280, and Jacopo da Voragine, *Ordinis predicatorum fratris Iacobi de voragine sermones dominicales per anni circulum predicabiles alphabetico ordine magistraliter registrati* (Ulm, 1484), 149va–150ra.

[197] *Sde* vi. 5, 296¹–297¹; Sermon 136, MS London, BL Addit. 24998. See Appendix Ib and Appendix II, which discuss a much more detailed list of pathologies.

[198] Epilepsy was used in religious discourse for other purposes as well. In order to demonstrate the ability to educate the young and reform their morals, Robert Holcot employs the Hippocratic clinical observation that epilepsy which strikes young people before the age of youth (*iuventus*) stops and vanishes. Robert Holcot, *In librum sapientie regis Salomonis prelectiones ccxiii* (Basel, 1586), *lectio* liiii, 192–3.

[199] Sermons 55 and 130, MS London, BL Addit. 24998, fols. 53rb–va, 187vb–188rb, employ Giovanni's knowledge of leprosy as appears in *Sde* vi. 10, 301¹–3. In Giordano da Pisa's sermons (Iannella, 'Malattia e salute', 189, 213) leprosy signifies mortal sin which turns the soul leprous and destroys it. For Vicent Ferrer, *Sermons* v. 15–20, leprosy is the incarnation of sin; each of its 7 symptoms corresponds to a different sin, and is vividly described.

[200] S. Sontag, *Illness as Metaphor* (London, 1978) and *AIDS and its Metaphors* (London, 1989). On the metaphorical representation of disease, see D. Lupton, *Medicine as Culture: Illness, Disease and the Body in Western Societies* (London, 1994), 54–71. On the attitudes to epidemics in general, see T. O. Ranger and P. Slack (ed.), *Epidemics and Ideas: Essays on the Historical Perception of Pestilence* (Cambridge, 1992).

typhus.[201] Yet the style some preachers chose to compare physical with spiritual disease is new.

Giovanni da San Gimignano makes an effort to describe meticulously the clinical symptoms of each and every such disease, and relies solely on Avicenna as his source for these pathologies (Appendix Ib). For example, the lethargic affliction which causes feverish fits is, according to Avicenna, caused by a putrefied phlegmatic ulcer (*apostemata phlegmaticum*) within the skull (fullness of the stomach, over-drinking, and excessive consumption of onions may trigger the process of putrefaction). Giovanni identifies this ulcer in the skull with sin in the soul accompanied by intemperance, exactly as intemperate fever accompanies lethargy. Secondly, lethargy causes unhealthy sleepiness (*dormitatio*). Similarly, sin is sometimes so well-established in the brain that it renders the sinner sleepy and immobile in the state of sin. Oblivion, which is the third symptom of lethargy and is caused by the cold humours which rise from the cerebral ulcer, is also common among sinners.[202]

Giovanni explains the resemblance between melancholy, which often appears in February and which has four accidental properties, and the vice of sloth.[203] Avicenna provides him with a framework to diagnose the slothful.[204] The melancholic person is solitary; he avoids the company of other living people and is attracted to tombs. Similarly, the sinner avoids righteous people and is attracted to the putrid elements of society. The melancholic is constantly agitated (*inquietus*), roams around day and night, and is usually drowsy. Similarly, the slothful person cannot stay in one place for more than an hour, and roams unaware of his whereabouts. The melancholic is inherently suspicious, as is the slothful when trying

---

[201] On the medieval environment as a universe of diseases, see K. Park, 'Medicine and Society in Medieval Europe, 500–1500', in *Medicine in Society: Historical Essays*, ed. A. Wear (Cambridge, 1992), 59–99, at 60–4; Y. Violé O'Neil, 'Diseases of the Middle Ages', in Kiple (ed.), *The Cambridge World History of Human Disease*, 270–9.

[202] *Sde* vi. 52, 334$^{2-4}$.

[203] *Sde* vi. 1, 292^4. This characteristic of *acedia* appears also in other preaching literature of the period. See e.g. Ramon Llull, *Liber de virtutibus et peccatis sive ars maior predicationis*, in *Opera Latina*, 205, eds. F. D. Reboiras and A. Soria Flores (*CCCM* 76; Turnhout, 1986), 235: 42–6. On the relationship between the medical, philosophical, and theological discourses concerning melancholy, see R. Klibansky, E. Panowsky, and F. Saxl, *Saturn and Melancholy: Studies in the History of Natural Philosophy, Religion and Art* (London, 1964), 67–123; S. Wenzel, *The Sin of Sloth* (Chapel Hill, 1967), esp. 191–4; and R. Jehl, *Melancholie und Acedia: ein Beitrag zu Anthropologie und Ethik Bonaventuras* (Paderborn, 1984).

[204] Avicenna, *Liber canonis*, iii. fen 1, 4.18–20 deals with melancholy, though there is no decisive evidence in the text that Giovanni directly used it.

constantly to hide his laziness. In a similar manner, avarice is equated with constipation, pride with dropsy, gluttony with the malfunction of the gullet and fatness, and envy with toothache.

In this language of disease Giovanni confines himself to the diagnostic phase only. Except for ways to alleviate headache, therapy performed by medical intervention is hardly mentioned. Recovery from a disease is always a result of a natural process, not the intervention of the physician: a boundary which he seems never to have crossed when he immersed himself in medical knowledge. From the religious point of view this is understandable, since precisely here lay the core of an insoluble tension between scientific medicine and the religious approach to disease. Giovanni thus avoided this danger, and used medicine meticulously up to the boundary established by his religious convictions.

The technical language of disease also infiltrated sermons. This was usually linked with verses of specific medical character. When Giovanni discusses paralysis in the context of Matthew 8: 6 ('my servant lieth at home sick of the palsy') he cites Avicenna for the explanation of the disease:

For paralysis, according to Avicenna, is some kind of softness of the nerves or the organs. It sometimes seizes the whole body except for the head, sometimes it affects one side, sometimes one organ. And in that part of the body where it sometimes concentrates, it removes the sensation that is the use of reason, as is evident especially amongst the lustful where reason is swallowed by the pleasure of flesh and wine.[205]

Luke 4: 38: 'Simon's wife's mother was taken with a great fever' is another biblical verse which invited the preacher to show off his medical knowledge. Giovanni discusses in a sermon for the third week of Lent the nature of the woman's disease (*qualitates morbi*). The fever with which she is afflicted represents the vices, he explains to his audience:

For fever, as Avicenna defines it, is extraneous heat which is kindled in the heart. It spreads from the heart to the whole body through the spirit and the blood and

---

[205] 'Nam paralysis secundum Avicennam, est quedam mollificatio nervorum sive membrorum; que quidem aliquando contingit toti corpori, preterquam in capite, aliquando in uno latere aliquando in uno membro; et in illa parte corporis ubi aliquando convenit, sensum tollit, scilicet rationis usum, sicut patet precipue in luxuriosis in quibus ratio absorbetur a voluptate carnis vel vini.' Giovanni da San Gimignano, *Convivium quadragesimale*, 22–3.

via the arteries and veins. In the body it creates a fire which harms the natural functions. All this generally fits sin.[206]

Every part of this medical definition is given its spiritual interpretation. Sin is that exterior heat which arises from non-natural and irrational desire in the heart or the mind, which affects the whole body through thoughts and desires, and which is expressed in words and deeds.[207] Giovanni returns to the medical foundation and says, 'Yet pay attention, that according to Avicenna, a certain kind of fever, such as hectic fever, spreads from the primary organs, another one, potentially putrefactory, spreads from the humours, and yet another one, such as ephemeral fever, spreads from the spirits.'[208] The first signifies avarice, the second lust, and the third pride.

Giovanni uses another medical authority in a sermon on a theme from John 4: 46 ('And there was a certain noble man whose son was sick'). The child suffers from fever, which is sin. According to Giovanni both cause inflammation, the first in the body, the second in the soul. This time he introduces Constantinus Africanus as his source for the definition of fever as excessive heat which goes beyond the course of nature and spreads from the heart to strike the body.[209] He then discusses the difference between the corruptive effects of two sorts of fever. Fever within the veins (*febris inter vasa*) signifies envy, because neither grants respite to the heart. Continuous fever signifies anger. According to Constantinus it putrefies the blood, burns up the interior

---

[206] 'Nam febris ut diffinit Avicenna, est calor extraneus accensus in corde, procedens ab eo mediantibus spiritu et sanguine, per arterias et venas in totum corpus et inflammatur in eo inflammatione que nocet operibus naturalibus; que omnia competunt communiter peccato.' Ibid. 329; cf. Avicenna, *Liber canonis*, iv. fen 1, 1.1, p. 393ra. On the academic debate at the turn of the 13th century about fever and its relationship with natural or innate heat, see the introduction to *AVOMO*, xv. 95–110.

[207] 'nam peccatum est homini extraneus calor, id est, non naturalis appetitus quia contra rationem accenditur concupiscentia sive in mente, sive in corde, procedens ab ea, mediante spiritu et sanguine, id est cogitatione et delectatione, per arterias et venas, id est per locutiones et opera, et impediens operationes naturales, id est, operationes virtuosas et rationales.' Giovanni da San Gimignano, *Convivium quadragesimale*, 329.

[208] 'Sed nota, secundum Avicennam quod aliqua febris procedit ex membris radicalibus, ut hectica; quedam ex humoribus ut putrida, quedam ex spiritibus ut ephemera.' Ibid. 329.

[209] 'Iste filius reguli designat peccatorem ratione inflamationis quia febribus tenebatur. . . . Febris igitur peccatum designat quia febris ut dicit Constantinus est calor innaturalis cursu nature supergradiens, procedens a corde in artarias corpusque suum ledens effectum. Ubi habemus febris defectum quia est innaturalis calor. Et sic peccatum potest dici quidam innaturalis aut inordinatus amor.' MS London, BL Addit. 24998, fol. 218^{ra-b}. See also sermon 73 on John 6: 1, ibid. fol. 76va, which twice cites Avicenna when explaining why the healthy need more food than those who have fever.

and exterior of the body and results from a combination of fever outside the veins (*febris extra vasa*) and inside them.[210] Part of the sermon revolves around the concept of *discrasia* (complexional imbalance) and discusses various ways in which it may cause a disease. Giovanni mentions six possible causes for *discrasia* (related to movement and rest, sleep and wakefulness, evacuation, and repletion—all elements of the six non-natural things). The third is immoderate sleep, and Giovanni cites Hippocrates' *Aphorisms* when he draws the comparison between the pathogenic medical result of excessive sleep (immoderate cooling down of the body) and the detrimental result of excessive interior sleep (sloth).[211]

Giordano da Pisa makes the same differentiation between fever that originates from within the veins and from without, the first being significantly more dangerous than the second, in a sermon on Matthew 8: 6 ('my servant lieth at home sick'). Giordano, who, in other sermons, substantiates his description of the causes, accidents, and effects of fever by referring to 'physicians' (*dicono i medici*), attributes his medical knowledge here to 'the sages' (*i savi*). He discusses Hezekiah's case in Isaiah 38: 1–6 as an example of the healing of the soul. Hezekiah suffers from fever, which is a disorder of the interior bodily heat that harms the natural heat, and is spiritually understood as sin and as the lack of love of God which deprives the soul of life. Giordano stresses that interior diseases are always more perilous and difficult to detect and heal. Thus sin which is hidden in the depth of the heart is most difficult to heal.[212]

Sociologists of medicine who deal with the relationship between the natural and cultural aspects of bodily disfunction distinguish between disease, which is some deviation from a biological norm, illness, which is the personal experience of unhealth, and sickness, which is a social role expressing the public dimension of unhealth.[213] In their medical writings

---

[210] 'Febris extra vasa' signifies anger 'quia continua, ut Constantinus dicit fit ex putrefactione sanguinis comburens utramque partem exteriorem et interiorem potest assimilari ei. Ira inquam est inflammatio sanguinis interius et exterius.' Ibid. fol. 218vb.

[211] Ibid. fol. 217ra.

[212] 'Onde dicono [i savi] che sono in due maniere le febri: *intra vasa et extra vasa*, cioè dentro al vaso e di fuori da'vasi. Vaso chiamano le veni che sono nel corpo, però che sono vasi ove sta il sangue. Quando la febre è *intra vasa*, dentro alle veni, nel sangue, or questa è la mala febre, e è detta febre acuta, ma quando è *extra vasa* si è leggieri e non è sì periculosa né sì molesta.' Giordano da Pisa, *Quaresimale*, 18: 66–72; cf. ibid. 221–5.

[213] B. S. Turner, *The Body and Society: Explorations in Social Theory* (Oxford, 1984), 206–7.

Arnau and Galvano use the terms *morbus* or *egritudo* when they discuss diseases, adhering to these terms when they speak of the spiritual aspects of diseases. This is a further indication of the medical approach to spiritual problems which characterizes our two physicians. However, in the spiritual context Arnau also uses the more general term *infirmitas* (rarely used in his medical writings), which one may translate as sickness. This term is overwhelmingly employed by clerics who were interested in disease's moral dimension rather than in its clinical aspects. Arnau and Galvano thus share with everyone else in that period the notion that disease is a system of signs which can be read and translated in a variety of ways. Each in his own way moves smoothly from speaking about disease to speaking about sickness; the very subtle difference between Arnau and Galvano and people like Giovanni lies in the direction of the movement and its spontaneity. While Giovanni is interested mainly in sickness (*infirmitas*), and his vocabulary of disease is only a metaphorical and artificial aid, Arnau's and Galvano's adherence to the term *morbus* even in the spiritual context is a symbolic sign of their conscious or unconscious effort to maintain and announce the link to their real medical background. Unlike Giovanni, Arnau and Galvano do not employ the analogies of disease merely as rhetorical devices. By introducing the vocabulary of disease into their spiritual writings, each in his own way, they extend their curative spheres from physical to spiritual disease, from body to soul.

In the light of the preachers' high-level medical language when they discuss the moral meaning of disease, what is specifically medical in Arnau's and Galvano's mode of employing medical language? Both use physiological metaphors in a spontaneous manner and fully intercalate them in the text. Physiological and anatomical metaphors and similes constitute by far the bulk of their figurative language. Though they share many metaphors with the clergy, they do not use encyclopaedias and other manuals from which to draw linguistic decorations. Thus, spontaneity should be added as a crucial variable when determining the level of medical language employed by a writer. Their medical background apparently provided them with the linguistic, analytical, and conceptual tools they needed comfortably to deliver spiritual and moral messages.

The language of Arnau and Galvano serves as a subtle pointer to the mechanism which induced them to theologize. As physicians they extend their interest from the human body and its pathologies to the spiritual body by means of a process Galvano calls *transumptio* (functional transference).

But does Arnau reveal his 'medical frame of mind' more explicitly than this? I have alluded to a notion shared by both physicians that they are divine agents, armed with superior knowledge and acumen and obliged to divulge it. Could this prophetic mood be related in any way to their medical profession? The next chapter will attempt to answer these questions.

3
Medicine as a Vehicle for Religious Speculation

So far my interpretation has been based on analysis of Arnau's language; it is now time to discuss his explicit references to the role of medicine in religious discourse, in a human world geared to participate in a divine plan of salvation or perdition. Does the scientific profession of medicine exert any influence on Arnau's religious thought beyond the linguistic links I have shown so far? Does the physician's daily encounter with the signs of decay and the automatic connection between sin and disease impel him (if he is pious) also to diagnose signs of disease and dangerous deviation in the body of the Church?[1]

Medical Knowledge and Theological Knowledge as Divine Gifts

I have already discussed the requirement that the perfect physician be loyal and faithful (*fidelis*), and linked this with the concept of medicine as a religious system. When he elaborates on this issue, Arnau reiterates one virtue—*caritas*—which creates another common denominator between the physician and the faithful. In his spiritual writings Arnau the wise, the prudent, and the humble lists among those who have access to the deeper divine knowledge, and then adds a fourth category, the charitable. *Caritas* is a prerequisite for receiving understanding (*intellectus*) of Scripture.[2] Yet *caritas* is also repeatedly cited as a most desirable characteristic of a physician in Arnau's medical treatises. Christian love, for example, motivates the author of *De venenis* (probably Arnau) to discuss theriac, the most powerful of all medicines. By so doing he is preventing it from being misused as a poison

---

[1] C. Crisciani, '*Exemplum* Christi e sapere. Sull'epistemologia di Arnaldo da Villanova', *Archives Internationales d'Histoire des Sciences*, 28 (1978), 284.

[2] 'Sciebant etiam, quod habentibus caritatem datur intellectus sacrorum eloquiorum, non habentibus autem aufertur etiam ille quem videntur habere.' *Presentatio facta Burdegaliis*, MS Vat. lat. 3824, fol. 257[va–b].

and is exposing its benefits.[3] If perfect physicians are by definition charitable, as Arnau asserts, then the door to divine knowledge is open to them. Though this is not explicitly said, it can be inferred from reading his spiritual as well as his medical texts.

Christian love (*caritas*) together with poverty (*paupertas*), humility (*humilitas*), and modesty (*pudicicia/castitas*) should be the pillars of those who aspire to live the evangelical life. Each of these ideals has a spiritual as well as a corporeal aspect. In order to persuade people to follow the way of truth, a man must adapt himself and his conversation to the habits of the ignorant and the infirm, who are the spiritually weak.[4] The best test for *caritas* or the lack of it is one's state of health. Arnau's chief criticism of false clerics and monks centres on their failure to promote *caritas*. In health they care more for their own temporal advantage and that of their next of kin and personal friends (by being obsessed with acquiring benefices and dignities) than for the honour of God. In times of disease they attend to their relatives and friends, but betray their vocation to cure the spiritually sick and are content to procure for their needy clients only corporeal treatment. When a member of their order falls ill, they abandon him totally; instead of helping him as they should, according to the rules of divine charity, they prefer leaving the monastery under the pretext of attending their parents.[5] Conversely, the perfect physician, who is by definition charitable, complies with an essential tenet of evangelical life.

Like Arnau, Galvano also creates a clear link between *caritas* and the divine source of the medical knowledge he possesses. The prologue to his treatise on digestion starts with passionate praise of compassion and *caritas* as a necessary and integral part of the physician's curing activity, stating that it should be universally applied whatever the type of the disease. The prologue thus labels his medical writing as an act of charity. In support of the contention that true virtue cannot be acquired without true piety and veneration of the Lord, Galvano refers to Augustine's *De civitate Dei*, v

---

[3] *De venenis*, in Arnau de Vilanova, *Opera* (Lyons, 1520), fol. 216[vb]; *Liber de vinis*, ibid. fol. 264[ra]; Crisciani, '*Exemplum Christi*', 274.

[4] On *caritas* in the context of evangelical perfection, see *De zona pellicea*, in O. Cartaregia and J. Perarnau, 'El text sencer de l'*Epistola ad gerentes zonam pelliceam*', *ATCA* 12 (1993), 25 ff., and J. Petratnau, 'Troballa de tractats espirituals perduts d'Arnau de Vilanova', *Revista Catalana de Teologia*, 1 (1976), 508–9.

[5] *Epistola ad priorissam de caritate*, in R. Manselli, 'La religiosità d'Arnaldo da Villanova', *Bullettino dell'Istituto Storico Italiano per il Medio Evo e Archivio Muratoriano*, 63 (1951), 65. Arnau devoted this treatise (condemned in 1316) to *caritas*. In it, illness and health are among the temporal things and serve as a focal point for the discussion of Christian love.

and *De catechizandis rudibus* and to John Chrysostom, and concludes: 'Truly, the pious love of the physician directly communicates to the needy the treasure of medicine. Indeed, there is no knowledge without piety.'[6]

Unlike Arnau, Galvano links the physician to a religious way of living marked by piety, and expands the role of the physician 'to the health of both men' (*pro salute hominis utriusque*), exterior and interior.[7] Galvano compares himself to the prophet Ezekiel (1: 1) and describes how the heavenly skies of medical knowledge were opened for him while he was studying Scripture, philosophy, and the medical authorities. His solemn prologue is formulaic in part, but it also provides the structure for the whole work. The first chapter in the treatise on digestion and stomach conditions is entitled: 'To Rouse Prelates in the Church of God and Faithful Magnates to a Healthy Care of their Stomach so that Consequently they will Healthily Live to a Great Age' (*Ad incitandum prelatos in ecclesie dei et magnates fideles ad salubrem custodiam stomachi ut per inde fiant sanitate longeui*). The last chapter of the treatise completes the circle, and is entitled: 'To Rouse Prelates of the Church of God and Princes of the Earth into Inspiring the Lord Jesus in the Stomach of their Souls' (*Ad incitandum prelatos ecclesie dei et principes terre ad incitandum dominum Ihesum Christum in stomacho animarum suarum*).[8] Although the text is largely medical, it allows Galvano to extract any possible spiritual implications that medical preoccupation with the stomach may have. Digestion, evacuation, appetite, nausea, the essential harmony between the receiving capacity of the stomach (*receptiva potestas*), the degree of appetite, and the digestive power—all, in his eyes, have clear spiritual and moral meaning.

The common virtue of *caritas* shared by perfect physicians and righteous clerics implies the physician's access to divine knowledge, and it is on this that I shall now elaborate.

The Divine Source of Medical Knowledge

In a recent article Robert Lerner has offered a possible explanation for Arnau's recurring appeal to direct revelation and miracles in his spiritual

---

[6] 'sane pia caritas medici inuentum medicationis thesaurum mox communicat indigenti. Nulla quidem sine pietate scientia.' MS Vat. lat. 2463, fol. 1[rb–va]. His citation from Augustine: 'istud constet inter omnes ueraciter pios neminem sine uera pietate—i.e. ueri dei culto ueram posse habere uirtutem' is accurate; cf. *De civ. Dei* v. 19, *PL* 41, 166.

[7] See also the prologue to the following treatise on catarrh in MS Vat. lat. 2463, fol. 70[r].

[8] Ibid., fol. 68[v].

texts[9] as being the conscious attempt of an unauthorized religious speculator to create legitimacy for his writings when his affairs were becoming
desperate and after he had realized that intrinsic merit would not suffice
to gain acceptance. This is why the claim to privileged insight appears in
Ars philosophiae catholicae of 1302 and not in *De tempore adventus
Antichristi* (*c.* 1288–1300). I shall suggest another possible (and less sinis-
ter) explanation for Arnau's use of the 'inspiration argument' in his spiritual writings, namely that it was a continuation of his belief that medical
knowledge could be the product of direct divine revelation.

According to Michael McVaugh, in most of his scientific works Arnau
developed a pragmatic instrumentalism when discussing the origin of
medical knowledge. Stressing the primacy of principles of practice (*doctrina operativa*) over knowledge of general scientific truths (*doctrina cog-
nitiva*), he emphatically tried to separate medicine from science, restrict
it to the realm of *ars*, and stress sense-knowledge rather than broad theoretical generalizations.[10] Paniagua's interpretation of Arnau's epistemology[11] also stressed the role of experimentation and rational reasoning and
played down the role of revelation. He based this view on Arnau's words
in *Speculum medicine*, where he had asserted that what is known through
revelation (*revelatio*) made apparent through particular properties
exceeds human skill and does not fall within the scope of the medical art.
No human teaching (*mortalis doctrina*) can provide the physician with the
desired certainty when he must determine the complexion of food and
medicines. Therefore knowledge acquired through experience (*experimentum*) is essential.[12] However, it is my contention that the context of this
utterance does not warrant a broad generalization that Arnau rejected
divine revelation as a possible source of medical knowledge. First, there is
the question of what exactly *revelatio* means here. As we shall soon see,
revelatio (literally 'uncovering') cannot automatically be translated into

[9] R. E. Lerner, 'Ecstatic Dissent', *Speculum*, 67 (1992), 33–57. On Arnau's failure to
acquire authority as a prophet see F. Santi, 'Arnaldo da Villanova. Dal potere medico al non
potere profetico', in *Poteri carismatici e informali: chiesa e società medioevali* (Palermo, 1991),
262–86.

[10] M. R. McVaugh, 'The Nature and Limits of Medical Certitude at Early Fourteenth-
Century Montpellier', *Osiris*, 2nd ser., 6 (1990), 68 ff.

[11] J. A. Paniagua, *El Maestro Arnau de Vilanova médico* (Valencia, 1969), 89–91, and
'Abstinencia de carnes y medicina', *Scripta Theologia*, 16 (1984), 323–4.

[12] 'Quod enim scitur revelatione facta per substantias separatas, excedit facultatem
humanam et sub arte non cadit. Sed constat quod nullius mortalis doctrina sufficit
medicum ubique certificare de viribus complexionatorum quapropter ad habendum de ipsis
certitudinem ubique necesse est ut ad propriam recurrat experientiam.' *Speculum medicine*,
in Arnau de Vilanova, *Opera*, fol. 22[rb].

the modern use of the word 'revelation'. Second, a careful reading of the text shows that Arnau merely suggests that the ways of reaching absolute knowledge of chemical complexion (*noticia de viribus complexionatorum*) cannot be rationally foreseen, but can be directly experienced through taste (*per considerationem saporum*) and by investigating the actual effect of the medicine on the body (*per considerationem impressionum quas relinquit in corpore*). This leaves no room for any other source of knowledge when the complexion of food and medicines is sought.

I argue that, concurrent with his basic instrumentalist approach, Arnau leaves some room for the notion that medical knowledge originates from a source of direct divine illumination. His placing of revelation beyond the boundaries of the medical art in *Speculum medicine* does not eliminate it, either when he discusses medical science or when he takes up more practical questions. Furthermore, this characteristic of his epistemology, if proved, should not shatter Arnau's image as a rational instrumentalist physician. His medical epistemology is found scattered throughout his writings (especially *Repetitio super canone Vita brevis*). For the purpose of my argument, I have selected only small sections of his discussions, which form an important common denominator in his spiritual and medical thought.

Physicians of Arnau's period employed a fundamentally Augustinian approach, insisting on a source of knowledge higher than experience or scholastic logic and expressing this in largely formulaic invocations of God and divine power. The author of *De epilepsia*, attributed to Arnau, opens his discussion of the preventive measures against infant epilepsy by saying: 'Lest I omit what divine grace has conveyed to me' (*ne omittam, quod gratia Dei mihi collatum*). This observation might be discarded as a rhetorical commonplace, did not the text provide further evidence for the author's belief in a close contact with the divine sources of knowledge. The author holds that, without God's consent, nobody can discuss remedies for epilepsy with certainty; and he entreats Christ, the supreme physician, to teach him how to destroy the abscess which causes the disease. As he continues to discuss the various forms of the illness and to offer remedies, it is clear that in his opinion the source of his medical knowledge is direct divine inspiration. The same attitude recurs later in the treatise when he discusses tertiary catalepsy. The author asks Jesus to shed the light of his divine knowledge and clarify the darkness of the physician's ignorance.[13]

---

[13] *De epilepsia*, ibid. fol. 312[ra], 314[vb]. See also the introduction to Arnau's *Contra calculum*, ibid. fol. 305[va].

Yet Arnau seems to be more specific than that. In *Medicationis parabole* he proves the divine origin of medical knowledge not only by the first verses of Ecclesiasticus 38, but also by James 1: 17: 'Every good gift and every perfect gift is from above, and cometh down from the Father of lights'.[14] As medicine is by definition good (since its end is good) it has to have a divine origin. When discussing the meaning of Ecclesiasticus 38 he declares that 'the Supreme Good has instructed him to write this teaching' (*ad hanc doctrinam scribendam fuit informatus a Summo Bono*). This divine source can be a general, common influence of God who is the source of every truth (*modum communis influentie vel generalis*). Thus it is obvious that whoever teaches any truth was taught by God: it is the instinct of the eternal truth that moves him. But equally, he could be instructed by the Superior Good, which can effect an individual influence. God, when he wishes to enforce the knowledge of some truth, enlightens a person's soul, so that he may be the promoter of that truth, like a water pipe extending from a well and supplying water to troughs and pools. The chosen one acts as a divine agent and minister of the Lord.[15]

Since the whole context of the discussion is the interpretation of Ecclesiasticus 38: 2 (*A Deo est omnis medela*) and the divine source of medicine, Arnau must be thinking of the physician. He declares that only eternal wisdom knows why this person and not another has been chosen for the task, and ends his commentary with an *exemplum* which explains the 'private influence' of God that induced him to write the *Medicationis parabole*. He describes a vision of a person sitting on a rock in a river-bed. He inserts a finger into the flowing water which parts to reveal a room full of treasures stored in various vessels. He picks a small basket heavily loaded with gold 'as many as are the aphorisms in this work' (*quot sunt in hoc opere amphorismi*). The next day, he starts writing with wonderful, incredible speed. And he concludes: 'Similarly it could happen to the author of this work; and if it did happen then the correct explanation would be that through a remedy he

---

[14] This is part of Arnau's commentary on the first canon in his *Medicationis parabole*: 'Omnis medella procedit a Summo Bono' in *AVOMO*, vi. 1, 29. Arnau then adds: 'Sumit autem exordium hic auctor ab Altissimo, scilicet, a primo fonte cuiuslibet boni quod est Summum Bonum.' *AVOMO*, vi. 2, 153–4.

[15] 'Potuit informari a Summo Bono secundum modum influentie particularis in qua Deus propria bonitate dignatur, cum vult imprimere notitiam alicuius veritatis et circa eam illuminare notabiliter mentem eius, ut sit minister veritatis illius et ut canalis a fonte propinans aquam pilis et alveis aut piscinis.' *Commentum super quasdam parabolas, AVOMO*, vi. 2, 154: 20–5; see ibid., 334–7 where Paniagua and Gil-Sotres link this exceptional spiritual outburst in Arnau's usually rational medical texts to his attested divine revelation in summer 1301 at the papal villa in Scurcola (H. Finke, *Aus den Tagen Bonifaz VIII* (Münster, 1902), pp. clx–clxi).

understood the science of healing which, avoiding ingratitude, he acknowledged he had duly received from the Supreme Good'.[16]

Arnau's occasional allusions to a divine source of medical knowledge could indeed reflect a commonplace shared by other physicians or a rhetorical convention applicable to all sorts of knowledge.[17] However, his picture of the physician as a chosen agent of God suggests that one should not easily dismiss these as an empty, formulaic rhetorical device. In *Parabola* I.16, which deals with the knowledge needed for effective pharmacology, he mentions revelation together with *experimentum*[18] as possible sources of knowledge when syllogism and reason do not provide a solution.[19] He defines property (*proprietas*) as hidden power (*virtus occulta*), since it must be known not simply by human reason, but by accidental experience or some kind of revelation.[20] His reference to this in at least three other medical treatises makes it impossible to dismiss it as the result of a momentary lapse of mind or as merely a rhetorical device.[21]

The question is, of course, what revelation means in this medical context. Arnau provides the answer in the commentary on the *parabole*, where he explains that the term *revelatio* encompasses two kinds of revelation.

---

[16] 'Similiter potuit auctori huius operis contigisse, quod si taliter contigit tunc recte posset exponi quod per medelam intellexit doctrinam medendi quam ad vitandum ingratitudinem digne cognoscit se recepisse a Summo Bono.' *Commentum super quasdam parabolas*, *AVOMO*, vi. 2, 155: 2–5.

[17] *De consideracionibus operis medicine* was written 'gratia revelante', *AVOMO*, iv. 267; *Antidotarium*, in Arnau de Vilanova, *Opera*, fol. 243^{va-b} ends a prologue loaded with religious messages asking the eternal wisdom to throw open the written avenues to his plentiful treasure. Cf. Ch. 1, n. 111.

[18] On the common medieval sense of *experimentum*—information derived purely from experience—see M. R. McVaugh, 'The *experimenta* of Arnald of Vilanova', *The Journal of Medieval and Renaissance Studies*, 1 (1971), 107–18.

[19] 'Proprietas incognita ratione vel sillogismo, revelatione vel experimento iuvantium et nocentium innotescit'. *Medicationis parabole*, in *AVOMO*, vi. 1, 31, no.16.

[20] 'nisi enim experimento casuali vel aliquo modo revelationis sciretur corallum habere determinatum aspectum ad stomachum non posset ullo modo ratione cognosci.' *Speculum medicine*, fol. 6vb when speaking of the effect of coral (*corallum*— an aquatic plant that hardens upon contact with the air) on the stomach.

[21] *Repetitio super can. Vita brevis*, in Arnau de Vilanova, *Opera*, fol. 276ra: 'Nam cum notitiam proprietatum non possit haberi per rationem, sed tamen experimento vel revelatione.' In *Antidotarium*, fol. 243vb God reveals the occult powers of composite medicines through experience: 'Experimento enim innotuit deus largifluus servis suis effectus aliquos compositi.' *Tractatus de sterilitate* ii. 7, frequently attributed to Arnau or to Raymundus de Moleris, describes the most efficient drug to increase fertility and determine the gender of the conceived child as 'divinitus revelato'. 'et sic poterit habere, domino adiuvante, masculum, quod non est omnibus revelandum sed secretis tantum, quia hoc est valde preciosum et certum.' A. de Vilanova, R. de Moleris, and J. de Turre (attr.), *Tractatus de sterilitate*, ed. E. Montero Cartelle (Valladolid, 1993), 138–40.

One is from God, and is granted to only a few; the other is human, and all physicians must pay attention to it. This human revelation is acquired by interrogating the patient and his attendants.[22] Thus, revelation as a source of general medical knowledge does not automatically make every physician into a divine agent, and the use of the term in *Repetitio super canone Vita brevis*[23] seems indeed to refer to human revelation, since Arnau introduces it in discussing the contribution of the *vulgus* to the physician's clinical knowledge.

It has been suggested that Arnau felt the need to distinguish between the two types in order to overcome the originally ambiguous formulation of *revelatio* which, in the case of medicine, denotes solely human information that the physician collects from the patient or people surrounding his bed.[24] However, in the light of Arnau's commentary on his first aphorism, which attests the revelatory circumstances under which the aphorisms were written, divine revelation remains a possible source of medical knowledge, especially where the hidden properties of compound medicines are concerned; hence the term is ambiguous.

Arnau sees the end of acquiring knowledge as spiritual. All sciences share one common aim (*utilitas*), which is the procurement of the soul's perfection and serves as a preparation for eternal beatitude. The usefulness of medicine, which employs other sciences, is qualified by the degree of perfect certitude it achieves. Unlike the logicians (*topici*) who deal with probable reasoning and merely produce suppositions (*opiniones*), and the sophists who want to be regarded as wise and are not really interested in the truth, physicians produce certainty (*certitudo*). Medicine relies on prior knowledge and learning of the natural sciences (arithmetics, geometry, and astrology in particular), yet its special merit lies in its superior excellence.[25]

---

[22] 'Et primus est revelatio, que prout fit a Deo paucis conceditur, sed prout fit ab homine debet communiter a medicis observari. Nam prudens medicus debet suum patientem diligenter interrogare vel assistentes ut ei proprietas indicetur illius. Tali etiam revelatione, humana scilicet, multarum medicinarum proprietates individuales multis innotuerunt.' *Commentum super quasdam parabolas*, *AVOMO*, vi. 2, 160: 6–12. García-Ballester and Feliu, 'La versió hebrea', in *AVOMO*, vi. 2, 126 and J. A. Paniagua and P. Gil-Sotres, 'Estudio de su contenido y notas al texto', in *AVOMO*, vi. 2, 282 hold the view that only the second type of *revelatio* is to be understood in Arnau's texts.

[23] Cf. n. 33 below. [24] *AVOMO*, vi. 2, 126.

[25] See Arnau's discussion of *scientia naturalis* whose subject is the physical human body in *Repetitio super can. Vita brevis*, fol. 276vb–277va at 277^{rb-va}: 'omnes scientie communicant in una utilitate, que est acquisitio perfectionis humane anime in effectu preparantis eam ad futuram felicitatem . . . intentio ultima in hac scientia est cognitio gubernationis Dei altissimi et cognitio angelorum spiritualium et ordinum suorum et cognitio ordinationis in compositione cellorum.'

Other sciences were sometimes regarded as gifts of God, based on Matthew 10: 8,[26] but in Arnau's view the divine origin of medicine gives it a status superior to all other sciences—a notion which was a stark deviation from the traditional medieval hierarchy of the body of knowledge.[27]

Does Arnau mean that every knowledgeable physician is by definition a chosen divine agent? Or that within the community of physicians there is a sub-group of the elect? The commentary on *Parabola* i. 16 specifically states that divine revelation is not a common source of medical knowledge;[28] and similar limitation appears at the end of a discussion of the ways of turning wine and various fruits into laxative medicines in *Liber de vinis*. The author (possibly Arnau) stresses that, though these ways are known to only a few people, they should not be admired as miraculous because nothing happens by chance (*nihil est forte*). The man who knows the nature and powers of simple things can produce effects which will seem miraculous. Thus only those ignorant of the medical teaching (*magisterium*) should be astonished by this type of concoction. The physician holds a powerful position over his clients; he can make it seem as if he performs miracles. And the author concludes:

Blessed therefore is that physician to whom God gives knowledge (*scientia*) and understanding (*intelligentia*) for he is nature's partner. And not unreasonably it says in *The Wisdom of Solomon*: 'Honour the physician etc. for God created him' (Ecclesiasticus 38: 1, 12). But alas, many are called but few are chosen (Matthew 22: 14) . . . Therefore it is correct to say that medicine is knowledge (*scientia*) which is unknown. But blessed God causes us to know and understand and act according to his good will.[29]

Hence only a few of those holding the title of physician have been elected by God.

Was medical knowledge regarded as open knowledge, that is, a body of transparent knowledge which could be learnt by anyone intellectually equipped for it? In *De simplicibus* Arnau determines that learned physicians

[26] G. Post, K. Giocarinis, and R. Kay, 'The Medieval Heritage of a Humanistic Ideal: *Scientia donum Dei est, unde vendi non potest*', *Traditio*, 11 (1955), 195–234.

[27] 'medicina scientiarum nobilissima . . . que ab altissimo creata necessitate sanationis corporis et anime mortalibus utilissima ac ipsa preciosior scientiis cunctis existens.' *Antidotarium*, fol. 243[va]; *Repetitio super can. Vita brevis*, 277[va].

[28] *AVOMO*, vi. 2, 160.

[29] 'Beatus igitur ille medicus, cui deus dat scientiam et intelligentiam, quia est nature socius. Et non absque causa dictum est in scientia Salomonis: 'Honora Medicum etc., etenim illum deus creavit.' Sed heu 'multi sunt vocati, pauci vero electi'. . . Ideo bene diffinit [sic] quidam dicens: Medicina scientia est, que nescitur; Deus autem benedictus faciat nos scire et intelligere, et secundum suum beneplacitum operari.' *Liber de vinis*, in Arnau de Vilanova, *Opera*, fol. 263[rb].

compose a closed group, not only in their control of a vast amount of human knowledge, but also in their possession of a secret element.[30] The secret element of medicine is divine, not magical knowledge; it is based on influencing the blood equilibrium of the body through quantitative alterations, and on affecting the passions of the soul (*passiones anime*) by creating confidence in the physician's ability to heal. Thus the very belief in the secret powers of the physician is a part of the therapy. This again conferred on secular medicine another element parallel to a religious phenomenon—confidence (*confidentia*). As with religion, medicine demands a belief in its power, and offers an accurate (*certus*) solution to disease (the equivalent of guaranteed salvation).[31] Mastering its secrets will enable the physician to offer better medical treatment for the physical side-effects of anger, love, fear, pleasure, hope, and despair, since medicine is much stronger than any passion of the soul. Here medicine converges with necromancy, divination, and augury; all have secret powers which affect the imagination and the judgement, and all employ their power to create trust among their clients.[32] Therefore it is not enough to read the books that prudent physicians have written in the past, for they have already acknowledged the secret aspect of medicine (and thus the limits of the medical knowledge in their possession).

Sometimes true knowledge concerning the quality of matter (*noticia proprietatum*) can originate from the people (*vulgus*) or the unlearned physician (*parvus medicus*) rather than from the sages (*sapientes*).[33] The physician faces a plurality of sources for the full medical knowledge he seeks. Reason or theoretical speculation must be supplemented by experience and revelation which are open to all, including the unlearned.

---

[30] *De simplicibus*, ibid. fol. 242$^{ra–b}$.

[31] Ibid. fol. 242$^{va–b}$. Arnau claims that John of Damascus and Galen said that, from the clinical point of view, one ought to maintain a minimal level of hope in the patient, for sometimes hope is the most effective cure. See above, Ch. 2, n. 25.

[32] *De simplicibus*, fol. 242vb.

[33] 'multa enim sapientes a vulgo recipiunt; sicut patet per Aui. in et per Rasim in experimentis et per Galienum in de simplicibus medicinis. Nam cum notitiam proprietatum non possit haberi per rationem; sed tamen experimento vel revelatione et experientia et revelationes sunt communes vulgo et sapientibus possibile est ut proprietatum noticie prius habeantur a vulgaribus quam ab aliis.' *Repetitio super can. Vita brevis*, fol. 276ra. On the broader context of this citation, see L. García-Ballester, 'Medical Ethics in Transition in the Latin Medicine of the Thirteenth and Fourteenth Centuries: New Perspectives on the Physician–Patient Relationship and the Doctor's Fee', in A. Wear, J. Geyer-Kordesch, and R. French (ed.), *Doctors and Ethics: The Earlier Historical Setting of Professional Ethics* (Amsterdam, 1994), 42–4. See also *Liber de vinis*, fol. 264va for a *parvus medicus* who can produce efficient cures despite his limited knowledge. Crisciani, '*Exemplum Christi*', 271–3.

Obviously, every piece of knowledge acquired from the *vulgus* should be examined by reason and experience before it is applied. Furthermore, the medical field is not fully open to outsiders. At least once Arnau appears as a learned physician, who is sealing the boundaries of his profession against the encroaching illiterate. This happens in Part I of the treatise *De cautelis medicorum*, which provides important practical background knowledge for the daily work of the physician and for his interaction with the patient. It deals with precautions physicians must take to maintain their position within society and to withstand the criticism that is constantly directed at them. In the thirteenth precaution the physician encounters an old woman (*vetula*) who attends the patient. She nags him to tell her exactly what kind of disease the patient is suffering from. As the most inferior of all medical practitioners, the *vetula* was for the learned physicians the incarnation of primitive superstition, ignorance, and neglect of natural reasoning and natural causes of diseases.[34] In the ensuing dialogue the physician creates an insurmountable barrier between himself and the woman, when he calls her and all those who cannot distinguish between fever and other sorts of maladies *laici*.[35] Here one should certainly understand *laici* as illiterate or inexpert rather than 'not in orders'. Arnau is insinuating that in the quasi-religious structure of the medical care system he belongs to the upper echelon of the 'medical clerics', who have access to superior knowledge.

The secret element of medicine, acknowledged by the medical authorities, creates a complex relationship between medical practice and medical learning. Arnau does not reject learning, but suggests that it must be fortified with a clear recognition of the hidden path which reveals the medical secrets so esssential to efficient cure. He calls those people fools who read the books of the authorities yet refuse to accept the occult dimension of medicine; they are far removed from the secrets of medicine, and are unable to accept the fact that medicine is more than healing a headache, abscess, or fever.[36] We know that Arnau was an

[34] On the image of the *vetula* amongst physicians and clerics, see J. Agrimi and C. Crisciani, 'Savoir médical et anthropologie religieuse; Les représentations et les fonctions de la *vetula* (xiiie–xve)', *Annales Économies Sociétés Civilisations*, 48 (1993), 1281–308.
[35] *De cautelis medicorum*, in Arnau de Vilanova, *Opera*, fol. 216ra.
[36] 'Insipientes cum legerint in libris prudentum medicorum et senuum qui sciverunt iam esse secretum medicine, cum vident eos facere bonum intellectum et facere prudentem et facere fidelem fortunatum valde derident eos et derisi valde elongati sunt a secretis medicine, et non volunt audire, nec credunt, quod ad medicinam spectet nisi curare dolorem capitis, aut apostema aut febrem. Et ipsi deberent prius curare seipsos de grossitie intellectus, donec possent intelligere ea, que nostri senes in medicina nobis scripserunt.' *De simplicibus*, fol. 242[va].

active member of the university system which limited the access of outsiders into the medical profession. When asked what should one do in order to become a good physician, three out of the four prerequisites he suggested were related to the academic context and the acquaintance of the physician with the authorities.[37] But by stressing medicine's secret element which is not automatically revealed by reading medical books, Arnau leaves an open door for a few unqualified people to make their own contribution to the curing process. This conviction that a physician has access to secret knowledge and to channels of communication which transmit such knowledge should not be ignored when we come to understand Arnau the spiritual activist who was convinced that as a divine agent he was transmitting a divine message.

Arnau consequently refers to Hippocrates in order to substantiate his claim for the existence of a secret part in the art of medicine which should not be readily divulged to the public. What is the key to this secret knowledge? Here Arnau is predictably less clear; from the viewpoint of someone who already has that special knowledge, he asserts that the wise investigator (*homo sapiens et investigans*) will find out for himself these secrets and share this gift of philosophy (*donum philosophie*) with those who already have it, provided that he is worthy of it (*dignus est*). Arnau gives no clear indication as to what this merit depends on. It seems that the intellectual capacity to search and understand these secrets is what renders the person fit to receive them. Consequently, Arnau rejects profit as a motive for study or acquisition of knowledge: those who learn in order to gain material profit are compared to an aborted child who was born to an imperfect end. The end of learning (in this case medicine) must be the knowledge of God (*cognitio Dei*).[38]

It is this belief in the divine origin of medical knowledge and the close relationship between God and the physician as his agent which links Arnau the physician with Arnau the spiritual mystic. For when the God/physician relationship is proclaimed, the ground for a broader definition of the physician's role and mission is prepared. Whilst one cannot argue that the content of Arnau's spirituality emanates from his medical profession, a substantial religious element was constantly present in his medicine. If, for him, reason, experiment, and revelation could coexist, attributing a divine source to his medical knowledge is not incompatible with his position as a primarily Galenist physician. This refinement of

---

[37] García-Ballester, 'Medical Ethics in Transition', 42.
[38] *Medicationis parabole*, *AVOMO*, vi. 1, 29.

his scientific and instrumentalist image introduces a common denominator between Arnau the physician and Arnau the spiritual prophet: both regarded themselves as divine agents, the former implicitly and the latter explicitly.

The Characteristics of Medical Knowledge

It would be wrong to conclude from the above discussion that an air of mystic piety engulfed Arnau's medical texts. The divine source of medical knowledge was supported by recognized medical authorities like Hippocrates and Galen, whose crucial importance Arnau could not ignore. In *Contra calculum* he remarked that the *prothomedicus*, Hippocrates, lived and wrote long before the coming of the supreme physician, Christ. He also hailed Galen as the prince of physicians,[39] and regarded the ability to read the Hippocratic and Galenic texts properly as a prerequisite for the physician who was following the way of the medical truth. Those who only read summaries of these authoritative texts are unable to discern the right path, and their ignorance leads them nowhere. Since the work of the physician has a definite final end, and it can be achieved only if he uses the laws and rules of the art as they have been conveyed from the divine source through the authorities, knowing the sources is essential.[40] Yet Arnau is fully aware of their fallibility. The test of the validity of a medical theory is not, therefore, the identity of its author, but its practical effects, which give the physician room for change and innovation, despite his basic conservatism. Thus experience, observation, and rational inquiry were more important than authority, as sources of medical knowledge.[41] Arnau preferred the first principle of all knowledge according to Galen's hierarchy of knowledge[42] (that is, rational reasoning) to other sources of knowledge. By reason, the true physician could isolate the cause of the disease, and thereby devise an appropriate therapy that would assure success. The physician could best understand each patient individually, and diagnose accordingly in an effective manner.

This approach towards the sources affected physicians' attitudes to innovation. On the one hand physicians normally prescribed as a major therapeutic device the maintenance of habits and customs (*consuetudines*)

---

[39] *Contra calculum*, in Arnau de Vilanova, *Opera*, fol. 306ra.
[40] *De consideracionibus operis medicine*, in *AVOMO*, iv. 133.
[41] *Contra calculum*, fol. 306ra.
[42] Galen, *De ingenio sanitatis*, in *Opera ommia*, x. ed. C. G. Kühn (Leipzig, 1825), 209.

governing not only diet but all aspects of everyday life. Habits were regarded as laudable, and should be adhered to even when unpleasant or not very useful. However, this adherence should not be obsessive, since there are cases in which habits must be changed.[43] In *Contra calculum*, Arnau conservatively discourages the faithful physician from indulging in new medical recipes (*nova experimenta*), because innovations tend to introduce danger. He pays tribute to the ancient authorities of the medical profession, Hippocrates and Galen, for nothing is more certain than ancient authorities and the proven truths of the past. Yet this does not preclude him from highly esteeming new scientific contributions by contemporary physicians. Despite his reverence for the *prothomedicus* Hippocrates and the *princeps medicorum* Galen, Arnau (who must legitimize his own medical novelties) recognizes that they may have erred; their experiments may have been faulty and the simple application of their results may thus be fatal. The passage of time creates defects in the doctrine of the *antiqui*, for, like the body, knowledge also ages and needs constant renewal. The work of the *moderni* is thus necessary and essential, and there is no cause for surprise when the *moderni* can achieve what the *antiqui* failed to do, using the experience of the ancient authorities and adapting it to the contemporary level of understanding.[44] For example, the traditional medical approach regarded sleep in the middle of the day as harmful for both the body and the mind. But while the 'first authors of medicine' (*primi inventores medicine*) rejected it, we, the *moderni*, says the author of the *Commentum super regimen Salernitanum*, think that daytime sleep should not always be disparaged. Five conditions are necessary in order to render sleep in the middle of the day acceptable. It must be habitual, it should not be immediately after a meal, the head should not be lowered, the nap should not be long, and the awakening should not be abrupt.[45]

Bernard de Gordon and Henri de Mondeville did not accept every word of Galen as part of an inviolable and absolute dogma. Arnau, therefore, was conforming to standard opinion among medieval physicians who adhered to an image of science that encompassed ideas of the 'new'

---

[43] Anonymous, *Commentum super regimen Salernitanum*, in Arnau de Vilanova, *Opera*, 142rb–va.

[44] 'Nec mirandum Christo vivente, si per modernos agitetur quod adimpleri non potuit per antiquos. Proinde ergo sic moderatis antiquorum experimentis, ac suis dogmatibus ad nostrum intellectum conversis . . . prelibate mee experientie ratione probate adhesi'. *Contra calculum*, fol. 306ra; Crisciani, '*Exemplum Christi*', 267–9.

[45] Anonymous, *Commentum super regimen Salernitanum*, fol. 130rb.

and of increase by organic accretion.[46] Like theologians, physicians saw themselves bound by the authorities of their science. But in the case of physicians this tie was somewhat looser. They not only accepted the notion that authorities could err, but also the conviction that the *moderni* could add to what the ancients had created. Furthermore, they were convinced that experience, observation, and rational scrutiny were the final tests of the validity of a medical theory, not the identity of its author. This meant that, despite their inherent conservatism, they kept the door open to change when necessary. This was true of medical knowledge; as we shall see, Arnau applied the rule to theological knowledge as well.

The Source and Character of Theological Knowledge

The discussion of the source and character of theological knowledge reveals more of Arnau's peculiar ideas and sheds more light on the causes for the tension between him and the Church. He offers a model of knowledge which differs radically from the prevalent view, challenging the magisterial authority of the Church and opposing its claim for a monopoly over theological thought. This model is strikingly similar to Arnau's model of medical knowledge.

Arnau agrees that knowing God through Scripture is necessary for eternal salvation. Reason and usefulness justify even innovation (*novitas*) such as the calculation of the exact time of the coming of the Antichrist.[47] Foreknowledge will ease the inevitable hardship accompanying this period, since everyone will be able to prepare himself properly by adapting his private behaviour to the special circumstances of the times, and also by creating the necessary defence against the cunning and fraud of the Antichrist and his servants. In the case of the ignorant and illiterate, this knowledge might be gained through the mediation of those who are learned in Scripture, namely the clergy. Yet those who are capable should study the texts themselves, for it is always better to be able to

---

[46] C. Crisciani, 'History, Novelty, and Progress in Scholastic Medicine', *Osiris*, 2nd ser., 6 (1990), 118–39 and esp. 125–7, 135–7 and '*Exemplum Christi*', 267–9; L. E. Demaitre, *Doctor Bernard de Gordon: Professor and Practitioner* (Toronto, 1980), 118–20; M.-C. Pouchelle, *The Body and Surgery in the Middle Ages* (Cambridge, 1990), 199–200. W. J. Courtenay, '*Antiqui* and *moderni* in Late Medieval Thought', *Journal of the History of Ideas*, 48 (1987), 3–10.

[47] 'novitas ratione suffulta et utilis non est horrenda sed pocius amplectenda,' Arnau says in his complaint to Philip the Fair, King of France, when he tells him of the event of 1300. *Protestatio facta coram domino rege Francorum*, in M. Menéndez y Pelayo, *Historia de los heterodoxos españoles*, iii (Buenos Aires, 1951), p. lxxxi. On the utilitarian approach, see *Carpinatio*, MS Vat. lat. 3824, fol. 195ʳ.

teach oneself and others than to be taught by others.[48] Arnau thus stripped from the Church one of its most sacred duties and privileges—the monopoly on teaching Scripture. Since *Dyalogus de elementis catholice fidei*, from which these notions were taken, is dedicated to James II King of Aragon for the education of his children, Arnau intends that the laity should read Scripture independently. If we accept Josep Perarnau's notion that the text was to be used as an introduction or initiation into the way of life of various groups of spirituals (Beguins, who were of lay origin) in Provence and Catalonia, then the import for the laity of the call for universal learning becomes even more significant. Arnau's message is not restricted to the upper echelons of society.

Engaging in theological matters is inextricably bound up with the question of authority. *Tractatus de tempore adventus Antichristi* was the main cause of Arnau's first collision with the faculty of theology in Paris and with Pope Boniface VIII. According to Arnau's (or one of his associates') testimony he was in a state of acute physical suffering (severe pain to the head and the legs as well as a chest condition) when the divine word was transmitted to him; it freed him from his physical feebleness, and induced him to write his treatise.[49] The main error of which he was accused was specifying the exact date of the coming of the Antichrist. Of all future events, Arnau regarded this as the most necessary and useful to know in advance, in order to acquire the capacity to counter the deception of the Antichrist. Superficially, this treatise has nothing to do with Arnau's medical background, yet it conceals a particular (though subordinate) subtext which derives from his medical career. The message in the treatise was more subversive than a mere prophecy of the exact date of the coming of the Antichrist. Relying heavily on biblical prophetic books, Arnau declares that God provides humans with watchmen (*speculatores*) who, by virtue of their ability to see and understand the perplexities of the

---

[48] 'Ex quo patet quod ad salutem humani generis necessarium est quod aliqui studeant diligenter in Sacra Scriptura. Et iterum etiam patet ex dictis quod melius est proprio studio habere noticiam documentorum Sacre Scripture, quam traditione alterius quia melius est se ipsum et alios posse instruere quam ab aliis instrui.' *Dyalogus de elementis catholice fidei*, in W. Burger, 'Beiträge zur Geschichte der Katechese im Mittelalter', *Römische Quartalschrift* (Geschichte), 21/4 (1907), 191–3 at 193; Burger, ibid. 163–73; J. Perarnau, 'Dos tratados "espirituales" de Arnau de Vilanova en traducción castellana medieval; *Dyalogus de elementis catholice fidei y De helemosina et sacrificio*', *Anthologica Annua*, 22–3 (1975–6), 548–53.

[49] On the medical circumstances of the vision which induced him to write this treatise, see *Tractatus quidam*, MS Rome, Archivio Generale dei Carmelitani, III Varia I, fol. 60[rb], and M. Batllori, 'Dos nous escrits espirituals d'Arnau de Vilanova', *AST* 28 (1955), 60–1; *ATCA* 13 (1994), 406–7.

future, should sound the trumpet to awaken drowsy souls. Possessing divine knowledge and thus the key to spiritual discipline (*regimen*) conferred upon them by individual or universal revelation, the watchmen are a channel through which the eternal teacher (*Doctor eternus*) supplies the most powerful remedy (*virtuosum remedium*) for the cure of humans.[50] They can cure the disease of ignorance by supplying men with the salutary knowledge communicated to them through Scripture. An important ingredient in the regimen which the *speculatores* introduce is rational fear of death. It has a salutary effect on the spirit of those who are affected by it, whilst the obstinate people who do not fear death are branded as mad.[51]

Who are these *speculatores* amongst whom he numbers himself? Ordinary watchmen are the prelates and those who possess cures of souls (i.e. priests); nevertheless, all those who preach and have some part in the Church of the prophets may be *speculatores*. In the *Presentatio* of Bordeaux in 1305 he expresses the same idea, but with a nuance which underlines the therapeutic effect of the pursuit of theology by non-qualified laymen. Even though guardianship (*custodia*) over the evangelical truth belongs by virtue of authority only to prelates and judges appointed canonically, the revelation and exposition of any wound or injury to the truth is entrusted to any of the believers without distinction of sex, age, or status.[52] In order to reveal the state of moral infirmity of any group of people, every faithful member of the Church is asked and ordered to speak out. Arnau thus opens the door for an alternative channel of learning besides the Church. All those who scrutinize Scripture are the Lord's watchmen even though they have not been appointed as preachers by due authority.[53] In one of his apologies, Arnau explicitly acknowledges the

---

[50] *Tractatus de tempore adventus Antichristi* in J. Perarnau, 'El text primitiu del *De mysterio cymbalorum ecclesiae* d'Arnau de Vilanova', *ATCA* 7/8 (1988/9), 164–5: 1322–3. See Ch. 2, pp. 103–4.

[51] Ibid. 138: 175–85.

[52] 'quamuis custodia ueritatis euangelice solum ex auctoritate conueniat prelatis et iudicibus canonice institutis, tamen denunciatio uulnerum et omnis lesure ipsius apud custodes communis est quibuscumque fidelibus, nulla differentia sexus uel etatis aut status uel conditionis aliquem eximente. Nam omnis fidelis habens usum rationis potest et debet catholico moderamine denunciare quoscumque falsarios uel aduersarios euangelice ueritatis.' *Presentatio facta Burdegaliis*, MS Vat. lat. 3824, fol. 260rb.

[53] 'Et licet speculatores ordinarii sint prelati et curam animarum habentes, unde et de apostolis, quorum vices prelati gerunt, ait beatus Petrus: "Speculatores facti sumus magnitudinis eius", nihilominus etiam speculatores existunt omnes missi ad predicandum, qui vices gerunt in ecclesia prophetarum . . . quicumque scrutantur sacra eloquia, speculatores domini sunt ad populum suo modo. . . . Unde, licet ad clamandum non sint ex auctoritate ordinaria destinati, quia tamen divine veritatis hauriunt cognitionem, per ipsam debitores efficiuntur Deo et proximo.' *Tractatus de tempore adventus Antichristi*, 135–6: 73–98.

position of the Church as universal spiritual authority and commits himself not to dispute it but to seek its judgement, like a boy who finds coins
and brings them to his mother for her to decide how much they are
worth.[54] However, the real implication of his words is a violent shake-up
of the ecclesiastical academic monopoly over learning and preaching.

In connection with the model of open theological knowledge that
Arnau professes, his tactic in the numerous declarations and complaints
he makes to various Church authorities should be observed: he constantly lures his opponents to an open debate. He stresses his sincerity, asks
for reaction, replies, and rebuffs, and commits himself to answering.
Every proclamation ends with a clause stating that it should be published.
And in his letter to Pope Benedict XI shortly after the death of Boniface
VIII, he urges him to oblige theologians to read and respond in writing
to all his treatises which have been misinterpreted under Boniface, since
this is the sole way of destroying their pride and revealing divine knowledge.[55] Thus common traits connect Arnau the physician, who believes
in the divine origin and usefulness of medical knowledge and who argues
for a partially open model of medical knowledge, and Arnau the spiritual speculator, who attributes exactly the same characteristics to theological knowledge.

The openness which Arnau preaches affects the very substance of theological knowledge. To indignant theologians who criticize the author's
lack of obvious authority, he says towards the end of his eschatological
work:

'The wise man instructs us to consider what is said and not who delivers it lest
we become like the man who inspects the ink rather than the meaning and essence
of the writing. And also [the wise man instructs us] that 'the wind bloweth where
it listeth' (John 3: 8) and that he who can make, when he wants it, mute animals
like Balaam's ass, speak out true and useful things can teach the humble people
the truth so that they may deliver it [to others] for his glory.[56]

The doors to the meaning of Scripture are open to everyone (as in medicine); the authoritative gloss does not contain all the meanings of
Scripture, a plurality of interpretations is accepted, and those directly

---

[54] *Protestatio facta Perusii*, MS Vat. lat. 3824, fol. 216vb–217ra.

[55] *De morte Bonifatii*, MS Vat. lat. 3824, fol. 213ra.

[56] 'sapiens monet attendere quid dicitur, non quis profert, ne similes videantur illi, qui
potius incaustum scripture quam vim et significationem eius considerat. Et iterum, quod
spiritus potest spirare, ubicumque voluerit et quod ille qui cum vult etiam muta facit animalia vera et utilia loqui, ut asinam Balaam potest parvulos de veritate instruere ut profer-
ant ipsam ad laudem eius.' *Tractatus de tempore adventus Antichristi*, 164: 1301–4.

illuminated by the Holy Spirit have better access to the truth than the exegetes.[57] The belief that the understanding of divine truth is the product of a divine concession helps him to reach this conclusion. Consequently, he can reject outright his opponents' repeated demand that he engage himeself in medicine and not in theology.[58]

Therefore it is not surprising that his models for imitation are St Peter and St John, who, though academically unqualified, received divine information about the end of the world, while the Pharisees, though doctors of the law, did not. Furthermore Balaam, St Mary Magdalene, and the children of St Philip the Apostle and St Francis were all outsiders who directly received the divine word. At least in this context, Arnau classified himself as one of the simple men, laymen, outsiders, who notwithstanding the opposition of professional theologians write and teach divine truth.[59]

While a personal conviction that one possesses the truth is a good enough reason to speak freely, Arnau also stresses that God never ordered that Scripture be interpreted once and for all, but that it be interpreted in a successive, accumulative way, at times established by Him.[60]

---

[57] Justifying his unique interpretation of key biblical verses, Arnau exclaims in *Protestatio facta coram domino rege Francorum*, in Menéndez y Pelayo, *Historia de los heterodoxos*, iii. p. lxxxii that 'nec est inconveniens aliter nunc exponi quam exposuerunt nostri patres. . . . Cum igitur Scriptura predixerit quod multi expositores transirent per eam multipliciter exponendo, tamen docti a Spiritu Sancto solum intelligent veritatem.' In *Gladius iugulans Thomatistas*, MS Vat. lat. 3824, fol. 183va he asserts that 'proprium priuilegium eloquiorum dei est quod sicut ipse uno intuitu uidet plurima sic uno eloquio uel sermone plurima significat, unde qui uolunt quod per sacra eloquia tantum unum intelligatur, bublericos potius quam theologos se ostendunt'. One of the main conclusions of *Carpinatio poetrie theologi deviantis* of 1304 (MS Vat. lat. 3825, fol. 200vb) is that 'glossa communis non continet omnes sensus scripture qui sunt de intentione dei sicut etiam omnes sacri doctores communiter clamant'. In *Antidotum*, MS Vat. lat. 3824, fol. 245va–b he says: 'sed scientia per que uerba docet expresse quod multos intellectus et multas expositiones poterat habere secundum rationem scientie que est sincera cognitio ueritatis.'

[58] 'Propterea dixi et etiam dico, quod quicumque diceret medico christiano: Intromitte te de medicina et non de theologia, non solum ostenderet se ignarum catholice ueritatis sed etiam falsarium et subuersorem ipsius. Nam sacra scientia communis est omnibus fidelibus secundum mensuram donationis christi et solum illi appropriant eam sibi.' *Presentatio facta Burdegaliis*, MS Vat. lat. 3824, fol. 260ra.

[59] *Raonament d'Avinyó*, in Arnau de Vilanova, *Obres Catalanes*, i. ed. M. Batllori (Barcelona, 1947), 209; *Epistola ad priorissam de caritate*, 75.

[60] 'nam deus non ordinauit quod intellectus et expositiones sacrorum eloquiorum simul et semel erumperent in ecclesia sed potius successiue secundum tempora statuta in eius mente.' *Antidotum*, MS Vat. lat. 3824, fol. 246rb; in fol. 246ra he speaks of the need to adhere to the 'regula expositionis catholice quam tradit Augustinus in principio super Genesim, scilicet quod et moribus non repugnet et circumstantiis litere consonet'. An identical idea is found in *Tractatus quidam*, MS Rome, Archivio Generale dei Carmelitani III Varia 1, fol. 57vb–58ra.

By showing that orthodox biblical commentators have added layers of inter-pretation throughout history he adopts a historical, incremental approach to the development of exegesis, using it as a foundation for his favourable atti-tude towards new interpretation. But confronted with the allegation that none of the authorities supports his interpretation of Scripture, he does offer a list of supporting authorities, and thus bows to pressure to link his ideas to an authority.[61] This concept of incremental knowledge is similar to Arnau's view of medical innovation discussed above.

Arnau does not claim that everything in the theological domain is open to question. For example, it is rash, erroneous, and illicit to doubt the primacy of the Roman Church. True investigation into theological questions should be motivated by *caritas*.[62] Scrutiny motivated by *curiosi-tas* or *superbia* is illicit and may radically damage a man's vision. Arnau describes those who are afflicted with *curiositas* as committing adultery against Scripture. They enjoy spilling words from their lips as adulterers enjoy spilling seed. They mix their fake theological language with vain philosophical and natural philosophical questions, and enjoy being called masters of divinity.[63] Arnau's ambivalent attitude towards philosophers as well as towards academic theologians is revealed here, and it appears throughout his writings. Yet it should be stressed that, despite his antag-onism for the Thomists and the theologizing philosophers and philoso-phizing theologians, he does not oppose the use of philosophy and the secular sciences in preaching and teaching, provided that they are not used to hide corrupt intentions or erroneous ideas.[64]

Arnau's perfect physician ascribes the source of his medical knowledge (*scientia*) to God. The extension of this link to other fields of knowledge, and religious speculation in particular, was potential and not essential. Whether this would happen obviously depended on other variables

---

[61] He mentions the following *antiqui* who support his Daniel commentary: Bede and his *Liber numerorum*, [pseudo-]Joachim's *De semine scripturarum* (M. Reeves, *The Influence of Prophecy in the Later Middle Ages* (Oxford, 1969), 58) and Gilbertus, *Super expositionem Cirilli* (perhaps the pseudo-Joachimist exposition of the *Oraculum Cyrilli* generally thought to have emanated from spiritual Franciscan circles 1280–90, Reeves, ibid. 57). The two contemporary supporters (*moderni*) of his commentary are Fr. Ferricus de Auria (possibly Ferricus de Metz who was regent master in 1300–2) and Fr. Iohannes Parisiensis (Jean de Paris (Quidort), regent master in 1304–5) both described as masters in Paris (Pelster, 'Die Questio Heinrichs von Harclay'; Reeves, *The Influence*, 315–16); *Antidotum*, MS Vat. lat. 3824, fol. 245vb–246ra.

[62] *Tractatus de mysterio cymbalorum*, in Perarnau, 'El text primitiu del *De mysterio cym-balorum ecclesiae*', 64–5, 67.

[63] Ibid. 69–70.

[64] *Raonament d'Avinyó*, 198.

connected to the personality of the physician and the cultural context in which he acted. But it certainly created a comfortable starting-point, for a physician who regarded himself as a divine agent with access to divine knowledge and to natural secrets, to assume the role of a divine agent on much broader terms. Arnau apparently took this step by way of his instinct to extend his curative knowledge and activity from the physical to the spiritual body and to diagnose and offer a safe and final therapy for a (spiritual) disease. His belief that medical knowledge may sometimes be open to the *vulgus* is transferred to the domain of spiritual medicine when he claims open access by the *simplex* to public religious debate on grounds of divine inspiration. Medical authorities can err, can fail to provide true knowledge, and need constant reassessment and adjustment; similarly, it is sometimes necessary to reassess or supplement theological authorities.

Arnau's medical frame of mind

In interpreting Arnau's language I have suggested that he perceived spiritual activity as a natural extension of his medical preoccupation. The proof of the existence of such a 'medical frame of mind' needs more concrete evidence.

Discussing the healthy mental composition of believers, Arnau offers the following signs by which they can be recognized: their language is salubrious, they remain immune to the poisonous words of pestiferous people, and they can heal the sick by the laying on of hands. Every true believer can participate in this act of healing by promoting the conversion of sinners through good example.[65] The sick are the non-believers, and the duty to heal them is entrusted to every believer. Arnau thus extends what was usually thought of as the priest's role to everyone.[66] Yet, despite these external signs of spiritual health, a serious problem of identification remains, since true believers (the righteous elect) and sinners (diseased people who ravage the city of God) coexist almost inseparably in this world. How is it possible to distinguish the healthy (*salubres*) from the infected (*pestilentes*) so as to prevent possible error, contagion, and lethal wounds?[67] Because it is a question

---

[65] 'sanatio egrorum per impositionem manuum, id est conversio peccatorum vel pravorum hominum per exempla bonorum operum.' *Dyalogus de elementis catholice fidei*, 174; cf. Mark 16: 17–18.

[66] *Glossa Ordinaria* on Mark 16: 18 in *Biblia sacra cum glossa ordinaria*, iv. 662 stresses that 'per hoc anime suscitantur non corpora', yet interprets the object of verses 17–18 as denoting Church officials only.

[67] *Ars catholicae philosophiae*, in J. Perarnau, 'L'*Ars catholicae philosophiae*: primera redacció de la *Philosophia catholica et divina*', *ATCA* 10 (1991), 57–9.

of life and death for the elect, this distinction must be demonstrative, infallible, and certain. It produces a kind of knowledge which is the opposite of sterile knowledge (*cognitio sterilis*). Arnau suggests two models to be imitated, the builder and the physician, both of whom work according to a rule which enables them to solve problems infallibly. The builder applies a rule to test the suitability of stones to a given construction; similarly, the physician uses the guiding notions of complexion and composition which enable him to measure accurately how far the patient conforms to or deviates from ideal norms. He thus is able to know without doubt whether a person has physically declined, and to recognize his qualities infallibly. Furthermore, he can prescribe treatment with a high degree of certainty. Using the concepts of complexion and composition he can accurately measure the value of every food and every medicine.[68] The stress on the absolute importance of correct medical diagnosis that can be attained through correct observation supported by the experience of medical authorities, and the search for certainty, are basic ideas in medical theory.[69] Knowledge and prudence are the foundation of the claim for the physician's certainty; Arnau creates here a parallel to the medical arena in the spiritual world.

Arnau the physician and Arnau the religious enthusiast who diagnoses the sickness of Church and society with absolute certainty are thus linked together. The spiritual zealot, as if extending the medical profession to the spiritual level, is using a rule, showing prudence and skill, and offering ways of judging how spiritually ill the patient is and what treatment may help. Arnau's insistence on calculating the exact date of the coming of the Antichrist should also be understood in this context. The basis of this claim for certitude is the superior knowledge he possesses, which gives his salutary spiritual art both a theoretical and a practical efficacy.

---

[68] 'Medicus etiam, tam in iudicio corporum sanabilium quam corporum salubrium pro canone directivo seu regula prestituit oculis sue mentis corpus in meliori formarum, ita videlicet quod illud corpus absque dubio fore dicit optime constitutum in compositione atque complexione, quod in omnibus illius circumstantiis conformatur eidem. Lapsum vero indubitanter cognoscit esse vel a temperamento complexionis vel ab elegantia compositionis vel ab utroque, quod eidem sensibiliter est difforme. Certus est etiam quod ille cibus aut medicina temperatam habet complexionem, cuius applicatio dicto corpori per se nullo tempore correpugnat. Et secundum maiorem vel minorem difformitatem corporum ceterorum ad illud aut maiorem vel minorem applicabilium repugnantiam, lapsum eorum a temperamento scit artificiali certitudine mensurare.' Ibid. 59–60: 31–43.

[69] *De consideracionibus operis medicine, AVOMO*, iv. 133–4. Visible causes of the illness (*evidens causa morbi*) and a clear knowledge of them (*manifesta cause eius cognitio*) are necessary even in treating epilepsy and leprosy—diseases which had strong religious overtones. *De epilepsia*, in Arnau de Vilanova, *Opera*, fol. 314[vb]; *Breviarium practice*, ibid. fol. 186[rb] ff.; V. Nutton, 'From Medical Certainty to Medical Amulets: Three Aspects of Ancient Therapeutics', *Clio Medica*, 22 (1991), 13–22.

Arnau's art of diagnosis and therapy for the spiritual infirmity of mankind also leads him to stress the real, practical consequences of the ideas he professes, paralleling his perception of physical medicine as one in which speculative science and practical art are inextricably bound together. The method employed by Arnau the physician and Arnau the spiritual eccentric is the same, the justification for acting is similar, the aim—health—is the same. Arnau believes he is therefore able to diagnose accurately the moral or religious complexion of people, whom he divides into three main groups: first, those who are healthy (*salubres*); second, those who are ill (*morbidi vel egroti*), who sin because of an imbalance in their moral/religious complexion and carnal infirmity or because of ignorance of the truth, and thus do not corrupt or infect anyone but themselves; and third, the pestilential people (*pestilentes*) who sin out of pure hatred towards Christ and infect others.[70]

The ability to talk about the soul using medical categories is directly connected to Arnau's acceptance of the Galenic theory of the soul. In *De diversis intentionibus medicorum*, which explains how philosophical and medical truth can be harmonized, Arnau presents four cases of apparent disagreement between Galen and Aristotle and then resolves the contradiction by showing that both approaches are acceptable since the presuppositions of the speakers are different.[71] Arnau defends Galen's definition that the power of the soul (*virtus anime*) is the complexion which emanates from the harmonious mixture of elements (*miscibilium armonia*). This approach, which links body and soul together into one physical entity, was rejected by Aristotle (and by many thirteenth-century theologians), yet it permitted the Galenic physician to treat the soul as well. Galen, of course, was interested in the effect of the soul on the functioning (*opus, operatio*) of the organs. For Arnau it is only a small step to go on to try to cure infirmities of the soul which have nothing to do with the well-being of the body. As a physician he knows what is necessary for the sustenance of corporeal life (a moderate consumption of food and clothing according to changing personal and seasonal circumstances). But as

---

[70] 'Qui enim delicto preveniuntur propter complexionis malitiam seu veritatis ignorantiam non pestilentes dicuntur, sed morbidi vel egroti.' *Ars catholicae philosophiae*, 73: 249. On the use of complexion, complexional debility (*infirmitas complexionis*), and melancholy in discussing behavioural flaws, see *De zona pellicea*, in Cartaregia and Perarnau, 'El text sencer, 31–2, and Perarnau, 'Troballa de tractats', 510.

[71] *De diversis intentionibus medicorum*, in Arnau de Vilanova, *Opera*, fols. 36[ra]–38[va]; 38[va–b] is the discussion about the nature of the soul. On the text see McVaugh, 'The Nature and Limits of Medical Certitude', *passim* and esp. 68–9.

one who claims to possess the key to understanding Scripture, he can naturally offer the way to spiritual health or even perfection; parallel to the use (*usus*) of food and clothing for the preservation of basic good health, he suggests the use of Scripture as the most essential path to perfection.[72]

Galvano, on the other hand, supplies more explicit evidence for the 'medical frame of mind' of the physician who engages with spiritual matters. In the third treatise in the Paris manuscript, entitled 'A Neophyte Observation concerning the Grace of God with Special Reference to the Human Body and its Preservative and Curative Regimen' (*Contemplatio de gracia dei neophyta gradiens super corpus humanum et ejus regimen conseruatiuum et curatiuum*), dedicated to the Dominican Mundinus de Papia, Galvano creates a total congruence between the conferral of grace and medicine. The presupposition for the discussion is the division of the human into exterior and interior persons. The text relies heavily on Augustine and John Chrysostom for its theological arguments and on Aristotle for the ethical arguments. I shall elaborate only on the medical track, which provides Galvano with the framework for his writing. Galvano's references to medical authorities throughout the manuscript are not merely ornamental: the names of the authorities are touched with red in the text and reappear in an abbreviated form in the margin. The reader is thus made fully aware of the citations and can easily detect a specific reference without reading the whole text.

According to Galvano, medicine is the necessary outcome of the Fall of man which introduced suffering, corruption, and death to the once-perfect human body: according to Ecclesiasticus 38: 4, it is an earthly necessity (*necessitas terre*).[73] The more scientific part of the definition of medicine relies heavily on Avicenna's discussion of death and refers also to Galen. As a physician, Galvano is happy to supply his readers with a

---

[72] 'Ad vite vero sustentationem est necessarius moderatus usus alimentorum et tegumentorum, secundum circumstantias personarum et habitationum et temporum. Ad spiritualem vero perfectionem, qua scilicet mens in Deum plenius erigitur, est necessarius usus divinarum Scripturarum.' *Ars catholicae philosophiae*, 126: 1041–5.

[73] 'Tam fideles quam infideles in hoc incedunt peritius quod corpus humanum ex illo protoplasto originatum post transgressionem originalis iusticie necessarie passibilitatis, mutationis, corruptionis, et mortis traxit naturam quantumcumque fuerit ex generatione optime ad iusticiam constitutum, propter quod deus statuens propter animam corpus ad supplendum indigentias hominis et potissime necessitates uite circa quam non modicam curam habet, creauit medicinam de necessitate terre et uir sapiens non aborrebit eam.' MS Paris, BN lat. 3181, fol. 14ra.

detailed description of the body's inevitable decay which creates the necessity of medical aid and a perfect correspondence between the medical authorities and Ecclesiasticus, between Christian and non-Christian texts. Medicine is an aid (*adiutorium*) for the preservation of the radical humour, lest it be consumed faster than it should. It fights elemental destruction and external wounds by regulating bodily heat and controlling the emission of bodily superfluities.[74] The benefit of abiding by the medical regimen is spiritual, not only physical: the healthy man can become wiser; influenced by the calm accompanying good health, he will abound in spirituality.[75] Medicine thus brings man physically and spiritually nearer to the ideal prelapsarian state.

The moral interpretation of medicine leads Galvano to the story of Adam, who also needed an aid (*adiutorium*), but for his soul rather than his immortal body. It was grace (according to the Augustinian teaching) which should have ruled his soul and directed him to obedience to the Creator (exactly like the desired relationship between the physician and the patient). As for the inevitable consumption of the radical humour (which explains the unstoppable ageing process among humans), this was solved by the tree of life which could reverse the process. Adam, with the aid of divine grace, had the aptitude (*aptitudo*) to carry on living a sinless, eternal life (*permanere in sua iusticia originali*), exactly like a patient who obeys the dietary rules of his physician. Both medicine and grace are divine gifts which enable the person who needs them to cope with his difficulties on condition that he obeys the prescribed regimen.[76] Thus Galvano creates a perfect congruence between physical medicine and grace, which is the source of

---

[74] 'Putasne sapientem non nosse quod natura corporis humani quantumcumque temperati secundum Galenum in libro de diffinitiua doctrina denunciat arte constituente indigere cum necessario, secundum eundem ibidem et secundum Auicennam in libro primo capitulo de necessitate mortis, mutetur et corrumpatur propter elementorum pugnam et dissolutionem, propter humidi radicalis consumptionem et propter extrinsecorum lesionem non seruans quam prius habebat consistentiam, adiutorio ergo indiget cooperante ad permanentiam sue uite cum sua optima consistentia usque ad terminum insitum sibi a deo . . . Si autem uult proficisci in sua optima consistentia ut perficiat suas operationes ordinate secundum exigentia speciei humane que dicitur sanitas ad iusticiam, secundum Auicennam indiget adiutorio medicinali artis conseruande, quod potest dici adiutorium operans, quia medicinale hoc autem est custodia humiditatis radicalis ne cicius quam secundum racionem exiccetur uel ne putrescat temperando dominium caloris extranei extrinseci et extranei intrinseci regulando quod in superfluitatum excussione completur.' Ibid. 14^{ra–rb}. Cf. Avicenna, *Liber canonis*, i. fen 3, 1 (Venice, 1507), 53^{ra–b}.

[75] 'sanus homo possit fieri sapiens et sub tranquillo sanitatis de diuinis contemplantes spiritualibus habundare'. MS Paris, BN lat. 3181, fol. 15ra.

[76] Ibid. 14^{rb–va}.

spiritual health. He confidently speaks of both using the same terms and logical constructs. From his starting point, the medical profession, he moves on to spiritual and moral matters, and the result is a convergence of medicine's two dimensions.

The last chapter of the treatise deals with the curative regimen of bodily diseases and its moral significance (*De regimine curatiuo infirmitatis corporis optime sani ex origine ad iusticiam et eius moralitate*), and is the chapter most saturated with medical issues. It starts with a discussion of the congruence between corporeal and spiritual life and between health of the body and that of the soul. This time, Galvano's analysis of health (determined by temperate complexion, balanced composition, and unity) is more specific when he defines the means to ensure cure; to the moderate use of food, drink, and air, he adds the generic term 'the rest of the six non-natural things'.[77] God, the universal agent (*agens universalis*) has provided the body with internal, natural mechanisms to regulate itself, but sometimes exterior intervention is necessary to maintain health and hence there is a need for the physician, who acquires the title of nature's servant (*minister nature*). Then follows a long discussion of medical ethics, or in Galvano's words 'the modes of which the correct help of the physician consists' (*modi in quibus consistit rectum adiutorium medici*). Galvano describes the desired characteristics of the physician and his relationship with the patient, relying mainly on Galen (*De ingenio sanitatis*, *Liber creticorum*, *Doctrina aforistica*, *Liber prognosticorum*, *De interioribus*, *Regimen sanitatis*, and *De virtutibus naturalibus*),[78] but also on Hippocrates (*Protocanon aforistico*, which is his first aphorism), on Aristotle's natural philosophy, ethics, and metaphysics, on Augustine, on John Chrysostom, and even on an unidentified treatise or aphorism

---

[77] 'Sicut uita corporalis hominis perfecta usque ad ultimum terminum eius producta, consistit in optima consistentia ad iusticiam ex generatione quod consurgit ex temperata complexione et equali compositione et debita unitate membrorum et in adiutorio necessario artis constituentis et conseruantis cuius materia est usus moderatus et congruus aeris cibi et potus et reliquarum rerum non naturalium.' Ibid. fol. 15va (the discussion continues until 16rb).

[78] *De ingenio sanitatis*, printed under the title *De methodo medendi; Liber creticorum* (elsewhere in medieval texts entitled also *De criticis diebus*) is printed as *De diebus decretoriis; Doctrina aforistica* is Galen's commentary on the Hippocratic Aphorisms; *Liber prognosticorum* is Galen's commentary *in Hippocratis prognosticon; De interioribus* is printed under the title of *De locis affectis; Regimen sanitatis* is printed under the title *De sanitate tuenda; De virtutibus naturalibus* is printed as *De naturalibus facultatibus*. I was unable to identify the *De diffinitiva doctrina* attributed by Galvano to Galen. Cf. R. J. Durling, 'A Chronological Census of Renaissance Editions and Translations of Galen', *Journal of the Warburg and Courtauld Institutes*, 24 (1961), 230–305, at 234 n. 24 and 235; García-Ballester, 'Arnau de Vilanova', 121–7.

entitled *cui cura* which he attributes to John of Damascus.[79] The Galenic books he refers to reflect an up-to-date academic medical knowledge; at the beginning of the fourteenth century they were incorporated into the standard textbooks for the study of medicine at the universities, and were included in the 1309 statutes of Montpellier.

Four conditions must be fulfilled to achieve the beneficial effects of the physician's auxiliary role. The physician should do all that is required when confronted by disease; the patient should be obedient and refrain from aggravating the physician and leading him astray; the physician should be competent and should avoid harming the patient by prescribing wrong or defective medicines; and the physician should refrain from over-emphasizing the importance of one symptom, since the causes are always various and complex.[80] The moral dimension of this medical speculation then follows: just as maintaining the complexion, composition, and unity of the physical body is a prerequisite for good health, so cultivating and preserving the three parts of the soul, rational, irascible (*irascibilis*), and desiring (*concupiscibilis*), is essential for the soul's health. Just as the ordering of the non-natural things dictates health or disease, so the ordering of free will can lead either to the freedom of spiritual health or to the servitude of sin.[81] Spiritual cure, like physical medicine, is a help (*adiutorium*), and God might cure at the moment of death those who are curable (*sanabiles*). By introducing this term Galvano links the common

---

[79] On the *Aphorismi Iohannis Damasceni*, a late eleventh- or early twelfth-century translation of Ibn Masawayh's (d. 857) aphorisms, see Yuhanna ibn Masawayh (Jean Mesue), *Le livre des axiomes médicaux (aphorisms)*, ed. D. Jacquart and G. Troupeau (Geneva, 1980), 13, 85–8.

[80] 'Sunt ergo quatuor modi in quibus consistit rectum adiutorium medici ad naturam infirmi. Primus est ut faciat medicus omne quod necessarie est facere. Secundus ut infirmus sit obediens medico in omni quod preciperit ei et non grauet eum et erret super se. Tertius modus est ut non erret super se aliquis ex hiis qui sunt ei presentes et non noceat ei per errorem uenientem ex eo aut . . . noceat ei per defectum quod sit ex eo in eis que preparantur ei omne quo indiget ante horam in qua indiget eo et eius decoctionem optimam faciat . . . Et modus quartus ex modis in quibus precipit ypocras considerationem esse, est ut non accidat accidens forte et appropriauit hoc genus totum in nomine uno et nominauit ipsum quod accidit extrinsecus.' MS Paris, BN lat. 3181, fol. 16[rb].

[81] 'sicut res naturate fabricam corporis immediate constituentium complexio, compositio et unitas si propriam naturam seruauerit faciunt sanitatem, et si propriam naturam dimiserint faciunt infirmitatem, sic positione anime rationalis, irascibilis et concupiscibilis si propriam naturam seruauerint faciunt sanitatem libertatis et beatitudinis et si propriam naturam dimiserint faciunt infirmitatem peccati et seruitutis . . . Et sicut materia rerum non naturalium est causa in ad aliquod ad sanitatem et egritudinem corporis humani ut dictum est, sic et usus liberi arbitrii . . . est materia in ad aliquod ad causam generalem sanitatis anime; nam usus liberi arbitrii bonus conseruat et stabiliter originalem iustitiam anime et proficisci facit in melius.' Ibid. fol. 16[va].

concept of medicine which cures the body as far as it is curable (*in quantum sanabile est*) to its spiritual parallel—the curable essence (*substantia sanabilis*) of the soul which is the sinner's will to be cured. The efficacy of the treatment in spiritual medicine, as in physical medicine, depends on the obedience of the patient to the physician's demands and on the patient's will and motivation to be cured.[82] The spiritual physician's role is to direct (*ordinare*) the soul to its final end (*finem ultimum*); Galvano used the same words in speaking of the physician whose role is to maintain the body until its naturally determined end.[83] The natural inclination of the body to resist anything that opposes its well-being is compared with divine grace, which is the main medicine to overcome sin and to direct the free will towards the Good. Just as, according to Galen and Hippocrates, the body is sufficiently capable of expelling all the harmful materials which invade it, so according to Augustine, grace is sufficient (*sufficiens*) to reject any spiritual affliction (as long as free will allows it to operate).

Galvano compares the gradual recovery from fever through the total expulsion of putrid humours until perfect health is restored to the gradual healing process of the diseased soul, which must undergo the infusion of grace, expulsion of culpability, contrition of the heart, and revival of free will before it reaches a state of perfect health.[84] As for the cure of spiritual disease, grace and the sacraments are obviously the key solutions. Just as curing an innate natural disease can be achieved only through exposing the body to material with the opposite complexion (*contrarium*), so correcting an innate sin like Adam's sin can be achieved only through the mystery of incarnation. The same parallel applies to the

---

[82] Ibid. fol. 18va.

[83] Ibid. fol. 17vb–18ra; there, God the physician brings health to mankind through the seven medicines of the sacraments, and all is tied to Ecclus. 38.

[84] 'Sicut natura corporis est morbo contraria ipsum destruens et salutem inducens ut dictum est, sic et ipsa diuina gratia est peccato contraria reuocans liberum arbitrium a malo excitans ad bonum. Et sicut natura corporis est sufficiens secundum Ypocratem in omni quod indiget in regimine eius et inest uirtus quam expellit omne quod est ei contrarium et quod refugit secundum Galenum libro 3° creticorum, sic et diuina gratia, secundum Augustinum, est sufficiens remedium contra peccatum licet non infundatur adulto nisi adsit liberi arbitrii consensus. Et sicut ad integram sanitatem inducendam in febriente ex putredine humorum requiritur digestio materie febris et eius totalis expulsio ex corpore, resumptio nutritiuam, et motus gradualis ad salutem perfectam, secundum Galenum et Auicennam ita quod digestio et expulsio materie morbi fit a natura reintegratio nutriens et motus gradualis eius ad salutis perfectionem ex consensu et uoluntate infirmi complentur, sic ad ueram curationem et perfectam sanitatem infirmi que fit per iustificationem quatuor concurrunt, scilicet infusio gratie, expulsio culpe, contritio cordis et motus liberi arbitrii.' Ibid. fol. 18va–b.

cure of fever and the cure of sins in general.[85] Yet, as with physical medicine, a preparatory stage is necessary so that the treatment can be efficacious. The prelate and the preacher pave the way for the real treatment; as a feverish body is gradually healed (sometimes aided by its innate powers of health), so also is a sinful soul. Like the corporeal physician who must be faithful (*fidelis*), so the spiritual physician must be *fidelis* and attend his patient diligently, with the utmost energy and devotion and out of pure love (*caritas*) rather than for any other reason.[86] Galvano devotes a long discussion to original sin and to the resulting fragility of the soul that is manifest in carnal lust. In doing this he fuses together Augustine's discussion of sin (which is the spiritual affliction that strips the soul of its form and ordered nature) and the medical concept of fever attributed to Galen, John of Alexandria (Johannitius), and Avicenna.[87] The sacraments which he describes throughout the treatise as medicines prescribed by the good or new physician are for him a means to expel spiritual affliction, to induce and restore good health, and to maintain it over a long period of time (*expulsio, introductio sanitatis, conservatio sanitatis inducte*). The terms employed to describe that proper spiritual maintenance are taken directly from the medical world; repletion and evacuation (*repletio simul et euacuatio*), which is one of the six non-natural things necessary for health, apply also to spiritual medicine.

Thus medicine provides Galvano with a whole structure for describing and explaining key moral issues along orthodox Christian lines. Galvano also analyses, in his peculiar way, religious questions from an undoubtedly medical frame of mind and his medical expertise is the infrastructure for the moralization. What Arnau only alluded to, Galvano does openly and fuses the two disciplines together. Each in his

---

[85] 'Uerum sicut correctio morbi corporalis innati unum habet modum scilicet per contrarium secundum Galenum in diffinitiua doctrina, sic et correctio peccati innati id est originalis unum habet modum scilicet per incarnationis misterium quod factum est.' Ibid. fol. 17[vb]. 'Item sicut curatio corporalis morbi ex tempore id est actualis unum habet modum quia per contrarium in eodem gradu secundum Galenum in libro de diffinitiua doctrina, sic et curatio morbi spiritualis actualis unum habet modum quia per contrarium in eodem gradu.' Ibid. fol. 18[rb–va].

[86] 'sicut ergo medicus corporis in curatione egritudinis debet esse fidelis ut dictum est, ita et medicus spiritualis debet esse fidelis profecto.' Ibid. fol. 20[ra].

[87] 'propter transgressionem originalis iustitie est quedam fragilitas illecebrosa carnis que est fomes peccati, id est morbi spiritualis qui secundum Augustinum est priuatio modi speciei et ordinis. Sicut ergo febris corporalis secundum Galenum, Iohannitium Alexandrii et Auicennam est calor naturalis mutatus in igneum procedens a corde per artarias per totum corpus suoque ledens effectu, sic et febris spiritualis anime est calor naturalis obedientie humilitatis suo redemptori mutatus in igne per rebellionem et aduersionem procedens a corde quod est origo cuiuslibet uitii.' Ibid. fol. 17[vb].

own way, both physicians thus suffused their spiritual writings with descriptive medical metaphors and with analytical medical categories which originated in their medical background. Their presupposition was the existence of a total congruence between their field of expertise, corporeal medicine, and the spiritual medicine they were offering in their texts.

Galvano's Medical Discourse about Christ

Galvano's writings provide some striking examples of the impact of his medical background on the way he speculates about the divine. Chapter 32 of the treatise *Ars nauigatoria spiritualis* deals with magnetic stones. It starts with a description attributed to chapter 376 of Serapion's *De medicinis simplicibus*, which discusses a stone named almagertes that is found near the coast of India.[88] When ships encounter it the effect is traumatic, for they are stripped of any metallic matter which is on board, including the nails which hold them together, so that ships sailing to that region must be built without metal nails but with wooden pegs. However, according to Dioscorides the stone has an important medical effect, which is at the centre of Galvano's discussion and which will be the link to its theological dimension.[89] The colour of the magnetic stone is described as celestial and its weight as moderate. Its power (*virtus*), apart from its ability to attract metal, is that when immersed in mead (*cum mellicarte*) it lightens thick and dense humours (*laxat humores crossos*). There are those who burn the stone to produce adamant from it, Galvano says, and he sets forth the alchemical and magical powers which were attributed to the stone and which were the main reason for the continued preoccupation of medieval scientists with magnetism. But its most frequent medicinal use is in the case of dysentery (*fluxus ventris*). Magnetic medicine which stops diarrhoea introduces to the body the same powers and qualities (extreme dryness) that enable it to extract (*transglutire*) the scoria of iron (*scoria ferri*). A meticulous description of the concoction of the magnetic stone follows (a process that involves boiling, cooling down, and pouring into another vessel, repeated four times). Galvano stresses

---

[88] Cf. Serapion, *De simplicibus medicinis* (Strasbourg, 1531), 260–1, *ch.* 384.

[89] On the medical use of magnets, see *Paulys Realencyclopädie der classischen Altertumswissenschaft*, xiv/1 (Stuttgart, 1928), 483–4; *Lexikon des Mittelalters*, vi. 95–6. Galvano mentions 'Dyascorides' as his source, yet his text is identical to Serapion's version, which also mentions Dioscorides as his source. Therefore it is most likely that Galvano did not use Dioscorides directly but via Serapion. Cf. Dioscorides, *De materia medica* (Basel, 1557), bk. v. cvii and cxi, pp. 474, 476.

that the stone should not and cannot be used as a medicine in its simple form, lest it lose its powers of attraction.[90]

This medicine represents Christ, who, like a magnetic stone, attracts sinners.[91] Like the magnetic stone which acquires a specific power or property (*virtus specifica*), so Christ also has a specific divine property and a whole and perfect form (*tota species*). By showing infinite mercy Christ attracts people to the Christian faith and brings spiritual as well as physical health, for example by restoring sight and enabling the lame to walk. By attracting and extracting human sins, Christ potentially cured every human. On the cross, He drank all the thick humours of pride (*humor crossus superbie*) and all the filth of evil (*omnis sordities cupiditatis*). He extracted malice from the soul of the faithful with mead (*cum mellicarte quod fit ex aqua et melle coctum igne*) and caused every poison and pollution to be expelled. The water involved in the concoction of magnetic medicine signifies tears, honey signifies the sweetness of grace, and fire is the heat of *caritas*. Like magnetic force, which depends on the distance of the attracted matter from the magnet, so the healing effect of Christ depends on the spiritual distance of the sinner. And like celestial aid in the form of the constellation of stars and the air as a medium, which are necessary for magnetism, Christ's healing effect also depends on celestial assistance. Like the magnetic needle which gives the right direction, Christ also shows the way to those who look to him for direction.

On two matters the magnetic Christ does not behave exactly like a magnet. First, he does not attract only the rigid sinner (*ferreum peccatorem*). In the totality of his attractive powers he resembles a vacuum which attracts everything.[92] Secondly, unlike in nature, the attracted person should play an active role if effective extraction of sin is desired. Effective attraction depends not only on the attracting power of the object, but also on the will of the attracted person. Unlike most other thinkers of his time, Galvano disregards the magnet's occult and magical properties, and treats it mainly from the medical angle. He is interested in the medical efficacy of magnetic power and not in its causes.

Another metaphor for Christ which derives directly from Galvano's medical background appears in a treatise entitled 'The Theriac of Spiritual Death Based on the Theriac of the Physicians' (*Tyriaca mortis spiritualis*

---

[90] MS Paris, BN lat. 3181, fol. 38[ra-b].

[91] 'Sane o reuerende minister hic lapis magnes christus est qui exaltatus in cruce, sicut lapis magnes trahit ferrum per uirtutem specificam sic christus trahit peccatorem ferro duriorem per suam uirtutem diuinam.' Ibid. fol. 38[rb].

[92] Ibid. fol. 38[vb].

gradiens super tyriacam medicorum). Theriac was the most famous drug compounded in classical antiquity. It was regarded as an all-purpose antidote which was highly effective against snakebite and all other poisons. At the basis of Galvano's text lies a full congruence between physical and spiritual death, the human reaction to both and possible treatment which may delay it. This congruence gives the physician who already possesses superior knowledge on the medical side of the equation a comfortable starting-point for discussion of theological matters.

Galvano starts with a meticulous description of theriac and the ways to produce it according to Avicenna (*testante Avicenna*).[93] Michael McVaugh has shown that the discussion of theriac exemplifies the growth of natural-philosophical ideas in medieval universities in general and in Montpellier in particular.[94] Galvano, about whose contacts with Montpellier we know nothing, shows how information flowed in the opposite direction. The concepts of natural quality (*proprietas*), simples (*simplices*), compounds (*compositus*), specific form (*forma specifica*), and form (*species*) which were essential to the discourse of theriac are intercalated into the spiritual discourse that follows almost naturally.

According to Galvano, the discovery of this medicine is attributed to the Greek warrior Andromachus, who for the benefit of mankind composed the most efficacious and precious medicine from spices (*res aromatici*), balsam-gum, the gum produced from mummies (*mumia*),[95] poppy juice (*opium*), serpents' flesh, honey, wine, and other composite medicines. This medicine could counteract every poison and overcome practically every known disease. Galvano's list includes: phlegmatic and melancholic diseases as well as fevers associated with them, violent flatulence (*ventositas maligna*), paralysis, apoplexy, epilepsy, spasm (*tortura*), shaking (*tremor*), talking to oneself, madness, and leprosy. In addition, it strengthens the heart and stomach, sharpens the senses and the appetite, regulates the pulse, and restores the spirits of the blood. It is useful against various kidney afflictions including the removal of kidney- and

[93] Galvano's description is almost identical to Avicenna's *Liber canonis*, v. Summa 1, 1, c. *De tyriacis et confectionibus magnis*, 507vb–508rb, and *De vir. cor.* Tract. 2, c. 4 (Venice, 1564), 340.

[94] M. R. McVaugh, 'Theriac at Montpellier 1285–1325', *Sudhoffs Archiv*, 56 (1972), 113–24 and especially McVaugh's introduction to *Epistola Arnaldi de Villanova de dosi tyriacalium medicinarum*, in *AVOMO*, iii. 57–73.

[95] On the medical use of mummies in the West, see A. Wiedermann, 'Mumie als Heilmittel', *Zeitschrift des Vereins für rheinische und westfälische Volkskunde*, 3 (1906), 1–38; K. Park, 'The Life of the Corpse: Division and Dissection in Late Medieval Europe', *Journal of the History of Medicine and Allied Sciences*, 50 (1995), 116–17.

bladder-stones; it cures intestinal ulcers and internal hardness (*durities*) of the liver and spleen. As an aid to nature it strengthens the innate heat (*innatus calor*) and the spirit. It is the only means of preserving the regular flow of the radical humour and of slowing down the inevitable physical decline which starts ten years after the stage of puberty in a warm climate and after twenty in a cold one. The overwhelming power of theriac is a result of the quality of its specific form, which follows the complexion of its simple components.[96]

Christ is the *divinus andromachus*, the supreme physician and celestial apothecary or spice-producer (*pigmentator celestis*) who wanted to be useful to mankind. To earn its salvation through his merits and deeds (the spices, the wine, and the honey), he was raised on the cross like a serpent; and by dying he produced from the gum of his blood and the opium of his death (*ex balsamo et mumia sui sanguinis et opio dormitionis*) the most sufficient and efficacious medicine offered to poisoned mankind—theriac.[97] Like the total effect of the physical theriac, the theriac of Jesus's death and resurrection (*tyriaca mortis et resurrectionis Ihesu*) influences all the members of the Christian body (including the just ones who lived before Christ) and its completion was gradual. Galvano describes at length the descent to hell, the resurrection, and the conferral of the Holy Spirit as a process which ended in the perfection of the spiritual theriac. This is congruent to the periods of fermentation at the end of which medical theriac is completed. Christ's age when he fulfilled his mission accurately corresponds to the minimum age specifications of between 30 and 40 which determine theriac's correct and ideal application. Spiritual theriac, like its medical replica, must be applied gradually and cautiously to those who have been properly prepared for it and have achieved the appropriate disposition.

As the preparation of theriac begins with simple but qualitatively very pure ingredients mixed in exact quantities, and results in the emergence of one compound body with a well-balanced complexion (*ydonea complexio*) and its own specific form, so the *divinus Andromachus* produced his holy theriac (*tyriaca sacrata*). The various simple ingredients from which theriac is composed are Christ's merits. The fire which is essential

---

[96] 'proprietas totius speciei eius sequens complexionem simplicium ipsius'. MS Paris, BN lat. 3181, fol. 40ra. Cf. Avicenna, *Liber canonis*, v. Summa 1, 1, *c*. '*De tyriacis et confectionibus magnis*', 507vb.

[97] 'sacratam et preciosam tyriacam composuit sufficientissimum et efficacissimum remedium humani generis uenenati et languidi et mortificati ab olim, multiplicitate uenenorum et langorum spiritualium.' MS Paris, BN lat. 3181, fol. 40ra.

for the production of theriac is, on the spiritual level, the fire of the suffering on the cross (*ignis passionis crucis*), and Galvano uses the same verbs to describe the production of theriac and Christ's suffering before the crucifixion (to prepare, *parare*, to thresh, *triturare*, to grind, *terere*, and to pound, *conterere*). The result was the creation of a new specific form, which is the Catholic faith.[98] In addition, Christ also provides the believer with a specific property (*virtus specifica*) according to which one should live, namely *caritas*. *Caritas* is the theriac of man's spiritual death, and through the sacraments it provides the opportunity for men to escape eternal death. And if Christ is theriac, it is not surprising to find in Galvano's writing Mary as 'the mother of our theriac' who lacks any 'humour of carnality'.[99]

While Galvano proudly presents himself as learned (*expertus*) in the laws of Avicenna,[100] he expresses the fear that, as a simple physician, he might be regarded as too *inexpertus* to moralize about quantitative aspects of the production of spiritual theriac. The passage from the medical to the theological domain would not necessarily be acceptable to his audience. To remove these doubts, Galvano offers a quantitative interpretation of spiritual theriac immediately after discussing the quantitative aspects of medical theriac.[101] Thus, in addition to the qualitative similarity between the medical and the spiritual theriac, there also is a quantitative congruence. As with medicinal theriac, the efficacy of spiritual theriac depends on its proper preparation, which must be based on accurate measurement of the various ingredients. The number seventy, as the product of multiplying ten by seven, encapsulates the spiritual theriac produced by the divine Andromachus to counter death. It quantitatively proves that Christ's death and resurrection fulfilled the Decalogue and introduced in its place the perfection of the law of the Gospel which is based on various combinations of seven, such as the seven sacraments, seven virtues, and seven divine gifts. This type of numerical moralization

---

[98] 'nouus pigmentator celestis descendens ad limbum, resurgens a mortuis et ascendens in celum in eum credentes in se transformans, unum corpus misticum inde constituit, eius est caput, et dans ei formam specificam et diuinam uiuendi scilicet fidem catholicam.' Ibid. fol. 40va–b.

[99] Ibid. fol. 58va.

[100] 'Fateor quippe expertus umbra medici ego imitator dogmatis auicenne in licitis.' Ibid. fol. 40va.

[101] 'Postremo ne dicatur me umbram medici moralitatis numeri ponderis et mensure rerum et aromatum componentium tyriacam andromachi fuisse inexpertem aut non solicitum, sufficiat mihi de moralitate numeri eorum ad incitationem fidelium aliquid balbutire.' Ibid. fol. 41rb.

(whose specific source is not stated) is not original; its context, however, is significant. By initiating his discussion of the aim of spiritual theriac on the foundation of medical knowledge, and by juxtaposing the efficacy and mode of production of both types of theriac, Galvano implicitly creates a link between medical and religious practice. His insight into theology originates in his professional background. For him, medical knowledge and practice fulfil a distinctive spiritual purpose which extends beyond their therapeutic function.

Is the use of theriac as a metaphor for Christ unique for theologizing physicians, or did preachers also employ it in their spiritual discourse? When discussing the spiritual medicines that Christianity offers (the word of God received through preaching or prayer), preachers and theologians throughout the fourteenth century occasionally used the metaphor of theriac as the ultimate spiritual cure. Confession, the sinner's fear, and the curative effect of the remembrance of Christ's passion are depicted as spiritual theriac.[102] However, I have not come across a specific comparison of Christ to theriac, and nowhere is there such a detailed scientific discussion attached to the metaphor of theriac.

The Theologizing Physician: A Defence

In reply to his opponents' frequent demand that he should devote himself to medicine and not theology, Arnau also makes some explicit declarations about the status of the physician within the religious debate. The arguments he uses occasionally differ, but all suggest that he, at least, failed to see a distinct boundary between the disciplines. In *Apologia de versutiis et perversitatibus pseudotheologorum et religiosorum* he concludes that to ask physicians to avoid theology amounts to blasphemy against God and Christ who incarnates the fusion between the two aspects of health. Forbidding physicians to engage with theology amounts to criticizing Christ, who was given by God as a medicine to humanity and who simultaneously performed acts of healing and expounded theology. Furthermore, Jesus never specifically excluded physicians from understanding scripture. On the contrary, one of the Evangelists (he implies

---

[102] Giordano da Pisa, *Quaresimale Fiorentino 1305–1306*, ed. C. Delcorno (Florence, 1974), 225, 336: 157–63, 383: 2–3; C. Iannella, 'Malattia e salute nella predicazione di Giordano da Pisa', *Rivista di Storia e Letteratura Religiosa*, 31 (1995), 209–10; Pierre Bersuire, *Reductorium morale super totam bibliam* (Venice, 1583), vi. 27, 108^2: 'de veneno'; Robert Holcot, *In librum sapientie regis Salomonis prelectiones ccxiii* (Basel, 1586), *lectio* cxciiii, 639.

that it was Luke) was hailed as a physician. Finally, he returns to the universal argument that by being organs of Christ's body, baptized physicians are infused with the Holy Spirit, which is the source of all knowledge and science and also of health.[103] Similarly, when in August 1305 Arnau approaches the newly elected Pope Clement V, he says that Christ did not exclude physicians from understanding Scripture, nor did any of the apostles tell Luke when he was writing the Gospel and the Acts to confine himself to medicine and not to engage with theology. Gaining full understanding of the divine word depends solely on divine will; he whom God deems worthy to know his secrets will know them. On the basis of John 3: 8 'The wind bloweth where it listeth' (*spiritus ubi vult spirat*) and 6: 45 'Every man that . . . has learned of the father comes unto me' (*omnes fideles sunt docibiles*) he conveys his attitude to universal learning.[104] As a married man, Arnau is also forced to rebut the contention that married men have no credibility in theological matters, declaring this to be an impious, abominable blasphemy not only against the sacrament of matrimony but also against Christ who conferred the primacy over the Church on a married man, Peter.[105]

Galvano also feels the need to justify his intrusion into the theological domain; his introductions at the beginning of each treatise reveal his unease. He introduces himself as 'formerly a physician of the bodies, in name only, but presently the worm of Christ, the tiny mound of earth before his feet' (*Galuanus de levanto ianuensis olim medicus corporum solo taliter nomine nunc vero autem vermis ihesu terre obsculum ante pedes*).[106] Elsewhere he adds to his attributes the name *in umbre medici* which has

---

[103] 'Illa enim blasphemia non uos tangit solummodo sed uniuersitatem sanctorum. Et primo deum patrem et spiritum sanctum, qui Christum exposuerunt humano generi ut medicinam et medicum, et qui de ipso dicunt: "Honora medicum quia propter necessitatem creauit ipsum altissimus' . . . Specialiter etiam hec blasphemia Christum uulnerat seu sagittat. Nam ipse ab intelligentia scripturarum medicos non exclusit cum inter euangelistas connumerauerit medicum cuius laus ut ait apostolus est per omnem ecclesiam in euangelio quod scripsit et actibus apostolorum. Nec minus ista blasphemia uituperat totum collegium electorum et etiam totam ueritatem misterii saluatoris. Clamat enim apostolus quod quicumque baptisati sumus in Christo membra, sumus unius corporis, scilicet Christi . . . Nam si medici baptisati de corpore Christi sunt, constat quod uiuunt per spiritum Christi, ait enim apostolus "si quis spiritum Christi non habet hic non est eius", quod si per spiritum christi uiuunt scientia et sapientia dei dantur eis secundum mensuram donationis Christi et non secundum uoluntatem et auctoritatem magistralis inflationis.' MS Vat. lat. 3824, fol. 147vb–148ra.

[104] *Protestatio facta Burdegaliis*, MS Vat. lat. 3824, fol. 257^{va–b}, 259^{rb–va}; see n. 52 above.

[105] *Tertia denunciatio Gerundensis*, in J. Carreras i Artau, 'La polémica gerundense sobre el Anticristo entre Arnau de Vilanova y los dominicos', *Anales del Instituto de Estudios Gerundenses*, 5/6 (1950/51), 55.

[106] MS Paris, BN lat. 3181, fol. 1ra.

led some historians in the past falsely to believe that he was a physician in Umbria. Galvano probably meant to say that he was in the shadow of a physician, thus stressing his medical past and at the same time his present distance from this profession.[107] Whether his humility was sincere or fake, Galvano's harping on his past career as a physician is noteworthy, for if a medical past were regarded as a liability it would be a mistake to emphasize it. His treatise 'A Neophyte's Teaching Concerning the Inferno, Purgatory and Paradise' (*Neophyta doctrina de inferno, purgatorio et paradiso*) adds another element to the introduction: after presenting himself as 'a useless worm of Jesus Christ' (*vermis inutilis Iesu Christi*)—a metaphor used also by others, including Arnau and non-Christian authors—he also tells us that he has been induced by the Franciscan Dominicus Albanensis to teach him the correct way of living (*vita recta*) which leads to the gates of eternal health. Dominicus was anxious to learn from the Physician who had descended from heaven to cure the sick and who wished to confer salvation and health without delay.[108] Galvano thus creates a religious legitimacy for his transgression of disciplinary boundaries, since he is merely imitating Christ's healing activity. As a divine agent, he is recruited to contribute to the spiritual health of the people. The source of his knowledge is the Holy Spirit, which has revealed to him its visceral secrets (a popularly used metaphor in that period, which receives a special meaning when we know of the author's medical background).[109] In a treatise devoted to Mary (*Tractatus alphabeti christifere marie*), when discussing the simplicity (*simplicitas*) of her conception Galvano speaks of the dearest of all physicians—Luke, John of Damascus, Cosmas, and Damian—who after having served as physicians of the body duly became followers of Christ, the supreme healer. Physicians were thus urged and perhaps also expected to develop a particular inclination to theologize by virtue of returning to God what they had received from him.[110]

---

[107] Leclercq, 'Galvano da Levanto', 404. MS Paris, BN lat. 3181, fol. 9rb.

[108] 'Tunc autem is idem frater ardentius institit in petendo. Dicens: O medice christiane disce a medico qui de celo descendit ut sanaret egrotos, ne differas, non enim est apud illum ulla perendinatio sanitatis, neque timeas, tuos enim supplebit defectus ad cuius uocem, Christi caritate accensus, et eiusdem gratia confisus, a quo uenit omne quod expedit.' Ibid. fol. 45rb.

[109] 'Dum spiritus sancti misterio reuelauerit mihi secretum neophytum in uisceribus uestris latens.' Ibid. fol. 45ra.

[110] 'quia cum omnia que habent fluant a Christo dignum est ut omnia redeant, in ipso letentur et corporis humani curantes si Christum pauperem et summum curatorem sunt sectantes ut Lucas carissimus medicus, Pantaleo, Johannes Damascenus, Cosma et Damianus fratres.' Ibid. fol. 58vb.

As for Arnau, nowhere does he assert that a physician should indulge in theology as a physician. In fact, he explicitly determines that it is unsuitable for a physician to deal with theology by virtue of being a physician. This notion appears in *Tractatus quidam*, where Arnau (or possibly one of his followers) recites the various arguments of the critics against him, his ideas, and the methods by which he divulged his message.[111] On the traditional argument that a physician should concentrate on medicine and not theology, the critics against whom the treatise is directed say, 'Just as it is up to the craftsmen to handle those things suitable to their crafts, so it is up to the physician to handle those things relevant to medicine' (*sicut fabrorum est tractare fabrilia . . . sic medicorum medicinalia*), thus echoing the notion that medicine should be classified among the mechanical arts. Arnau agrees that 'it is not suitable to the craftsman while he is such and to the physician while he is engaged in medicine to handle divine things' (*fabro ut faber est, et medico ut medicus est, non convenit tractare divina*), but stresses that they both have the right to deal with divine questions as faithful Catholics, who are organs of Christ's body. One could argue that this puts an end to my quest for links between Arnau's medical background and his spiritual activity. Yet could Arnau have provided another argument that would have satisfied his critics? Surely he could not concede that he claimed the right to theologize because he was a physician—an unacceptable argument to any fourteenth-century clerical audience. Thus when read in the context of his defence, this sentence, whether uttered by Arnau or only reported by one of his associates, cannot be interpreted as an unequivocal denial of any relationship between Arnau's medical background and his spiritual activity.

Moreover, from what follows in the text, Arnau does provide arguments that it is religiously acceptable for physicians to theologize. He cites the medical dimension of Christ's activities as conveyed in Ecclesiasticus 38 and similar precedents among authorities of the early church. In addition to Luke he also mentions Fabianus and Sebastianus as physicians who dealt with theology.[112] He then attempts to prove that

---

[111] MS Rome, Archivio Generale dei Carmelitani, III Varia I, fols. 62vb–63ra (also in Batllori, 'Dos nous escritos', 62–3). A unique argument was that as a Catalan he was a member of a contemptible nation and therefore should not deal with theology; others referred to him being married, ignorant, uneducated (*illiteratus*), a fantasizer (*phantasticus*), and a dreamer (*sompniator*).

[112] The medical background of Fabian is not part of his recognized Life. It seems that he was introduced in this context because according to Eusebius, *Hist. Eccl.*, vi. ch. xxix, Fabian was elected as Pope in spite of being a layman and a stranger. His feast-day (20 January) is shared with Sebastian, who is also a patron against the plague.

denying physicians the right to treat theological matters because they are physicians amounts to a blasphemy against the whole Church, which even accepted the prophecies of a person like Balaam who was an infidel, a soothsayer, and impious. Claiming that a moral flaw which stains God's minister renders the content of his utterance objectionable, however true, is equivalent to accusing the Church of having committed grave errors in accepting these prophecies. Thus, Arnau thinks that the identity of the prophet and even his religious convictions should be wholly irrelevant to the validity of the prophecy.

Arnau even regards this transgression of boundaries as a divine commandment. Through an allegorical interpretation of Genesis 12: 1 (God ordering Abraham to leave his home and country), Arnau advises leaving the secular sciences into which one was born and by which one was nourished, and turning to theology. To deny that universal right by promising to honour and praise the physician who avoids theology is to contradict evangelical teaching and to act out of zeal for corporeal rather than spiritual profit. These people erroneously honour someone for his physical rather than for his spiritual occupation. St Paul, who graduated from a school that all would agree was more distinguished than the school of Paris, recommended that everyone study the Gospel. He never restricted the study to medicine only, and his example should be followed.[113]

The Boundaries of Medicine

To understand why Arnau transgressed the apparently clear boundaries of medicine, we must comprehend his perception of these boundaries. Defining cure or remedy (*medela*) as 'the service of a medicament offered to the living who is in a state of some [complexional] flaw—either corporeal service should the flaw be corporeal or spiritual service should the

---

[113] 'Nam qui debuit ut vir evangelicus dicere: egredere de domo tua . . . hoc est: relinque omnes sciencias seculares, in quibus natus es et nutritus et intende sacris eloquiis, dixit: intromitte te de medicina et non de theologia et honorabimus te, quibus verbis non solum pervertebat evangelica documenta, set ab agro theologie parvulos Christi nitebatur excludere, cupiens ipsum agrum singulariter cum gigantibus possidere. Palam etiam confitebatur quod non zelus Christi vel salutis animarum set corporum regnabat in eo, cum ob commodum corporum et non spirituum ministro communi sponderet honorem. Simulque sprevisset exemplum Pauli qui Magistratus in theologia sublimiori scola quam parisiensi commendavit omnes studium evangelicum, neque suasit ei potius studium medicine corporalis quam theologie.' *Interpretatio de visionibus in somniis* in Menéndez y Pelayo, *Historia de los heterodoxos españoles,* iii. p. lxxi.

flaw be spiritual',[114] Arnau undermined the clear-cut boundary between the physician of the body and that of the soul. Both cures, which at first sight seem to be separate, have a divine cause and are applied to the living person. Yet these cures are linked in a way which implies potential access of the physician to the domain of spiritual cure. Literally the teaching (*doctrina*) contained in *Medicationis parabole* applies to physical flaws. Its object is the living human body; but living includes both the physical and the spiritual aspects of life. Hence it is implied that the medical text may be relevant for the cure of the soul and that the physician may contribute to its well-being. Of course, by providing spiritual cure, Arnau did not claim to bring spiritual salvation to the patient, as did the priest. He merely hinted at the potentially spiritual level of a medical text (*Medicationis parabole*) and the possibility of adapting it for the cure of spiritual flaws. As we shall see, the spiritual aspects of medicine were usually limited and never transcendental. They were largely determined by the concept of 'accidents of the soul', which was the last of the six non-natural things to be regulated by the physician; hence the health of the soul would be of interest to the physicians only as far as it affected the health of the body. However, the notion that medicine could be useful for the health of the soul was bound to create ambiguity as to the exact boundaries between spiritual and physical medicine.

Medical theory itself warranted the physician's access to certain aspects of the human soul. Galen concentrated on a conception of disease which only took into account its somatic element. As far as the soul is concerned, he maintained a somewhat agnostic attitude, not because he doubted its existence, but because he did not consider speculation on its nature, substance, or characteristics as helpful to the solution of therapeutic problems which preoccupied him as a physician. He also established a clear separation between the things that relate to the natural state of the body and are of interest to the physician, and those things concerning only the virtues of the soul which are of interest to the philosopher. Nevertheless, Galen affirmed that there was some connection between the powers of the soul and the power (*krasis*) of the body, and even a dependence of the soul on the body. But he left the nature of the connection rather vague. By making medicine the foundation of the physical, psychic, and ethical life of man, he placed the physician at the

---

[114] 'beneficium sanationis quod viventi exhibetur in aliquo lapsu, vel corporale si lapsus fuerit corporalis, vel spirituale si lapsus fuerit spiritualis'. *Commentum super quosdam parabolas*, *AVOMO*, vi. 2, 153. See also the proemium to *Antidotarium*, fol. 243va, which describes medicine as divinely created 'necessitate sanationis corporis et anime'.

top of all professional activities.[115] On this basis it is not surprising that Arnau the Galenic physician adopted a broad definition of medicine which stretched far beyond bodily physique.

Arnau's treatise *De simplicibus* (largely dedicated to adapting simple medicines to specific organs and conditions) gives a broad definition of the science of medicine. Since illness exerts influence in a hidden (*occultus*) or a natural mode not only upon the body but also upon the mind and the soul, the art of medicine relates to all three fields, whether directly or indirectly. Medicines thus influence the disposition of members of the body, the memory, the sight, the intellect, and even the feelings such as love, since 'the art of medicine is inclined to affect everything'.[116] To illustrate the wide-ranging effects of the art of medicine, Arnau mentions the useful effect of medical treatment on the good quality of understanding (*bonitas intellectus*) which follows the excellence of the body's digestive, nutritive, and purgative functions. By keeping the brain free of superfluous humours and unhealthy vapours, and by purifying the blood and spirits, the physician strengthens the brain and the sensitive powers and thus enhances the faculties of the soul. That medicine influences the soul goes without saying, but Arnau goes beyond the usual idea of medicine as a protection against indispositions of the soul such as melancholy, phlegm, and heroic love. Among other things, he introduces a medicine which causes the patient to cheer up (*medicina letificativa*) and offers clinical treatment which will have an effect on the character of the patient and will endow him with the ideal traits of mercy, piety, gentleness, and benignity, and thus indirectly can lead him to paradise (as metaphorically understood).[117]

---

[115] L. García-Ballester, 'Soul and Body, Disease of the Soul and Disease of the Body in Galen's Medical Thought', in *Le opere psicologiche de Galeno*, ed. P. Manuli and M. Vegetti (Naples, 1988), 117–52, esp. 119, 129; on accidents of the soul, see M. R. McVaugh, *Medicine before the Plague: Practitioners and their Patients in the Crown of Aragon, 1285–1345* (Cambridge, 1993), 146–7.

[116] 'Si vis scire que faciunt bonam memoriam, bonum intellectum, bonum visum et que faciunt amorem secundum viam naturalem aut via occulta, ad omnia enim ars medicine habet ingenium.' *De simplicibus*, fol. 242[rb].

[117] 'Audivisti etiam quod quedam medicina vocatur letificativa, quia aggregat omnia confortantia membra principalia, et sanguinem clarificantia, et generantia bonum sanguinem et spiritum. Secundum hoc etiam potes dicere, quod quedam medicina ducit ad paradisum, quia est composita ex disponentibus sanguinem ad misericordiam et pietatem et mansuetudinem et benignitatem, quibus mediantibus sequitur bonus appetitus ad bona opera; et quedam incitat amorem, quia auget sanguinem laudabilem clarum in quanto et in quali, et privat ipsum a melancholia et flegmate, que sunt cause sollicitudinis, que prohibet conversativam et curabilitatem et amorem; sanguis vero multus clarus facit omnia contraria'. Ibid. fol. 242[va].

Medicine can cause people to love and to be loved; by purifying the blood it ignites the appetite and mutual desire. But medicine can also influence the religiosity of the patient and is regarded as a major tool for those who lead a monastic life. Hence it is not only the moral philosopher who is concerned with the production and expression of psychological states; physicians, though usually studying the emotions in so far as they lead to physiological, sensible changes pertaining to the health of the body, have the knowledge and the power to affect the accidents of the soul on a much broader front.[118] Here lies a potential point of friction between the physician and the priest, for the physician intrudes into monastic territory not as an agent who heals accidental or natural illnesses, but as an outsider who offers an alternative route to becoming properly religious. Religiosity can be attained through medical pharmaceutical intervention as well as through contemplation, learning, or simple obedience.[119]

The power of the physician to influence the character of the patient for good or bad renders him theoretically omnipotent in regard to all other humans. He can make the avaricious wasteful, the chaste lustful, the timid audacious. By altering the complexion of the patient's blood he necessarily changes all the inclinations and qualities of the patient. This extraordinary power is enhanced by the secret aspects of medical knowledge.[120]

This was doubtless an approach which was potentially at odds with the orthodox Christian attitude which regarded the soul as the domain of the priest. Though there is no evidence that Arnau's medical ideas became an issue in his strife with the Church, it provides us with important circumstantial evidence for explaining his natural inclination to join moral and spiritual debates.

---

[118] McVaugh, *Medicine before the Plague*, 147.

[119] 'quedam facit castum, religiosum, quia inclinat sanguinem ad frigiditatem et paucitatem, quo facto non appetit coitum, nec mulieres, nec ludum nec cantus nec similia, et ut generaliter dicatur, potes cum medicinis scire dispositionem sanguinis ad quamcunque qualitatem, et tota differentia morum hominis fit ex sanguine calido, frigido, humido et sicco, et cum medicinis predictis scis etiam facere circa hominem omne quod vis . . . Radix ergo agendi secreta medicinalia circa corpus est ut attendas circa sanguinem minuendum aut augendum et operaberis omne quod voles.' *De simplicibus*, fol. 242va. On the primary status of blood in pharmaceutical medicine, see ibid. fol. 240ra.

[120] 'Facit igitur medicus de avaro prodigum, de casto luxuriosum, de timido audacem et generaliter, sicut mutat complexionem sanguinis necesse est mutare sequentes inclinationes et complexiones ipsius; et hec sunt secreta ipsius ultima artis medicine.' Ibid. fol. 242va. Cf. the apocryphal *Regimen sanitatis*, in Arnau de Vilanova, *Opera*, fol. 68vb.

In *Speculum medicine* Arnau devotes a long discussion to the accidents of the soul. In addition to the four passions mentioned above, which were of particular interest to physicians, he also elaborates on distress (*angustia*) and shame, which are subspecies of sadness and fear respectively.[121] Let us look at the medical explanation of anger, which, incidentally, is also one of the seven deadly sins. In his *Regimen sanitatis ad regem Aragonum*, Arnau says that accidents of the soul which affect the physical body should be medically treated when their influence is harmful. Anger, which causes overheating of all the organs and of the heart in particular, confounds reason and rational behaviour. It thus should be avoided unless it is directed against unlawful matters and actions. Sadness (*tristitia*) cools down and dries out the organs and thus is also detrimental to good health. It should be avoided and neutralized, unless it is part of a penitential process (this is another example of the influence of Christian ideas on medical therapy). Licit pleasure (*gaudium*) and honest comforts are therefore useful to relieve and rejuvenate the soul.[122]

Hippocratic medicine was psychosomatic in so far as conditions of the body were recognized as affecting and being affected by mental states. Hippocrates, together with Plato and other philosophers, served as authorities for Galen's *That the Faculties of the Soul Follow the Temperament of the Body*. Thus the claim that diet could change every accident of the soul, including the intellect, can already be found in Greek medicine.[123] Discussion of the physical effects of the various accidents of the soul was an integral part of many medical textbooks in the Middle Ages. Occasionally it consisted only of practical advice, but it could include a more ambitious attempt to legitimize the physician's jurisdiction in this field. The scope of the passions of the soul relevant for discussion constituted one of the major differences between physicians and philosophers, who were equally interested in the topic. The strictly physical interest of the physicians reduced the passions relevant for medical treatment to the four principal ones: happiness and sadness, which reflected a disorder of the concupiscible appetite,

[121] *Speculum medicine*, fol. 23^V–25^V.

[122] *Regimen sanitatis ad regem Aragonum*, *AVOMO*, x. 1, 436. Cf. a fuller medical discussion of anger in the apocryphal *Regimen sanitatis*, fol. 68vb–69ra.

[123] Galen, *Quod animi mores*, 9 in *Opera omnia*, iv. ed. Kühn, 807–8; O. Temkin, *Hippocrates in a World of Pagans and Christians* (Baltimore and London, 1991), 8–17; García-Ballester, 'Soul and Body, 137–52 and especially 141, 142–5, 147.

and anger and fear, which reflected a disorder of the irascible appetite.[124]

Bernard de Gordon found in psychosomatics a justification for his concern with ethics, and applied psychosomatics in explaining and treating diseases. Though apparently a deeply pious man, he often based his ethical thinking on psychosomatics and natural reasons rather than on authority or pious considerations. Thus he gave a medical rather than an ascetic argument against drunkenness, and explained monastic silence by the need to concentrate on eating. Similarly, it is possible to detect an interdependence of body and soul in Henry de Mondeville's writing.[125] Arnau's psychosomatic approach was therefore neither original nor unique in his time; but it is another factor which could explain why, in his time, a physician who regarded his profession as transcending the body might encroach on the clerical domain.

Medical Knowledge at the Service of Religious Debates and Questions

The Medical Aspect: Arnau's Defence of Carthusian Vegetarianism

The symbiotic relationship between medicine and religion also has a practical dimension. One of its facets is the input of physicians (directly, or through the diffusion of medical knowledge) to clerical debates on moral, philosophical, or theological questions. Arnau provides us with such a case in his 'On the Eating of Meat' (*De esu carnium*)—the first full-length treatise in the Latin West devoted to vegetarian diet (*c.*1302–5),[126] and an example of the use of medical knowledge in support of one party in a religious conflict between the monastic orders. The broad context of the treatise is the debate over monastic abstinence. By the early thirteenth century the Carthusians had acquired notoriety for being harsh and cruel, refusing meat even to their sick members. The specific target of Arnau's treatise may have been Dominican friars who entered a Charterhouse pretending to be postulants and complained loudly to

---

[124] P. Gil-Sotres, 'Modelo teórico y observación clínica: Las pasiones del alma en la psicología medica medieval', in *Comprendre et maîtriser la nature au Moyen Âge: Mélanges d'histoire des sciences offerts à Guy Beaujouan* (Geneva, 1994), 181–204; at 188–92 Arnau's contribution to the medical discussion of the topic. See also id., 'La higiene de les emocions', in *AVOMO*, x. 1, 337–61.

[125] Demaitre, *Doctor Bernard*, 166–8; Pouchelle, *The Body and Surgery*, 116–17.

[126] See D. M. Bazell, 'Christian Diet: A Case Study Using Arnald of Vilanova's *De esu carnium*', Ph.D. thesis (Harvard, 1991). I have used the critical text which has been edited by Bazell: ibid. 190–213.

higher ecclesiastical authorities about the Carthusian practice of abstaining from meat. Since nothing definite is known concerning the specific historical context of the debate,[127] I shall confine my discussion to Arnau's medical argument and to the apparent ease with which he moves from medical to religious reasoning.

The treatise starts with the accusation of critics of the Carthusian Order that the constitution (*status*) of the order is detrimental to religious life and to life in general (*periculosus*), for by not allowing the consumption of meat by those who are dying it endangers the life of its followers. The prohibition to consume meat appears for the first time in the Order's ancient statutes (*statuta antiqua*) of 1259. The new statutes (*nova statuta*) of 1368 repeat literally the prohibition of 1259, but add a long punitive clause against the transgressors.[128] The critics argue that Carthusians run the risk of eternal damnation, because they lack the virtue of Christian love (*caritas*). Arnau's response is conveyed at first in religious language, and if one were unaware of his medical background one could mistake him for a member of the Carthusian order defending his brothers. He labels the criticism as inherently false, profane, imaginary, and deceptive, and refers to it as heretical depravity (*heretica pravitas*).[129] The premise of Arnau's first argument is the notion that the product of supreme love cannot diminish love. The Carthusians in a general statute deny meat to all those subjected to the rule out of the love of God, and not because of hatred towards their neighbours. Any assertion that they oblige themselves to do it for reasons other than the love of God is rejected as illogical, ridiculous, and abusive.[130]

Arnau then proceeds to his assertion that the critics' notion is heretical and therefore profane. By holding such ideas they form a new doctrine (*novum dogma*), because they run against the Church's enthusiastic approval of the constitution of the Order. However, this approval is enshrined both in recent statutes and in more ancient ones. Therefore, he who rejects these statutes, consequently rejects the approval of the Roman Church, and must be her enemy.[131] This argument is weak, since the early statutes of the Order (including the constitution of Guigno) did not mention the prohibition, perhaps in order to shelter the young Order from attacks by critics. As late as the seventeenth century, members of

---

[127] Paniagua, 'Abstinencia', 327–30; Bazell, 'Christian Diet', 128–9.

[128] Bazell, 'Christian Diet', 121–6. On vegetarianism as a sign of heresy and heretical groups, see ibid. 144–65. On the statutes of the Carthusians, see *Annales Ordinis Cartusiensis*, i (Correira, 1687) [*PL* 153]. The *statuta antiqua* of 1259 are at p. 124.

[129] 'in se falsa . . . et profana and fantastica et mendosa'. *De esu carnium*, 193.

[130] Ibid. 193–4.   [131] Ibid. 194–6.

the Order had to cope with the accusation that the prohibition was a later addition and repeatedly expressed their conviction that this abstinence was inspired in St Bruno by God.

However, the attackers are creating a new doctrine also in another sense. Tacitly they claim that in denying meat to a dying monk, the Carthusians expose him to the danger of death. The critics who teach this are not only religiously heretical, but also medically wrong. Arnau analyses both types of error under the heading of heresy, again conferring on medicine the air of a religious system based on truths and dogma, which demands adherence to authorities. Then he reverts to a medical discourse which is the core of his treatise.[132] The medical question is about the kind of food that should be given to a dying person in order to try to revive his vital force or power of living (*virtus vitalis*). According to Arnau, if the person is starving then naturally meat could strengthen his body and his vital force. However, to strengthen the vital force (which is the only way to stop death), other food is equally effective—indeed, aromatic wine and soft egg-yolks are much better.[133] Moreover, meat and its juices have an excessive fat content and thus are useless, if not damaging, for purifying the blood. Therefore the medical effect of meat in the case of dwindling vital force is nil at best, and one should use the better alternatives. The falseness and fanciful nature of the critics' opinion is demonstrated by Hippocrates, the most illustrious prince of the physicians, and by Galen; and those who tacitly assert the opposite invent a novelty (*novitas*), which may be the result of maliciousness (*malitia*). They are like the Jews, who oppose the manifest truth owing to their hatred towards Christ. Again we witness here a digression to religious language; the Jews are portrayed according to the traditional stereotype, and Arnau's negative attitude towards novelty is reminiscent of religious discourse.[134]

Arnau digresses briefly to introduce an argument from moral theology which he attributes to Aristotle.[135] The opinion of those who are motivated by the desire (*concupiscentia*) for meat is as valid as the opinion of the gluttons and incontinent concerning temperance. They are compared to the stupid and incompetent physician who mechanically prescribes for his patients what he has found useful for himself. Then Arnau returns to his medical argument to fill in the logical gaps. Each of the three forces that affect the body—the vital, the animate, and the motive—represent a

---

[132] Ibid. 196–206.

[133] Arnau employs here the Hippocratic distinction between food and drugs discussed in *Speculum medicine*, c.xv–xix, fol. 6rb–8rb; Paniagua, 'Abstinencia', 336–7.

[134] *De esu carnium*, 201: 118.

[135] Ibid. 201–2.

different quality of the blood. This quality can be influenced by the appropriate food; for example, since the motive force is strengthened when the blood is dense and thick, fatty food should be given to the patient. As compared with wine and egg-yolk, meat is obviously more adequate and useful for strengthening weakened organs, since it renders the blood denser and more tenacious. But, as Galen says, the strengthening of the motive force of a person confined to bed is unnecessary; hence he does not need meat.[136] It is up to the skilled physician to distinguish between the three forces and to know how and when each of them should be strengthened. As for the critics of the Carthusians, it is obvious that they are ignorant of these differences, and Arnau ridicules them for this. Their opinion therefore is fantastic 'since the teaching of physicians who particularly possess the truth on this topic opposes it'.[137]

After having shattered the medical premise of the critics' argument, he goes on to neutralize its possible religious premise. Had meat been medically necessary, the Bible would have said so explicitly, as it does for herbs according to Romans 14: 2—'who is weak eateth herbs'—and for wine in Psalms 103: 15 [104: 15]—'And wine that maketh glad the heart of man'. Furthermore, nowhere in Scripture is meat mentioned in connection with healing powers. In I Samuel 30: 10–12 David offers bread and water to the dying Egyptian servant; and Jesus does not offer meat to those whose vital force is withering away, but bread and fish (Mark 8: 2). Arnau further argues that the advanced age of people in the early biblical period and the extended life-span of Carthusian monks, who, he claims, regularly reach the age of eighty and even a hundred while keeping their intellect and bodily powers intact, should be ascribed to their vegetarian diet. The treatise finishes with praise of the Carthusian Order and way of life, and calls upon those who do not wish to climb that mountain of joy and eternal pleasure to get on with their own lives and leave the role of judging others to him who sees everything.

Dianne Bazell has called Arnau's medical argument weak because he did not positively advocate abstinence *per se*, and merely demonstrated why consumption of meat is not necessary for the maintenance or restoration of health.[138] But Arnau did not advocate vegetarianism for

---

[136] *De esu carnium*, 205: 170; cf. Galen, *De methodo medendi*, in *Opera Omnia*, x. ed Kühn, 635–6, 839–40.

[137] 'cum sit eis contraria doctrina medicorum quibus convenit specialiter in hac materia veritatem'. *De esu carnium*, 206: 178.

[138] Bazell, 'Christian Diet', 185–6, and '*De esu carnium*: Arnald of Vilanova's Defence of Carthusian Abstinence', in *ATIEAV*, ii. 247; also in *ATCA* 14 (1995).

everyone, since there was no medical justification for doing so, and he himself prescribed meat as a remedy for his patients. By confining himself to demonstrating that meat is not necessary for the restoration of health, Arnau remained absolutely loyal to the medical theories which he propounded. In this respect, *De esu carnium* was written by a sympathizer of the Carthusian Order or perhaps by an opponent of the Dominicans, but it was first and foremost a medical treatise consistent with Arnau's practical medical works. This treatise joins other sources which suggest that the wisdom of the monastic orders was close to being a 'profane' and naturalistic discourse on man and to carefully measured needs already worked out in medieval medicine.[139]

Bazell's observation that in *De esu carnium* Arnau never made reference to the theoretical framework of humoral physiology (as was introduced by Isaac Israeli's *Liber dietarum universalium* and *Liber dietarum particularium*, transmitted by Peter of Spain together with their twelfth-century commentaries) can be explained within the broad question of the use of medical authorities in non-medical contexts. For *De esu carnium*, which sometimes appears in medical collections,[140] originally targeted a non-medical audience. It was included in MS Vat. lat. 3824, which assembled many of Arnau's spiritual writings written by 1305, and it was intended to provide a clerical audience (presumably made up of Carthusians and Dominicans) with arguments to be used in a religious debate. Under such circumstances an explicit reference to Isaac Israeli would seem problematic merely by virtue of his name. Moreover, when looking at the use of medical authorities by clerics in a religious context, one must conclude that Arnau conforms to the rhetorical norm which made Galen, Hippocrates, Constantinus Africanus, and Avicenna the conventional authorities to be cited in such a context. Thus in order to convince and impress a non-medical audience with a scientific medical argument, Arnau's citing of Galen and Hippocrates in *De esu carnium* was entirely adequate.

How was Arnau's medical argument received by the clerics who disputed the topic? That twenty-four manuscripts containing this text survive (at least three more manuscripts are now lost) proves its popularity, probably among Carthusians and those who sympathized with

---

[139] P. Camporesi, 'The "Stupendous Abstinence" ', in *The Anatomy of the Senses: Natural Symbols in Medieval and Early Modern Italy* (Cambridge, 1994), 64–92, esp. 79–92.

[140] See e.g. MS London, BL Harley 3665; from 1509 onwards it was printed in all the editions of his medical works.

their cause. Yet popularity was not the whole story. In *c.*1397 Jean de Gohenans (Gousanus), a nobleman who had joined the Carthusians twenty years earlier, addressed Pierre d'Ailly (1350–1420), then the Bishop of Cambrai, and asked for his refutation of the anti-Carthusian allegations according to which the Carthusian rule and especially its dietary code endangered the life of members of the Order. The sixth and last argument in Pierre d'Ailly's reply, known as 'In Favour of the Carthusians that they Reasonably Abstain from the Eating of Meat' (*Pro Cartusiensibus quod rationabiliter abstinent ab esu carnium*), cited Arnau's medical thesis in *De esu carnium*.[141] The unconvincing reply of Pierre induced his successor, Jean Gerson (1363–1429), in his capacity as Chancellor of the University of Paris, to use a public lecture on Mark 1: 6 (John the Baptist's abstinence) for formulating an alternative reply at the beginning of the academic year 1401/2.[142] The public exposition was edited in the form of a letter addressed to Jean de Gohenans and was sent in December 1401. Gerson cited Arnau's argument (which he may have learnt via Pierre d'Ailly's earlier reply) but expressed his reservations about it. For him, Arnau's medical argument did not completely eliminate the tension between the Carthusian rule and the duty to maintain life in extreme emergency (*in extrema necessitate*). For what should one do, he asks, when in a case of extreme physical necessity, the patient cannot consume wine and yolk because he immediately vomits them up? It seems that Gerson made a special effort to waive Arnau's argument—a strange move, because by doing so he renounced an important support for the Carthusian cause he was defending. At the end of his letter he cautions physicians not to endanger patients' souls by their therapeutic devices, and asks them to subject medicine to theology. In the context of the Carthusian debate he might be implying that many physicians are generally regarded as opponents of extreme abstinence, and that he is dissatisfied with their meddling in spiritual questions. If this is so (and it deserves more evidence, which I cannot provide) then Arnau's attitude was not common among physicians.[143]

---

[141] P. Tschackert, *Peter von Ailli* (Gotha, 1877), 266 and Appendix VII, 28.

[142] On the incident see P. Glorieux, 'Gerson et les Chartreux', *RTAM* 28 (1961), 117–20; C. Burger, *Aedificatio, Fructus, Utilitas: Johannes Gerson als Professor der Theologie und Kanzler der Universität Paris* (Tübingen, 1986), 167–73.

[143] Jean Gerson, *Oeuvres complètes*, iii. ed. P. Glorieux (Paris, 1972), 80. Cf. *Annales Ordinis Cartusiensis*, 125 (c.44 a.4 of the ancient statutes), where the seventeenth-century commentator ridicules the *opinio medici* on abstinence.

The Clerical Aspect: Speaking about Gluttony and its Cure, Abstinence

Arnau's medical contribution to the debate on Carthusian vegetarianism did not occur in a vacuum; clerics also employed medical reasoning when they spoke of abstinence. In general, medical theory and practice rejected extreme abstinence. Did the medical discourse on fasts influence the clerics at a time when religious writers were busy defining exactly who should fast and when, urging spiritual rather than physical abstinence, and stressing the need for moderation in observance?[144]

Lenten sermons often discussed the justification for fasting and incorporated medical arguments. Giordano da Pisa devotes a whole sermon in his *Quaresimale* to proving the benefit of fasting.[145] He maintains that Christ disproved the opinion of the Epicureans that fasting was a harmful act of self-inflicted damage, an opinion still upheld by physicians, who in opposing abstinence represent lust and carnality. According to him, physicians claim that fasting is medically harmful, and compare the digestion without food to a burning fire without wood, arguing that an empty stomach consumes its substance and its healthy and essential humours.[146] Giordano says that fasting may harm the health (using an *exemplum* about the relationship between the socks or shoes and the leg which they are supposed to defend, even though they are worn out by performing this duty), but it saves the soul, since eating and drinking cause various vices (lust in particular), harm the judgement, and dim the mind. The physical dryness caused by fasting and thought to be harmful by physicians is essential for a clear mind. Here he might have reinforced his point, but did not, by referring to a prominent physician like Bernard de Gordon, who recommended fasting and scourging against concupiscence.[147]

However, medical therapy rejected gluttony, and hence medicine was used to support the opposite argument. Thus the Franciscan Bertrand de la Tour argues that fasting is necessary 'for obtaining the cleanliness of heart and body' (*ad cordis et corporis mundiciam obtinendam*). The four

---

[144] C. Walker Bynum, *Holy Feast and Holy Fast: The Religious Significance of Food to Medieval Women* (Berkeley, 1987), 42.

[145] Giordano da Pisa, *Quaresimale*, 44 ff.

[146] 'E questo non veggono ancora i medici, com'egli è buono e santo, anzi 'l contradicono, dicendo che se nello stomaco non è il cibo, e 'l fuoco, pur essendovi, non avendo legne che arda, sì ·ssi converte agli omori dell'uomo e consuma de la substanzia sua, e diventano secchi e asciutti.' Ibid. 44–5: 17–25.

[147] Demaitre, *Doctor Bernard*, 26.

elements of which the human body is composed correspond to the forty adverse impulses (*illiciti motus*) which must be curbed, and therefore a forty-day fast is needed. The number forty is also connected to the forty-day period of the formation of the male foetus 'as say the philosophers' (*ut dicunt philosophi*).[148] Fasting is needed not only for the purification of the soul, for expelling guilt, for avoiding punishment, or for procuring grace, but also for the cleanliness of the body. Since fasting originates not only in spiritual but also in physical needs, it is not uncommon to find corporeal benefits among the reasons for the need to fast in Lent: he who fasts in Lent will not be ill after Easter.[149]

Ramon Llull offers another variation on this, connecting gluttony with lust because both inflame the flesh. The flame caused by fat is shared by the kidneys, which produce the sperm which is then driven to the genital organ to excite it. This is Llull's utterly medical explanation within a sermon which describes the biology of erection:

And indeed this flame is born from fatness which distributes it through the kidneys. From the kidneys the flame is distributed to the productive organs which are bodies and spirits and in which the sperm bubbles and boils. From the productive organs exit both dry and humid hot vapours and heat, which heat and enlarge the penis.[150]

Llull also employs his medical knowledge to scare his audience off gluttonous eating and insatiable drinking. He describes the brain damage caused by excessive eating and drinking and exposes his audience to a meticulous description of the structure of the brain. Excessive garlic and strong wine destroy that part of the brain situated above the forehead responsible for receiving the impressions of the imagination (*phantasia imaginabilium*). The same destruction takes place in the anterior parts of the brain, where understanding takes place (*impressiones intelligibiles*), and in the rear parts of the brain, where memory is situated. The heat and dryness of this food disturbs the cold and humid complexion of the

---

[148] Bertrand de la Tour, *Sermones quadragesimales epistolares* (Strasbourg, 1501/2), fol. I[r-v].

[149] Giordano da Pisa, *Quaresimale*, 8; Vicent Ferrer, *Sermons*, v, ed. G. Schib (Barcelona, 1984) 115–16/158.

[150] 'Que quidem flamma nascitur et derivatur a pinguedine, participante cum renibus; de quibus derivatur ad genitiva, que sunt corpora et spiritus, in quibus bullit vel fervet sperma, a quibus egrediuntur vapores et calores calidi et sicci et humidi, qui calefaciunt et augmentant virgam.' Ramon Llull, *Liber de virtutibus et peccatis sive Ars maior praedicationis*, in *Opera Latina*, 205, ed. F. D. Reboiras and A. Soria Flores (*CCCM* 76; Turnhout, 1986), 245: 22–7.

brain.[151] Thus medical knowledge could be and was recruited to support abstinence in two ways: as something to confront and discard in favour of true religious argument, or as something congruent with orthodox religious argument, which could hence support it.

The Franciscan Servasanto da Faenza (d. *c.*1300) from the Province of Bologna, a contemporary of Salimbene who had especially preached in Tuscany and Florence, was in the vanguard of the invasion of preaching by philosophical arguments which he delightfully integrated into his sermons,[152] and his discussion of abstinence and gluttony shows that he knew how to do the same with medical arguments. In his 'Book Concerning Natural Examples' (*Liber de exemplis naturalibus*)[153] he examined gluttony and its cure, abstinence, in terms of their medical effects. He seems to have believed that this would be the effective way to convince his audience, and he shows that Franciscans also employed secular knowledge in their sermons. Aristotle and Constantinus Africanus are his authorities for describing fat as the product of undigested blood which causes diminution in bodily blood and endangers life. Fatness, according to Constantinus, suffocates the natural heat of the body by reducing the blood in the body, blocks the channel of the spirits, and makes the body more vulnerable to disease.[154] This constitutes a warning to avoid obesity for medical reasons.

[151] 'Qui continue comedit multa allia et bibit uina fortia, corrumpit cedulam existentem super frontem in locis, ubi participant cerebra ante et retro. In qua quidem cedula fiunt impressiones phantasiarum imaginabilium. Et hoc idem de cedulis anterioribus, ubi fiunt impressiones intelligibiles. Et hoc idem in cedula que est retro, ubi fiunt impressiones recolibiles. Et propter hoc ob nimium calorem et siccitatem turbatur cerebrum quod est frigidum et humidum. Propter quam turbationem homo est stultus et facit stultitias, propter nimium comedere et bibere.' Ibid. 246: 76–84.

[152] On Servasanto, see J.-Th. Welter, *L'Exemplum dans la littérature religieuse et didactique du Moyen Âge* (Paris, 1927), 181–6; *DTC*, xiv. 1963–7; D. L. D'Avray, *The Preaching of the Friars: Sermons Diffused from Paris before 1300* (Oxford, 1985), 76–7, 155, 158, 160 and 'Philosophy in Preaching: The Case of a Franciscan Based in Thirteenth-Century Florence (Servasanto da Faenza)', in *Literature and Religion in the Later Middle Ages: Philological Studies in Honor of Siegfried Wenzel*, ed. R. G. Newhauser and J. A. Alford (Binghamton, NY, 1995), 263–73.

[153] M. Grabmann, 'Der *Liber de exemplis naturalibus* des Franziskanertheologen Servasanctus', *Franziskanische Studien*, 7 (1920), 85–117; L. Oliger, 'Servasanto da Faenza OFM e il suo *Liber de virtutibus et vitiis*, in *Miscellanea Francesco Ehrle—Scritti di storia e paleografia*, i. *Per la storia della teologia e della filosofia* (Studi e testi, 37; Rome, 1924), 148–89. I shall quote from MS London, BL Arundel 198, MSS Paris, BN lat. 2338, 3436, and 3642, and MS Paris, BN nouv. acq. lat. 259.

[154] 'Pinguedo enim ut Aristotelus et Constantinus dicunt ex sanguine indigesto in corporibus animalium generatur. . . . Et ideo quanto amplius pinguedo in corporibus augetur tanto in eiusdem sanguis minuitur. Quare in hominibus ualde crassis est ualde modicus sanguis et cum in sanguine sit maxime vite hominis est per consequens in talibus uita breuis.'

In 'Antidote of the Souls' (*Antidotarius animarum*)[155] Servasanto devotes a substantial part of the thirteenth tractate, entitled 'On Fasting' (*De ieiunio*) and divided into thirteen chapters, to the physical aspects of fasting. After having discussed fasting as an instrument for diminution of lust, he moves on to advocate moderate fasting as an important means of conserving and prolonging life. When done in a rational way, it expels superfluities from the body, eases the digestive process, renders the consequent distribution of digested food more efficient, and prevents any putrefaction from taking place. He also cites Seneca, Cicero, and various *exempla* in support of the link between austerity and longevity.

Servasanto then leaps into the spiritual field, defining fasting as the privilege of those wishing to correct their ways (*venie impetrativorum*), since opposing things are cured by their opposites (*contraria contrariis curantur*). He cites Ambrose that there is no sin, even the gravest, which will not be purged by abstinence or extinguished by alms. But within the spiritual discussion he also cites Galen, who allegedly proclaimed that 'abstinence is the mother of all medicines, since the root of all afflictions is excessive fullness', thus fusing together spiritual message and medical authority. Galen serves here in a double role. He is the source of a metaphor which links spiritual and physical medicine, and he also provides concrete evidence for a logical argument. On the basis of Galen, Servasanto concludes: 'Therefore, if you wish to be spiritually cured, it is necessary that you impose upon yourself a suitable diet.'[156]

In chapter 10, which deals with the necessity to maintain a temperate diet (and hence advocates moderate fasting), Servasanto cites Aristotle when he discusses the putrefying effects of undigested excess food in the body. On the other hand, shortage of food is also detrimental to health,

---

Unde dicit et addit philosophus libro XIII° animalium non est utile pinguedinem augmentare. Et Constantinus dicit pingua corpora et nimia adipe plena sunt pessima et morbis pessimis preparata eo quod calor naturalis cuius fomentum est sanguinis sepe in talibus suffocatur et uia spirituum pinguedine clauditur et ergo ad regimen corporis spiritus influencia denegatur. Et addit quod corpora omnia pinguia propter superfluam humorum habundantiam incurrunt sepe infirmitatem prolixam et tardissimam curam'. *Liber de exemplis naturalibus*, MS London, BL Arundel 198, fol. 81[r–v]. Cf. Servasanto da Faenza, *Liber aureus qui antidotarius animarum dictus est* (Leuven, *c.*1485), fol. 44[r–v] on the dangers of fatness; Aristotle, *De Part. Anim.* 651b, 1–17.

[155] B. Kruitwagen, 'Das Antidotarius animarum', in *Wiegendrucke und Handschriften: Festgabe Konrad Haebler* (Leipzig, 1919), 80–106.

[156] 'Nonne dietantur egroti ut corpore fiant sani? Sicut Galienus ait: Omnium medicinarum mater est abstinentia quia omnium morborum materia est repletio nimia. Ergo si tu spiritualiter curari desideras, necesse est ut tibi dietam congruam imponas.' Servasanto da Faenza, *Antidotarius animarum*, fol. 199[ra].

since it causes the natural heat to consume the radical humour, and exposes to death by hectic fever. All this happens because food, according to Constantinus, is a substance convertable into the substance of the body (*substantia convertibilis in substantiam corporis*), and even when it is absent, natural heat will continue its permanent consuming activity.[157] Servasanto employs Avicenna's discussion of the phases of digestion to explain how to maintain an equilibrium between the intaken food and its effective digestion. Avicenna calls chewing 'primary digestion'. Masticated food then enters the digestory site, where it is boiled and cooked, and the pure is separated from the impure, converted into liquid, and transported to the liver. Finally it is distributed through each and every organ of the body and assimilated into it. For proper and healthy digestion, food should be of uniform composition and mixing diverse types of food simultaneously should be avoided. Avicenna and the *opinio medicorum* support this when they warn that stomach-aches, flatulence, nausea, vomiting, suffocation of the natural heat, spasm and contraction of nerves, ulcers which become abscessed (*ulcera apostemata*), scab, tremor, paralysis, acceleration of old age, and death may result from the excess intake of food. Conversely, lack of food debilitates nature and dims every sense. It may generate baldness and putrid fevers, it may weaken and desiccate the body and, in general, it may cause worse *passiones* than excess of food.

Servasanto devotes part of his discussion to the practical rules of fasting. Old people will always fast more easily than young ones since, according to Hippocrates, the young need to take in more food in order to balance and restore their bodily substance lost due to excessive innate heat. This also explains why less food is needed by those who are resting than by those who are physically active. Different metabolisms characterize choleric and phlegmatic people (according to Avicenna), and since metabolism is subjected to seasonal changes (according to Hippocrates), seasons specifically affect different people's abilities to cope with fasting.[158]

---

[157] 'Cibus enim si fuerit nimius dum ab insito calore non coquitur nec perfecte digeritur putrescit in stomacho et magnorum fit causa morborum. . . . Sed si fuerit nimis paucus mox a calore consumitur sic calor dum in quo agat non invenit humidum radicale consumit in quo tota vita consistit et ideo ad ethicam mortem disponit. Nam cibus ut Constantinus ait est substantia convertibilis in substantiam corporis qua deperdita restauratur calor naturalis instar ignis continue agit semperque aliquod continuatione consumit.' Ibid. fol. 200ra.

[158] Ibid. fol. 200^{r–v}; see also fol. 151^{r} and MS Paris, BN, lat. 2338, fol. 55vb–56^{v}, where Servasanto adduces medical justification for fasting, since it preserves and even prolongs life.

What is the point of all this meticulous discussion of food and digestion, which relies so heavily on medical knowledge and attempts to stick
to known medical authorities? Fundamental is the belief that it is
metaphorically useful for the physician of the soul when he attempts to
convey spiritual messages. Preachers thus felt impelled to dip into the
pool of medical knowledge which they shared with physicians of the
body. According to their belief, penance should be adapted to the spiritual complexion of the believer as diet should fit the physical complexion
of the person. It is thus perfectly acceptable to discuss a moral practice
which has religious implications and motivations from a natural viewpoint. In the opening sentence of his discussion of the virtue of temperance, Servasanto declares that 'the virtue of temperance is not only pleas-
ing to God but is also very much nature's ally for the salvation of man'.
Consequently he bases his discussion on natural reasoning.[159] It is nature
which provides the body with humid matter to compensate for the matter consumed by the incessant burning of natural heat, and moderate diet
is therefore needed to temper natural heat. Servasanto presents various
examples of nature's temperance which should be imitated by man: in
addition to astronomical and mineralogical examples he also employs
anatomical analogies.[160]

Yet Servasanto seems to have used medical knowledge also for practical purposes. At the end of the medical part of the treatise on fasting, he
says that the priest should take medical knowledge into account when he
imposes fasting on the penitent, for he should know that when all other
variables are equal, fasting furthers spiritual satisfaction among the
young more than among the old.[161] In the chapter entitled *De continencia
secundum gustum* Servasanto also relies on Hippocrates for the contention
that fat bodies in those who have terminated their growing phase might
incur paralysis and even graver afflictions unless their excessive matter is
quickly eliminated. Galen is subsequently his authority for saying that
those who suffer from superfluous blood will not live long and their souls

---

[159] 'temperantie uirtus non solum est deo grata sed nature multum amica saluti hominis.' *Liber de exemplis naturalibus*, MS Paris, BN lat. 3436, fol. 145[r].

[160] For example, ibid. MS Paris, BN lat. 3436, fol. 145[r]–146[v]: 'Item secundum medicorum doctrinam sanguis enim aliis humoribus mixtus est eorum maliciarum frenatiuus et
uoluntati temperatiuus.'

[161] 'Et nota quod omnia iam supradicta debet medicus animarum attendere dum imponit
penitentibus ieiunare ut sciat cui magis cui minus etiam sit ieiunia ferre quia ceteris paribus,
plus satisfacit iuuenis ieiunando quam senex quia sibi est difficilius eo quod assumentem
calorem fortiorem patiatur interius.' *Antidotarius animarum*, fol. 200[vb].

will not be healthy, since, as if burdened by excessive fat, their minds are prevented from contemplating celestial things. Such people are doomed to carnality and gluttony.[162]

There were twelfth-century thinkers who employed medical knowledge to back an ethical or moral argument. Thus Alain de Lille defined fasting as 'medicine to soul and body. It preserves the body from disease, the soul from sin. About its medicinal effects earthly and heavenly philosophy agree.'[163] Yet Alain does not cite the medical authorities as Servasanto does, and his discussion is significantly less detailed. As for Servasanto, medical examples are not the only or even the main source for his natural analogies.[164] The world of animals, mineralogy, and even history frequently provide him with vivid images; and the use of medical reasoning should be seen as part of this growing openness to nature and natural philosophy.

The above examples hint at a growing tendency to stress utility when speaking of abstinence: one should fast in Lent, for example, because it is physically and not only spiritually healthy. It is thus possible to suggest that the period around 1300 was an embryonic stage in a process which would ultimately lead to medicine replacing religion as a social guardian of morality.[165] At this early stage, medical subject-matter receives a growing role as an instrument to convince the believers that the ecclesiastical control over their bodies rests on a scientific foundation.

---

[162] *Liber de exemplis naturalibus*, MS Paris, BN lat. 3436, fol. 155[r].

[163] Alain de Lille, *Summa de arte predicatoria*, c.34 ('De jejunio'), in *PL* 210, 178A. Jerome in *Adversus Iovinianum*, *PL* 23, 300–1 refers to the Hippocratic Aphorisms as the source for the notion that an excessively fat body may cause paralysis and other grave illnesses unless one quickly lost the excess weight. In this context he also refers to *Exhortatio medicine* of Galen, who allegedly claimed that the relatively short life of wrestlers or athletes in general was the result of their fat-rich diet. H. Musurillo, 'The Problem of Ascetical Fasting in the Greek Patristic Writers', *Traditio*, 12 (1956), 17 (for Ps.-Athanasius's medical reasons for fasting); Bynum, *Holy Feast and Holy Fast*, 36–7.

[164] In MS Paris, BN lat. 3436, fol. 122[r] Servasanto cites Galen as the source for the description of the harmonious relationship between the arms and the heart. He extends the love between the organs of the physical body to *caritas* between the organs of the spiritual body. On conjugal continence, see Ch. 5, n. 159 below. See MS Paris, BN nouv. acq. lat. 259, fol. 2[rb], 106[va–b], where the discussion of the peace and unity amongst Christ's organs involves allusion to the relation between the heart and the bodily organs which received from him motion and life and served him in return.

[165] B. S. Turner, *The Body and Society: Explorations in Social Theory* (Oxford, 1984), 163–5, and 'The Discourse of Diet', in *The Body: Social Process and Cultural Theory*, ed. M. Featherstone, M. Hepsworth, and B. S. Turner (London, 1991), 157–69.

The Clerical Aspect: On the Use of Medical Authorities
by Scholastic Theologians

Servasanto enthusiastically introduced medical authorities into his preaching manuals. Yet a different approach to the use of medical texts in religious context and by clerics was possible. Ramon Martí (d. 1285) in the first chapter of *Pugio fidei* castigated the *naturales* (all those who rely on the evidence of the senses) as the second of three schools of error. The leader of this group which disregards God and morals is Galen. His denial of the immortality of the soul makes him the 'prince of the great crowd' of naturalists and physicians whose pernicious doctrine Ramon Martí boasts he has strangled. For Ramon Martí, the prominence of Galen in Islamic disputes attested his importance as an adversary to be addressed by a Christian apologist.[166]

An 'anti-Galen mood', which reduced Galen almost to silence in the extended disputes about the human soul, is one of the reasons for his exclusion from Thomas's writings. Galen's notion of the soul as complexion was incompatible with Aquinas's notion of the soul's immortality and its definition as a substantial form. It has been asserted that Aquinas knew very little medicine beyond what he had learned from Albertus or picked up from Aristotle and his commentators.[167] Mark Jordan describes Albertus and Roger Bacon, who retained Galen as an interlocutor, as exceptions to most contemporary theologians, who excluded medical authorities owing to ignorance, belief in the superiority of philosophy over medicine, or their desire to reduce the range of permissible authorities. The exclusion of Galen was reinforced by the overwhelming popularity of Avicenna's *Liber canonis*, which many perceived to be a much simpler and clearer text, by the growing distance between faculties of medicine and theology, and by the assimilation of Aristotelianism, which caused a reorganization of the hierarchy of scientific discourse. The lack of a medical treatise among Aristotle's *libri naturales* was a major reason for medicine's exclusion from fundamental natural philosophy and hence from philosophical and theological discourse.

However, the use of medical knowledge by academic theologians of

---

[166] Ramon Martí, *Pugio fidei adversus Mauros et Judaeos* (Leipzig, 1687), 1.1.7 (pp. 192–4 at 194) and 1.4.10 (p. 206). For anti-Galen attitudes see Thomas Aquinas, *Summa contra gentiles*, ii. 63, which rejects the idea of the soul as complexion. William of Auvergne, *De anima* 1.1 in *Opera omnia*, Suppl. (Paris, 1674), 2, 66a.

[167] M. D. Jordan, 'The Disappearance of Galen in Thirteenth-Century Philosophy and Theology', in *Mensch und Natur im Mittelalter*, ed. A. Zimmermann and A. Speer (Miscellanea Mediaevalia 21/2; Berlin and New York, 1992), 703–13, and 'Medicine and Natural Philosophy in Aquinas', in *Thomas von Aquin—Werk und Wirkung im Licht neuerer Forschungen*, ed. A. Zimmermann (Miscellanea Mediaevalia, 19; Berlin, 1988), 233–46; E. Paschetto, 'La natura del moto in base al *De moto cordis* di S. Tommaso', ibid. 247–60.

the late thirteenth and fourteenth centuries deserves further study. How typical was Aquinas's approach towards Galen? Did he extend his 'anti-Galen mood' to other medical authorities? In the above-mentioned example Ramon Martí denounced Galen in a very specific context—the question of the immortality of the soul. The friar explicitly limits his critique to this particular question when he says, 'Many physicians or medical practitioners who find Galen the most skilled in medicine, disregard the fact that he was ignorant on *this* issue.'[168] Does that mean that in other fields which are relevant to theology it is permitted to rely on Galen and other medical authorities? Servasanto's example and the other preachers discussed in Chapter 4 suggest that some clerics did not exclude medical authorities, even Galen, from their religious arguments.

We know that humoral theory and theories of generation and embryology were three fields which were extensively used by theologians as sources of arguments and analogies in a variety of scholastic debates. Medical knowledge in general and knowledge about the radical humour in particular was essential when discussing generation, the transmission of original sin, the ageing process, prolongation of life, death, resurrection, and immortality.[169] For example, is a child killed in his mother's womb by some persecutor of the Church automatically baptized by the baptism of blood (*baptismum sanguinis*) and thus purged of original sin? This is one of over fifty questions sent to Ramon Llull from Arras by the canon, Master of Arts, and Doctor of Medicine Thomas le Myésier, designed to try out the practical applicability of Llull's Art.[170] Llull replied in a short work of July 1299. The answer to this particular

---

[168] 'Multi quippe physici seu medici invenientes illum in medica peritissimum, ignorant ipsum fuisse in hac parte imperitum.' *Pugio fidei*, 1.4.10, 206.

[169] See e.g. the *questiones disputate* concerning the transformation of human nature from Adam, presided over by the eighteenth regent master of the Oxford Franciscans, Nicholas of Ockham, in 1287/8. Nicholas de Ockham, *Quaestiones disputatae de traductione humanae naturae a primo parente*, ed. C. Saco-Alarcón (Rome, 1993).

[170] Thomas le Myésier, *Questiones dubitabiles super quattuor libris sententiarum cum questionibus solutiuis magistri Thome Attrabatensis* (Lyons, 1491). On Myésier, see J. N. Hillgarth, *Ramon Lull and Lullism in Fourteenth-Century France* (Oxford, 1971), 150 ff. and esp. 158–64; E. Wickersheimer, *Dictionnaire biographique des médecins en France au Moyen Âge* (Geneva, 1936), 763. Extensive biomedical knowledge was needed for answering *Questio* 52: *Queritur utrum aliquid extrinsecum transeat in veritatem humane nature per actum generative; Q.*53: *Utrum aliquid extrinsecum transeat in veritatem humane nature per actum nutritive* (both in ii); *Q.*34 (ii), which deals with the corruptibility of bodies of those summoned to heaven by angels and the biological mechanism of putrefaction; among the short questions at the end of the book, *Q.*26 about the aging process; *Q.*27 about the possibility to prolong human life artificially; *Q.*29 and 35, concerning the relationship between the seminal humour and the *substantia* of the foetus; *Q.*36, on the necessity that the woman emit sperm in generation.

question necessitated a detailed analysis of the sharing by mother and embryo of the nutritive humour which passes via the umbilical cord. The will of the mother compensates for its absence in the unborn child, who is purged because of the biological bond between the two (*ratione copule*).[171] In another question Thomas le Myésier is interested to know whether Adam and Eve could have had sexual intercourse before they had eaten anything. This question was pertinent, since medical theory regarded semen as the most subtle form of digested food. Llull's affirmative answer was based on the belief that the perfect nature with which they were furnished also included the desire to generate offspring (*appetitus ad generandum*) without the need of food. This in turn demanded an explanation of how it was possible to combine generation and lack of corruption.[172]

Biblical stories also raised questions which demanded from preachers and commentators some medical knowledge for their solution. Thus Ramon Llull describes the effect of the vinegar which Jesus tasted prior to his death (John 19: 30) as allegorically signifying a change of his complexion to melancholic—the complexion of death, since it is cold and dry.[173] And Giordano da Pisa describes in one of three sermons dedicated to Luke 1: 28 ('Hail art thou that art highly favoured') Mary's miraculous conception without a seed (*sine semine*), and introduces scientific terms (natural philosophical rather than purely medical) to his audience. In order to stress the miraculous character of the conception and the fact that nature is too weak to cause such an event, he describes the natural way of conception and uses concepts like passive and active matter, elemental theory, and humoral system. Examples of plants (palms) and animals are employed to prove that male presence and contribution of active matter is necessary for any kind of conception. Out of the 84 lines of the sermon, 67 are dedicated to the scientific discussion of natural conception, and they culminate in the conclusion that the Holy Spirit played the role of the father as an active agent (*fattore*). The Galenic theory of conception seems to have provided a useful foundation for a slightly more elaborate explanation of Mary's conception. For Giordano does not ask

---

[171] Wickersheimer, *Dictionnaire biographique des médecins en France au Moyen Âge* iv. *Q*.2.

[172] Ibid. ii, *Q*.44.

[173] 'Acetum habet quattuor proprietates, scilicet circulationem, amaritudinem, penetrationem et fortitudinem. . . . et quando est vinum in acetum alteratum, tunc acetum est frigidum et siccum. Iesus autem gustavit acetum; et acetum suam complexionem mutavit, illam in melancholiam transmutando. Que quidem est de complexione mortis; que quidem est sicca et frigida, allegorice loquendo.' Ramon Llull, *Liber de praedicatione*, in *Raimundi Lulli Opera Latina*, 118, ed. F. Stegmüller (Palma de Mallorca, 1961–3), 239.

his audience simply to believe in the miraculous conception: he also tries to make them understand it by anchoring it to the natural world. Thus, seed was involved in the Virgin's conception—namely, her own. As the factor responsible for the formation of the body of Christ it was the purest of its kind, since it originated in her blood which is the purest and most essential of all humours in any living creature.[174]

How did more learned biblical commentators cope with similar questions? Some commentaries also served as vehicles for transmitting medical knowledge which was usually popular in character. Thus Psalms 37: 8 [38: 7] ('For my loins are filled with a loathsome disease and there is no soundness in my flesh') allows the exegetes to discuss the loins as the seat of carnality and lust because the kidneys, the source of sexual appetite, are fixed in them. And 1 Timothy 5: 23 ('Drink no longer water but use a little wine for thy stomach's sake and thine often infirmities') enables Nicholas of Lyra to add to the commentary that excessive drinking of water is detrimental to the body whilst modest quantities of wine do not contradict the precept of chastity and are useful for health. Earlier, Ambrose is cited to the effect that the verse's purpose was to avoid the need to look for the opinion and advice of physicians.[175]

Albertus Magnus, whose extensive medical knowledge may have been gleaned through private reading, provides us with more examples of the use of medical knowledge when glossing the Bible, as in the following selection. When he refers to paralysis in his commentary on '[M]y servant lieth at home sick of the palsey' (Matthew 8: 6), he gives a long scientific description of the paralytic humour which attacks the nerves, and justifies his exposition by the need to clarify the severity of the disease and thus the magnitude of divine power in curing it.[176] His discussion of fever in the commentary on '[H]e saw his wife's mother laid and sick of a fever' (Matthew 8: 14) clearly relies on Avicenna's definition of the condition, and portrays Albertus's Aristotelian approach to the role of the heart as the principal organ.[177] Similarly in his commentary on '[A] woman which was diseased with an issue of blood twelve years' (Matthew

[174] 'Il sangue è il più puro omore e 'l più generale e necessario: collera è sangue troppo cotto; flemma è sangue mal cotto; meninconia è feccia de sangue. Il sangue non ha questi difetti, del quale si fanno l'ossa e le membra e le nerbora e la carne'. Giordano da Pisa, *Quaresimale*, 355–7 at 357: 61–5.

[175] *Glossa Ordinaria* on Ps. 37: 8, in *Biblia sacra, cum glossa ordinaria*, iii. 693–5; *Glossa Ordinaria* on 1 Tim. 5: 23.

[176] Albertus Magnus, *Super Matth.*, in *Opera Omnia* XXI/1, ed. B. Schmidt (Münster, 1987), 279: 2–20.

[177] Ibid. 285: 40–5; cf. Avicenna, *Liber canonis*, iv. fen 1 tr.1 c.1.

9: 20), he elaborates on the woman's haemorrhage in order to stress the gravity of her condition. His explanation includes an explicit reference to Galen's commentary on the Hippocratic aphorisms, and shows his effort to provide a scientific explanation.[178]

Albertus's scientific interpretation of medical phenomena in Scripture leads him to a quasi-natural explanation of the effect of demons on the human soul. In so doing he follows Avicenna's approach to the ancient problem of whether melancholy could come from evil demons. Stressing that he teaches medicine (*physica*), not metaphysics, sceptical Avicenna leaves the question unanswered; but he determines that if a demon causes melancholy disease it does so by affecting an imbalanced complexion which is the immediate cause (*causa propinqua*) of the disease.[179] In his commentary to '[T]hey brought unto him many that were possessed with devils: and he cast out the spirits with his word and healed all that were sick' (Matthew 8: 16), Albertus explains that the demon affects the human body through the humours in a natural way. Unnatural humour diffused throughout the organ impedes its operation. Sometimes the humour's quality or its material cause the impediment, as Galen asserts, and, in a similar way, the demon hinders bodily operations through the operations of the humours or their qualities.[180]

In his commentary on Matthew 4: 12, Albertus explains the rational order in which the sacraments are presented in the Gospel (in Matthew the Eucharist appears only in chapter 26) through a medical example. No medical treatment is effective unless it is connected to the natural heat of the body: the same principle applies to the sacraments of Christ and the Church, none of which will be effective unless it is connected to the soul through confession and devotion.[181] Thus, to Siraisi's list of three contexts in which Albertus uses his medical knowledge, a fourth should be added: biblical exegesis.[182] Though Albertus, with his outstanding intellectual

---

[178] Albertus Magnus, *Super Matth.*, in *Opera Omnia* XXI/1, 311: 65–73; cf. Galen, *Hippocratis Aphorismi et Galeni in eos commentarii*, in *Opera omnia*, xviii/1. ed. Kühn, 43–4, no. 29.

[179] Avicenna, *Liber canonis*, iii. iv. fen 1, 1.1.

[180] 'Sed sicut nos videmus, quod humor innaturalis diffusus in membro impedit operationem membri, et aliquando facit hoc qualitas sive materia humoris, sicut dicit Galenus, ita facit daemon per operationes humorum vel qualitatum quarum novit semina in corpore, impediens corporis operationes, applicitus membris et inviscans ea talibus seminibus.' Albertus Magnus, *Super Matth.* 8: 6, in *Opera Omnia* XXI/1, 288: 40–7.

[181] Ibid. 4: 12; ibid. 93: 10–15.

[182] On his medical knowledge, see N. G. Siraisi, 'The Medical Learning of Albertus Magnus', in *Albertus Magnus and the Sciences*, ed. J. A. Weisheipl (Toronto, 1980), 379–404: Albert the Great, *Man and the Beasts—'De animalibus'*, 25–37.

capacity and scope, should not be regarded as typical, he proves that the study of the Bible could profit from medical knowledge.

These are just a few examples of another contact between religion and medicine which enhanced the symbiotic relationship between the two. They highlight the need for a systematic study of the topic in order to find out whether, in that period, as it seems from the examples cited above, medical knowledge indeed played an important auxiliary role in religious discourse,[183] in corroborating orthodoxy and also, sometimes, as an argument to be refuted if orthodoxy was to be preserved. In Chapter 4 I shall attempt to substantiate this hypothesis by discussing the use of medicine amongst preachers who use a more popular level of religious language.

[183] See e.g. P. Biller, 'Views of Jews from Paris around 1300; Christian or Scientific', in *Christianity and Judaism*, ed. D. Wood (Studies in Church History, 29; Oxford, 1992), 187–207, which shows the infiltration of medical scientific terms (mainly the concept of a melancholic complexion) into the discussion about the Jews in the literature of the 'quodlibets', and 'Introduction: John of Naples, Quodlibets and Medieval Theological Concern with the Body', in P. Biller and A. J. Minnis (ed.), *Medieval Theology and the Natural Body* (York, 1997), 3–12.

4

Medicine for the Preachers

Introduction

Thus far I have concentrated on the writings of physicians. Occasionally, I have juxtaposed Arnau's language and that of clerics who employed medical language and knowledge in their religious discourse.[1] It is now time to examine more systematically the use of medical matters by those outside the medical profession, and to assess the second control for Arnau. Because I have already presented much of the relevant evidence, this section will be mainly interpretative, and is necessary in order to contextualize Arnau and Galvano and to find out how, if at all, their mode of employing medical language and subject matter differs from that of clerics active in the same period.

My decision to concentrate on preachers' manuals for the purpose of comparison needs justification. It might seem more suitable to compare Arnau and Galvano with their academic peers in the faculties of theology—a path which offers interesting results. However, since neither Arnau nor Galvano was involved in high-level theological debate, since their spiritual writings were not produced in the university context, and since both lived as laymen who had no solid theological training, I preferred to start my inquiry with preachers' texts which reflect similar characteristics. Moreover, since I am attempting to describe the broad linguistic context in which the two physicians acted, preachers' texts provide a better starting-point than theological writings, because they were not limited to the closed scholastic environment and thus reflect more widespread modes of expression.

I largely devote my discussion to three religious authors: the Dominican Giovanni da San Gimignano (d. *c.*1332), the Franciscan Servasanto da Faenza (d. *c.*1300), and the Benedictine Pierre Bersuire (d. 1362), who produced texts[2] which belong to the same literary genre of

---

[1] See the discussion of generation, the use of organic similes, and the language of disease in Ch. 2, and that of abstinence in Ch. 3.

[2] Giovanni's *Sde*, Servasanto's *Liber de exemplis naturalibus* and *Antidotarius animarum* (Leuven, *ca.* 1485), and Bersuire's *Reductorium morale* (Venice, 1583).

moralized *exempla*. These are encyclopaedic texts, compiled towards the end of the thirteenth and the first half of the fourteenth centuries as preachers' manuals to help those who were composing sermons for the laity in predominantly urban settings. Their clerical authors received university training in the last decades of the thirteenth and the beginning of the fourteenth centuries. The essential question which I confront in studying these texts is that of what their authors did in practice communicate to the audience they intended to address. How, if at all, is the link between medicine and religion expressed in such texts? Is it a matter of shared contents, or of common analytical language? And, if either, what does it mean for the status of medicine and of the learned physician in that period? How can we interpret the dissemination of medical subject-matter and medical language into non-medical religious discourse? In Chapter 3 I argued that, despite rumblings of opposition, many clerics did not exclude medical authorities, even Galen, from their religious arguments. In what follows, I will substantiate this hypothesis and argue that in the late thirteenth and fourteenth centuries technical medical material was incorporated into religious discourse at various levels, and that this phenomenon served to make medicine a significant cultural agent.

Since this chapter is mainly about the use of language, some preliminary definition of terms is necessary. In what follows I shall mainly speak of similes (in their medieval usage of *similitudo*—similarity or likeness) which are tropes of comparison and are identifiable within speech through the presence of a 'like' or an 'as' or an occasional 'not like' (in the medieval context introduced by the verb *assimilare* and the conjunction *sicut*). This was one of the more popular tropes used by clerics throughout the middle ages to render abstract messages intelligible.

In the fourteenth-century context, the following distinction, attributed to Isidore of Seville, was reproduced in various preachers' manuals: 'The difference between *exemplum* and *similitudo* is that *exemplum* is a narrative (*historia*) whilst *similitudo* is demonstrated by the thing itself (*re adprobatur*).'[3] As a preaching instrument *similitudo* had an explanatory

---

[3] C. Brémond, J. Le Goff, and J.-C. Schmitt, *L'"Exemplum"* (Typologie des sources de Moyen Âge occidental, 40; Turnhout, 1982), 31, 154–8. On the foundations of early medieval theories of metaphor and figurative language, see M. Irvine, *The Making of Textual Culture: Grammatical and Literary Theory, 350–1100* (Cambridge, 1994), 104–7, 182–6, 225–34. For the late medieval context and a general classification of metaphors used in medieval preaching literature see J. Huizinga, *The Waning of the Middle Ages* (London, 1955), 192–221; H. Martin, *Le Métier de prédicateur à la fin du Moyen Âge 1350–1520* (Paris, 1988), 427–84.

role, and it was usually introduced in the sermon by an *auctoritas* (often a biblical citation which conveyed the theme of the sermon). Similes show us what the preachers knew about the particular signifying object, what they saw fit to transfer to their audience, and the manner in which this communication was undertaken. I shall demonstrate this with examples from Giovanni, Servasanto, and Bersuire, who compiled their manuals in a period characterized by a passion for similitudes and comparisons of all kinds.[4]

Figurative modes of expression envelop the discourse to make spiritual reality accessible. These constructions are flexible instruments that can always be revised; they can be simply an ornamental substitute for a literal expression; they can be aids to persuasion, attention-catching, or memory- enhancing. They can be agents for the supply of knowledge and ideas which are not necessarily directly connected to the subject under discussion. In a theological context, they introduce an element of realism to the speaker's words by linking God causally to the world.

It is accepted that the theological realist who uses figurative language of any kind does not want to claim privileged knowledge. However, what happens when a theologizing physician employs medical analogies, similes, or metaphors in a religious context? Will the speaker and the audience assign more weight, or at least a different kind of meaning, to his words because he is a physician? One can only speculate about the reaction of the audience in the middle ages and tentatively propose that the audience would indeed take the message more seriously when uttered by the expert, or if it were at least based on scientific authority.

There are two points fundamental to the underlying assumption of this chapter. First, since one of the aims of figurative language is to revitalize religious language or to render it relevant to the audience, it also may provide us with further insight into the 'people's mind'. Hence, approached judiciously, it is a particularly direct pointer to the deeper layers of belief of the speaker and his audience. Secondly, the use of figurative language, however banal it may seem, reflects the experience of the user and the intellectual environment in which he functioned. Metaphors and similes are not merely a device of the poetic imagination and the rhetorical flourish: they also structure what we perceive and play a central role in defining our everyday realities. Moreover, they reflect everyday collective experience and are grounded in physical and cultural

---

[4] D. L. D'Avray, *The Preaching of the Friars: Sermons Diffused from Paris before 1300* (Oxford, 1985), 9.

reality. Thus a full understanding of the codified information which lies hidden within the language of any speaker is important for a better understanding of his motivation and the intellectual world to which he belongs.

Let us look at the construct 'Christ is the True Physician' which appears so often in religious language throughout the middle ages.[5] Both principal (Christ) and subsidiary (physician) subjects bring with them their own associations. The speaker and the listener have a body of shared knowledge or assumptions about them. The efficacy of the metaphor does not depend on the accuracy of these associations, but simply on the fact that both speaker and listener make them. An intercourse of thoughts is created; the two associations interact in such a way as to produce a new unit of meaning. This unit of meaning causes the principal subject to be affected by the meaning of the subsidiary subject and vice versa.[6] Huizinga tells us that Dionysius the Carthusian (1402–71) reminded the people in vain that it was but for the sake of comparison that he called sin a fever or a cold and corrupted humour.[7] It is plausible to assume that the imagination of a late-thirteenth- and early-fourteenth-century individual functioned in a similar mode and that the 'material conception'[8] of religious and moral categories fused together the sign and the signified object. Thus, extensive use of metaphoric language tying Christ, priests, and spiritual well-being to physicians, medicine, and physical health was likely to mark physicians with some kind of spiritual aura.

An isolated analysis of individual tropes would therefore be misleading, since it would diminish the broader picture. When single banal metaphors are put together, they may create a more elaborate structure and hence may acquire another layer of meaning. The texts of Giovanni, Servasanto, and Bersuire provide a good starting-point for a thorough study of the medical language employed in religious discourse. As we shall see, they put into practice a rhetorical principle which Ramon Llull propagated in the same period, that medicine can be applied in religious

[5] Here I borrow terms from Max Black's interactive theory as summarized in J. M. Soskice, *Metaphor and Religious Language* (Oxford, 1985), 38 ff. Though she rejects his theory at least in part, I have still found some of his terms useful for my discussion.

[6] Soskice, when discussing the construction 'man is a wolf', cites Black saying, 'If to call a man a wolf is to put him in a special light, we must not forget that metaphor makes the wolf seem more human than he otherwise would.' Ibid. 41.

[7] Huizinga, *The Waning of the Middle Ages*, 221.

[8] Ibid. That is, understanding abstract ideas through images of tangible, concrete objects or phenomena.

discourse. In the epilogue to his *Ars abbreviata praedicandi*, Ramon Llull says of this preaching guide: 'It is a book to which law, natural philosophy, medicine and the liberal and mechanical arts could be applied.'[9] He advocates preaching in a knowledgeable way (*scire predicare scientifice*) and giving diverse examples which can include profane wisdom.[10] In this respect it is important to note that medicine does not hold a unique position, for Llull mentions law, physical sciences, and liberal and mechanical arts as branches of knowledge which can also be applied in preaching, although these are not disciplines which concern us here.

The Evidence

A detailed summary of the medical information in Giovanni's *Sde* and Bersuire's *Reductorium morale* is in Appendices I and II.[11] In what follows I offer a synthesis of this information. I have divided the evidence into five categories: the medical model, the vocabulary of disease, the anatomy of the Christian faith, the anatomy of the Christian body, and the anatomy of the mind and the intellect.

Similes which portray the relationship between God and his ministers and the believer in terms of the relationship between a physician and his patient[12] form the medical model, on which all the other four categories depend. As a dominant metaphor with staying power it offers a general framework for describing and explaining abstract notions. This 'conceptual metaphor' organizes a system of metaphors and other tropes which are all derived from it.[13] According to this model, Christ, priests, confessors, and preachers appear as physicians, the sinners appear as patients,

---

[9] 'Est autem liber, cui leges, physica et medicina et liberales artes et mechanice poterunt applicari.' Ramon Llull, *Ars abreviata praedicandi*, in *Opera Latina*, 208, ed. A. Soria Flores, F. D. Reboiras, and M. Senellart (*CCCM* 80; Turnhout, 1991), 155: 808–9.

[10] Ibid. 157.

[11] The original text of *Sde* is alphabetically arranged according to the signified topics; it starts with *Acedia* and ends with *Unitas membrorum*. In App. I, I have chosen to introduce the data according to the signifiers in order to stress the medical dimension of the text. Appendix II maintains the original order of appearance of the medical topics in Bersuire's *Reductorium*. It starts with medical theory, continues with anatomy from head to heel, and concludes with pathologies.

[12] On the desirable physician–patient relationship from the medical viewpoint around 1300, see L. García-Ballester, 'Medical Ethics in Transition in the Latin Medicine of the Thirteenth and Fourteenth Centuries: New Perspectives on the Physician–Patient Relationship and the Doctor's Fee', in A. Wear, J. Geyer-Kordesch and R. French (ed.), *Doctors and Ethics: The Earlier Historical Setting of Professional Ethics* (Amsterdam, 1994), 38–71.

[13] G. Lakoff and M. Johnson, *Metaphors We Live By* (Chicago and London, 1980), 3–9.

the soul is represented by the body, and every stage in the curing process, from diagnosis through prognosis to therapy, represents a stage in the process of spiritual cure. At its basis is the belief in the existence of a perfect analytical similarity between body and soul. This similarity allows and even invites the use of medical language when speaking of the healing of souls. It is explained by the two concepts of outward man (*homo exterior*) and inward man (*homo interior*) which tie in with 2 Corinthians 4: 16 ('though our outward man perish, yet the inward man is renewed day by day'). The body, which is the exterior dimension of the human being, is by definition corruptible; the soul, which is the interior dimension of the human being, is renewable. Yet this dichotomy between decay (*corruptio*) and renewal (*renovatio*) permits complex ties between body and soul. The relationship can be of enmity; Giovanni does not ignore the view of the human body as a dangerous enemy (*periculosus hostis*), a pernicious plague (*perniciosus pestis*), and a penal prison (*carcer poenalis*)[14] to the soul. Yet in his sixth book, he dwells on an alternative relational model—partnership, comradeship, and shared existence epitomized in the concept of companion (*comes*) and partner (*consors*). The soul needs the body as the craftsman (*artifex*) needs his tools, as form needs matter (the soul being *forma vite* or *actus vite*). The soul acts through the organs of the body; the body permits the sensual perception which is the root of intellectual perception, and is thus sometimes called metaphorically the eye of the soul (*oculus mentis*). The body needs to check the soul and repress its tendencies towards uncontrolled elation and pride (2 Corinthians 12 is prominent in supporting this point). Giovanni regards the mirror image of the relationship between soul and body as the door to the world of medicine; for if the body functions as a model for the regulation of the soul and thus may teach it the proper spiritual regimen, then every organ and every disease can teach us something about the disposition of the soul.[15]

Sermon literature of the period is saturated with allusions to the role

<hr>

[14] On this Platonic notion, see P. Ricoeur, *The Symbolism of Evil* (Boston, 1972), 283–9.

[15] 'habet anima corpus velut exemplar quoddam, ex quo homo in sui regimine informatur et regulatur. Nam ipsa dispositio corporis, atque membrorum figura patenter ostendunt homini, qualiter membra eadem ab anima sunt regenda. . . . In diversis quoque corporis membris naturales reperiuntur virtutes, spirituales virtutes anime per quandam similitudinem designantes. Accidunt et varii morbi in diversis partibus corporis, qui diversis anime viciis plurimum assimilantur. Nihil que reperitur in corpore humano, quod vel vacuum fit ab officio, vel vacans ab exemplo.' *Sde* vi, *Prol.*, 292[2] (at 290[3]–292[3] the philosophical foundation of *Sde* vi).

of Christ and his ministers as physicians.[16] It was from the pagan philosophers who called themselves physicians of the soul that the Church
fathers adopted the concept of the physician–patient relationship.
Preachers employed the traditional image of Christ or God the
Physician,[17] and reinforced it with medical imagery of the nature of sin
and analogies between the physical and mystical body. Christ is portrayed as the all-merciful physician who visits the sick in 'the hospital of
this world' and cures them through his art and wisdom.[18] Sermons depict
him checking the pulse, diagnosing grave infirmities (even performing
the urine check for sin), inducing the sweat of contrition, prescribing the
plaster of devout prayer, and ordering a regimen which included diet
(fasts) and medicines (sacraments) in order to revitalize the body's natural heat by infusion of *caritas*, and to purge the soul of evil spiritual
humours.[19] Just as in phlebotomy the physician adjusts the quantities of
blood extracted to the strength of the patient's body, so God extracts
more blood (in the form of tribulations) from the devout according to
how patient they are. The Dominican Martin von Troppau even
described Christ's passion as an act of phlebotomy.[20] Christ, who showed

---

[16] L.-J. Bataillon, '*Similitudines* et *exempla* dans les sermons du XIIIe siècle', in *The Bible in the Medieval World: Essays in Memory of Beryl Smalley*, ed. K. Walsh and D. Wood (Studies in Church History, Subsidia, 4; Oxford, 1985), 191–205 at 203–4, and 'Les images dans les sermons du xiiie siècle', *Freiburger Zeitschrift für Philosophie und Theologie*, 37/3 (1990), 330–4; Martin, *Le Métier*, 452–4. On the expression of the 'medical model' around 1200, see J. Agrimi and C. Crisciani, *Medicina del corpo e medicina dell'anima: Note sul sapere del medico fino all'inizio del secolo XIII* (Milan, 1978), 36–59 and esp. 36–9.

[17] L. Edelstein, 'The Relation of Ancient Philosophy to Medicine', *Bulletin of the History of Medicine*, 26 (1952), 299–316. On the use of medical metaphors by early Christian writers, see A. Harnack, 'Medizinisches aus der ältesten Kirchengeschichte', in *Texte und Untersuchungen zur Geschichte der Altchristlichen Literatur* VII/4, ed. O. v. Gebhardt and A. Harnack (Leipzig, 1892), 37–147 at 132–43; A. S. Pease, 'Medical Allusions in the Works of St Jerome', *Harvard Studies in Classical Philology*, 25 (1914), 73–86.

[18] Bonaventura, *Sermons De Diversis*, ed. J. G. Bougerol (Paris, 1993), i. 354–5 no. 26.3. Vicent Ferrer, *Sermons de Quaresma*, ed. M. Sanchis Guarner (Valencia, 1973), i. 72–6.

[19] Giordano da Pisa, *Quaresimale Fiorentino 1305–1306*, ed. C. Delcorno (Florence, 1974), 8: 6–7 expressed the belief that 'quasi sempre, le 'nfermitadi dentro de l'anima sono cagioni de l'enfertadi del corpo.' Hubertus de Sorbonientibus, who preached to the Beguins of Paris in 1272/73, described God as *bonus/sapiens medicus* (quoting Ecclus. 38) who pro-hibits the patient from eating meat and drinking wine (allegorically representing carnal delights) and prevents him from falling 'in frenesim mortalis peccati'. N. Bériou, 'La Prédi-cation au béguinage de Paris pendant l'année liturgique 1272–1273', *Recherches Augustiniennes*, 13 (1978), 208–9. Antonio da Padova, *Sermones dominicales et festivi*, i. ed. B. Costa, L. Frasson, and I. Luisetto (Padua, 1979), 59.

[20] Martin von Troppau, *Sermones Martini ordinis predicatorum penitentiarii domini pape de tempore et de sanctis super epistulas et euangelia* (Strasbourg, 1483/4), sermon cclxxxiii (on Luke 5: 31); *Fasciculus morum: A Fourteenth-Century Preacher's Handbook*, ed. and tr. S. Wenzel (University Park, Pa., 1989), 206. The anonymous English author of this text was

the utmost patience, had thus to undergo the worst tribulations, and his death offered the ultimate, universal medicine. The longer and the more widespread an illness is, the more effort the physician spends in finding a cure for it. Since original sin started at the beginning of the world and will last until its end, the medicine of Christ necessitated tremendous toil and suffering.[21] Christ provided men with a perfect example of voluntary poverty, like the good physician who first tries the medicine himself in front of the patient, so that he may take it without fear.[22] The spiritual medicines that Christianity offers (the word of God received through preaching or prayer) are also described as theriac, namely, the ultimate cure with the most extreme powers.[23]

The medical image of Christ was extended to his ministers. Martin von Troppau pictured the priest in a sermon centred around John 10: 11 ('the good shepherd giveth his life for the sheep') as a physician who checks the patient's pulse, heat, sweat, and appetite in order to detect diseases.[24] He compared confessors to midwives, since secrets are revealed to both. Others exhorted confessors to scrutinize the conscience of the sinner in confession as a physician scrutinizes wounds. Some even compared the confessor to the phlebotomer (*minutor*): both should not be too harsh (*durus*), should know how to find the vein, and should be careful when opening it.[25] Priests who do not fulfil their duties, who kill souls instead of curing them, are described as unskilled physicians. Just as physicians never amputate a more important (*nobilius*) organ for the preservation of a less important one, so the body suffers for the soul and not vice versa. Since the righteous do not suffer from a particular spiritual disease, the

probably a Franciscan who possibly lived at the time of Edward I. S. Wenzel, *Verses in Sermon: Fasciculus morum and its Middle English Poems* (Cambridge, Mass., 1978), 27–8.

[21] Giovanni da San Gimignano, *Conciones funebres* (Paris, 1611) 535. He concludes: 'ad penitentiam que medicina est, debet confugere infirmus, quia per eam nobis passio Christi applicatur.'

[22] *Fasciculus morum*, 386: 6–12.

[23] See Ch. 3, p. 148.

[24] 'Debet enim tamquam medicus diversitatem noscere pulsuum id est motuum cordis utrum scilicet penitens habeat validum et forte propositum cavere ab peccato. Si fortis est in eo calor caritatis an debilis. Si sudor lacrimarum multus aut paucus. Si universaliter id est omnia membra rigans ut scilicet pro omnium membrorum peccatis lugeat. Debet etiam invitare egrum ad spiritualem cibum ut cum appetitu recipiat'. Martin von Troppau, *Sermones*, sermon cccxxi D.

[25] *Astesana*, as quoted in Amundsen, 'Casuistry and Professional Obligations: The Regulation of Physicians by the Court of Conscience in the Late Middle Ages', *Transactions and Studies of the College of Physicians of Philadelphia*, n.s., 3 (1981), 27 (the analogy includes also the judge who scrutinizes a case); Gérard de Mailly in Bataillon, 'Les images', 359.

tribulation which affects them is preservative (*medicina preservativa vel confortativa*) rather than curative medicine.[26] Jean Gobi's *Scala Coeli*, compiled between 1323 and 1330, equates the ideal characteristics of preachers with those of physicians.[27] Like the physician, the preacher should be perceptive (*discretus*) and use common sense; both should occasionally frighten their clients in order to achieve satisfactory results by their treatment. Both should be sometimes stern and sometimes kind towards their patients (*firmus, amicus*). In the article on Pride, the author of *Fasciculus morum* cites Augustine and argues that, just as the physician's illness is no obstacle to the effect and power of his medicines, the moral wickedness of a priest should not reduce the efficacy of the sacrament he administers. In both cases the work performed is always pure, even if the performer is impure.[28]

Employing the similarities between the role of priests and physicians was not unique to preachers. Scholastic analysis of simony discussed the right of the physician to receive money for his treatment, which was perceived to be a product of a divine gift. The same arguments were applied to physicians and clerics and thus linked the two professions.[29] Physicians found it useful to do likewise when expressing themselves on non-medical issues. Such was the case with Marsilio da Padova, another four-teenth-century thinker with a medical background, who, like Arnau de Vilanova, developed a second career which became his main one. He found the priest/physician analogy most helpful in conveying his view that it was necessary to limit clerical jurisdiction and to submit clerics to lay authority.[30] For Marsilio, both the physician and the priest are professional, independent experts who can diagnose, advise, teach, admonish, and even frighten, but who have no coercive power and who are ultimately subject to the secular authority. Priests are expected to detect the first sign of spiritual or ecclesiastical offences, since according to divine law they are bound to separate people so afflicted from the community of the faithful so that others will not be infected. This is compared to the duty of physicians in times of contagious disease. But as the power to

[26] Giovanni da San Gimignano, *Convivium quadragesimale hoc est conciones et sermones tam sacri quam suaves singuli totius quadragesimae feriis et dominicis* (Paris, 1611), 130–1.

[27] *La 'Scala Coeli' de Jean Gobi*, ed. M.-A. Polo de Beaulieu (Paris, 1991), 463–4 no. 690–3.

[28] *Fasciculus morum*, 82: 32–5.

[29] Bonaventura, *In quartum librum sententiarum*, in *Opera Omnia*, iv. (Quaracchi, 1889) iv, dist xxv, art. ii. q. 1, 648.

[30] G. Rosen, 'The Historical Significance of Some Medical References in the *Defensor Pacis* of Marsilius of Padua', *Sudhoffs Archiv*, 37 (1953), 350–6; N. G. Siraisi, *Arts and the Sciences at Padua: The Studium of Pedra before 1350* (Toronto, 1973), 165.

expel the leper belongs to the community itself and not the physicians, so the priesthood has no power to punish individuals for offences against divine law even if the carriers of these suspect ideas are diagnosed as heretics. Like the physician who has no authority to compel anyone to take any action for his health, so also is the priest limited. Marsilio's analysis of clerical or priestly jurisdiction in *Defensor minor* limits the powers of the priestly office to the instrumental or managerial level 'whether speculative or practical, just like those which the physician exercises in counselling and treating healthy and ill persons'.[31] Spiritual power should not be understood as jurisdiction or authority in the sense of the coercive punishment of people in the present world, but as that kind of instruction or exhortation which does not have the effect of a law. And he concludes:

Just as physicians have learning and practical experience in accordance with the precepts of the medical arts in order that the health of the body may be conserved or its well-being recovered so they cannot compel anyone to observe a suitable diet, nor to avoid a harmful one, by imposing some punishment on the persons or property of patients. In this way, also, priests who are physicians of the souls cannot restrain anyone on the basis of Scripture, by punishment in the present world.[32]

The priest/physician analogy is also useful when Marsilio discusses priestly power to loose and bind. This power does not simply depend on knowledge of Scripture, and arises from authority specifically conceded to the person by God. In this respect, the priest's position is similar to the physician's, for without licence from the appropriate authority the physician, no matter how skilled he is, will be punishable for transgressing human law.[33]

While priests are depicted as physicians, sinners are depicted as patients. Bonaventura, for example, also strengthens the patient/physician model by describing the behaviour of extremely devout people who actively search for God as patients who are obsessed with the physician's coming and yearn for his arrival.[34] Similarly, Ranulphe de la Houblonnière (a secular master who died in 1288 as Bishop of Paris), whose sermons are saturated with references to blood, humours, and

---

[31] Marsilio da Padova, *Defensor minor*, iv.3, in Marsiglio of Padua, *Writings on the Empire: Defensor minor and De translatione Imperii*, ed. C. J. Nederman (Cambridge, 1993), 10. Cf. *Defensor pacis*, Disc. ii. 7.4 and 9.3.

[32] Marsilio da Padova, *Defensor minor*, xiv. 2, 51.

[33] Ibid. v.17, 18. See also 33, 47 for further allusions to physicians.

[34] Bonaventura, *Sermones*, in *Opera Omnia*, ix (Quaracchi, 1901), 351a.

other bodily fluids, describes the three Marys in search of Christ (Mark 26) as seeking a physician.[35]

However, Ranulphe's sermon shows that the physician/patient model was also used inversely; namely, Christ the Physician was sometimes shown as everything the human physician was not. Thus, unlike worldly physicians (*isti medici*), Christ feels compassion towards his patients; this has impelled him to offer himself as a cure. He undertakes a forty-day fast, swallows bitter medicine of vinegar mixed with bile (*acetum felle mixtum*), is tied and flogged—binding (*ligatio*) being a therapy for madness (*phrenesis*)—undergoes phlebotomy on the cross, and is totally washed (*balneatus*) by his blood, thereby washing all humanity. Similarly, Giovanni also occasionally contrasts the true physician with human physicians. In a sermon on the theme of John 4: 46 ('And there was a certain nobleman whose son was sick'), Giovanni describes Christ conferring three kinds of remedies on the sick child: one prognosticates, another cures, and the third causes conversion (*prognosticativa, curativa, conversiva*). The uniqueness of Christ lies in that he pronounced his prognosis without seeing the patient—a practice inconceivable among physicians and unacceptable to medical theory.[36] In another sermon, Giovanni contrasts Christ's love with that of the human physician. While human physicians usually are not very charitable and do not visit the sick unless they are called to do so, Christ came to save mankind without being asked.[37]

The medical model enabled the preacher to describe the disordered soul, diagnose its mental religious disposition, and prescribe sensible treatment as if it were a body. The Dominican Pierre de Reims (d. 1257 as Bishop of Agen) expressed the state of mental readiness to accept grace during Lent in terms of the prerequisites for a successful physical cure. This depends on an adequate supply of medicine (*habundantia medicine*), the physician's competence (*peritia medici*), and humoral preparation (*humorum preparatio*). The parallel concepts of medically bad or imbalanced humours (*mali humores*) and bad morals (*mali mores*) enables him to medicalize his discussion of the human soul.[38] For Bonaventura, an

---

[35] N. Bériou (ed.), *La Prédication de Ranulphe de la Houblonnière*, ii. (Paris, 1987), 132.

[36] 'quod alii medici facere nesciunt nisi audiant condiciones infirmi vel videant quedam signa ex quibus medicus ut ponit Ypocras in suis pronosticis potest pronosticari de sanitate vel morte infirmi.' MS London, BL Addit. 24998, fol. 218vb–19ra. The discussion is followed by an analysis of the signs which enable the physician's prognosis according to *Sde* x. 74, 485³–487⁴.

[37] MS London, BL Addit. 24998, fol. 195[rb] sermon 134.

[38] Bataillon, 'Les images', 370–2.

imbalance is the explanation for both physical and spiritual diseases; whilst a humoral imbalance causes the first, an imbalance of four dispositions (hope, fear, joy, and love) brings about the second and more harmful disease.[39]

According to Giovanni, discussion of the medical effects resulting from seasonal changes in weather is useful in describing and explaining the four conditions of the soul (*status anime*) that lead to its perfection.[40] The state of tribulation (*status tribulationis*), in which a person starts to repent and to direct himself to moral good, is represented by winter for three reasons. Winter is characterized by the increase of phlegmatic humour which is cold and moist; similarly, in time of spiritual tribulation the burning heat of carnal desire cools down, and the humour of tears becomes abundant.[41] The second reason is more scientifically grounded. Giovanni says that people of choleric complexion (such as the young, who are warm and dry) can sustain the vicissitudes of winter better than those of phlegmatic complexion (such as the old and decrepit, who are cold and dry). Diseases which originate in phlegm (such as quotidian fever, *febris quotidiana*) are more frequent than diseases which originate in choleric humour, like tertian fever. He then infuses this scientific model with religious and moral messages. Those who lament their sins, yet are not inflamed with celestial love, are like the phlegmatic who, in winter time and, in times of tribulation and temptations, succumb easily to corruption of their minds. Their immune system breaks down like the person whose corrupt phlegm makes him particularly susceptible to quotidian fever; from the corruption of their mind comes a continuous inflammation of the flesh.[42] However, those of fervent spirit who are devoid of the humour of the flesh (carnal desire) can resist these phlegmatic diseases. The third reason why the state of tribulation is represented by winter is that dietary norms (*discretio cibationis*) prescribe eating warm and dry food in winter to counteract the wintry complexion, which is cold and wet. As for the soul, love for eternal things can

[39] 'Nam sicut inequalitas humorum est causa infirmitatis corporalis, sic infirmitas spiritualis causatur ex inequalitate sive inordinatione quatuor affectionum que sunt hae, scilicet spes, timor, gaudium et amor.' Bonaventura, *Sermones de tempore*, in *Opera Omnia*, ix. 232.

[40] *Sde* i. 74, 92⁴–94². See a similar debate from the twelfth century in Hugues de Fouilloy, *De medicina anime*, PL 176, 1183–95.

[41] 'in tribulatione refrigescit ardor carnalium desideriorum, et abundat fletus et humor lachrymarum.' *Sde* i. 74, 92⁴.

[42] 'Ex propria enim mentis corruptione provenit continuus ardor carnis quasi ex corruptione phlegmatis quotidiana febris.' Ibid, 93¹.

kindle fire in it and dry the humours of carnal desire which corrupt it.

Similarly, spring corresponds to the state of conversion (*status conversionis*). Density of the blood (*augmentum sanguinis*), which may cause a continuous fever called *synnochus*, signifies the tumour of pride that grows out of excess elation and joy which characterize the first stage of conversion. At this stage old and decrepit people are in a better position than the young, because old people can better withstand the temptations which accompany conversion. The medically recommended diet for spring—cold and dry food—is spiritually interpreted as fasting and hard labour.[43] The meteorological instability of springtime corresponds to spiritual inconstancy and the excessive temptations to which the new converts have been exposed.

Abundant summer heat links summertime to the third state of the soul, which is influenced by the heat of love (*sub fervore dilectionis*). The heat signifies anger (*ira*) towards sin. A diet of cold and moist things (spiritually, tears) should neutralize the tremendous heat or the arid tumour of pride.

Autumn describes the state of perfection and ripe judgement (*sub maturitate discretionis sive perfectionis*). The increase in melancholy which characterizes autumn signifies sadness over sins committed (*tristitia de peccatis*). At this stage youths, who are of sanguine complexion, are better off than the old melancholics. The recommended diet, which includes warm and moist things, should dry up the humour of desire, cool down the heat of the vices, yet keep the penitent also slightly moist by contemplating the supreme things.

In using the seasons to illuminate spiritual states, Giovanni was conventional. Servasanto da Faenza, who describes man as a microcosm (*minor mundus*) because he is governed by the soul as is the macrocosm (*mundus maior*) by God, draws a parallel between the seasons and the four ages of man. In doing so, he openly prefers the philosophers' approach to child psychology over that of St Jerome. According to Servasanto, spring corresponds to childhood (*pueritia*) because it is warm and moist and decorated with flowers that signify the innocence and purity of the child. He cites Avicenna, who believed that childhood was not an appropriate time for learning. The child quickly absorbs anything new, yet forgets it as

---

[43] He concludes: 'Ne enim per desiderium vane glorie fervor sanguinis ebulliat, necesse est ut animus frigus tentationis et sterilitatem siccitatis ad memoriam reducat.' *Sde* i. 74, 93².

quickly and can only focus on one thing at a time. The threatening presence of the master is not sufficient to ensure long-term learning. Children may be well-disposed to learning, but disposition to knowing (*dispositio scientie*) must become a habit of knowing (*habitus scientie*) before real learning can begin; this does not happen in childhood. Here, however, Avicenna disagreed with Jerome, who had held that 'what a new jug holds will last longer' and thus believed that early learning assured better reception. By allowing Avicenna and Aristotle to conclude the debate, Servasanto shows clear preference for the philosopher's interpretation.[44]

Giovanni also equates certain healing procedures with stages on the path to salvation:[45] plastering represents the word of God, inducing sweat signifies the fear of God (*timor Dei*) that repels sin from the mind, baths are compunction, vomit is confession, diet is abstinence from sin, and amputation represents Job's tribulations. Finally, medical unction depicts devotion and piety which serve to soothe the soul. Other preachers add cauterization, phlebotomy, enema, sleep, and exercise to this list, and allot them a spiritual meaning.[46] Therapeutic physical exercise represents exercises of penitence which lubricate the soul and prevent it from rusting. The shame involved in the practice of enema portrays the conscience, through which sins must be expelled. The last phase of physical cure involves purgation; after the preparatory syrup, the physician gives the patient purgative medicine which he wraps with white biscuits to disguise its taste. Christ does the same; once the person has performed the necessary penance at the end of the Christian therapeutic path, Christ offers and provides him with Holy Communion.

Hippocrates' nine signs for efficient medical prognosis help Giovanni to simplify a more complex spiritual-religious message.[47] Sweat is the ninth indicator of health, and good sweat enables the body to purge itself of disease. It can be identified by an equal purgation in every member.

[44] Servasanto da Faenza, *Liber aureus qui antidotarius animarum dictus est* (Leuven, *c.*1485), fol. xxi[r]. Adolescence corresponds to summer, youth to autumn and old age to winter.

[45] *Sde* x. 53, 479[1–2].

[46] Vicent Ferrer, *Sermons*, iv. 115–20, and *Sermons*, v. 15–20 no. 145; *Fasciculus morum*, 254–6; Bataillon, 'Les images', 358–62 (for Gérard de Mailly); John Bromyard, *Summa predicantium* (Nuremberg, 1518), *Sanctitas*, ii. fol. cccxliii[va], who likens holiness (*sanctitas*) to health (*sanitas*).

[47] *Sde* x. 74, 485[3]–487[4]. Cf. an identical description (attributed to Galen's *De prognosticis*) in Hugues de Fouilloy, *De medicina anime*, *PL* 176, 1195–8; Aldobrandino Cavalcanti (OP, d. 1279 as Bishop of Arezzo) in Bataillon, 'Les images', 354–5 mentions seven indicators of good health which do not correspond to Giovanni's division.

Purgation of the soul is achieved by the sweat of confession (*sudor confessionis*), which, like real sweat, must be total and include all misdeeds.[48] When only one organ is sweating (usually the head) it is a sign of pathological disfunction (*membrorum debilitas*). This evil sweat signifies a person who confesses his deeds yet praises his intention and thus consciously excuses himself; this person is culpable, and should be damned.[49]

In the last years of the thirteenth century the Franciscan Servasanto da Faenza frequently used the concept of medical priests (*presbyteri medici*) in his moralistic treatises. On the basis of the belief that 'the same should apply to the physician of the souls and to the physician of the bodies',[50] he repeatedly employed the medical model. The tenth tractate in his *Antidotarius animarum* deals with the last stage of penance, satisfaction. Its first chapter is entitled: 'What Should the Physician of the Souls be Like?' (*Qualis esse debeat medicus animarum*),[51] and it maintains that satisfaction can be achieved by imposing penance according to the principle that a condition is opposed by its opposite (*contrarium contrario opponitur*). This principle, used so frequently in the medical/pharmaceutical context, initiates here a meticulous discussion of the resemblance between the priestly and medical professions. The physicians of the body and of the soul must share the same characteristics when diagnosing an affliction and prescribing therapy. They must be wise, careful, prudent and cautious, discreet and discerning, and fully committed to finding a cure. Servasanto asserts that health (*salus*) can only be safeguarded by the experience, true knowledge, and caution (*scientia et circumspectio*) of physicians. Failure (due to inexperience, ignorance, or indiscretion) which results in the death of the diseased patient would result in a criminal charge being brought against the physician.[52] The physician of the body should be pleasant, humble, accessible (*tractabilis*), kind (*benignus*), and pious. In practice, he is expected conscientiously to approach the patient's bed, inquire about the disease and its causes, touch the patient's organs, and avoid showing any sign of abhorrence. He should comfort the patient with kind words and promise him hope of health, since often

---

[48] For more examples of the spiritual meaning of purgation, see Bataillon, 'Les images', 366–7 for Gérard de Mailly; MS Paris, BN lat. 15956, fol. 42vb–44va, 132^{r}–134^{r} for Guillaume de Mailly; Bériou, (ed.) *La Prédication de Ranulphe de la Houblonnière*, ii. 48.

[49] *Sde* x. 74, 486^2.

[50] 'circa animarum medicum est notandum quod talis esse debet qualis et medicus corporum'. Servasanto da Faenza, *Liber de exemplis naturalibus*, MS Paris, BN lat. 3436 fol. 82^{v}.

[51] Servasauto da Faenza, *Antidotarius animarum*, fol. 149^{r}–150^{r}.

[52] Servasanto da Faenza, *Liber de exemplis naturalibus*, MS Paris, BN lat. 3436, fol. 82^{v}.

hope is more useful than the treatment itself. The same attitude is expected from the physician of souls, since in the realm of spiritual disease only hopelesness (*desperatio*) brings death.

The function (*officium*) of both physicians is identical. Invigorative medicine (*medicina confortativa*) which is essential for convalescence is provided spiritually by visiting the penitent. Such visits, like those of a doctor to his patient, mitigate the effects of the radical change (*mutatio*) which the penitent undergoes. Here Servasanto introduces Hippocrates to reinforce his belief in the necessity of visiting the penitent. Like the body, the soul does not tolerate sudden changes, and the penitent should be treated slowly and gradually lest shock-treatment utterly destroy his soul.[53] When necessary, the physician of the body should pleasantly advise cauterization or incision, and he should counteract the bitterness of the medicines he prescribes by tender ('sweet') and pleasant words, and even taste the prescribed medicine in front of the patient, thus fulfilling the biblical saying, 'Who is weak (*infirmatur*) and I am not weak?' (2 Corinthians 11: 29).[54] The compassionate physician of the body, unlike the foolish physician (*stultus medicus*) who applies unnecessarily harsh therapies, should always prefer the pleasant (*dulcia*) therapy to the bitter (*amara*), and thus should refrain from surgery when plastering will help. The pious physician should be careful not to destroy nature while destroying the disease. However, when the patient needs it the physician must maintain the rules and even be severe, strict, and harsh (*iustus*, *severus*, *rigidus*). He should thus be prepared to order the amputation of one organ for the preservation of the whole body, and to quarantine the sick, since sometimes kind words will not cure. This should be done only after all other remedies have failed. In these circumstances the physician should not heed the patient's copious tears, lest while undeservedly sparing one organ he harm the whole body. The parallel here is excommunication. Thus, for Servasanto, the physician/priest analogy based on compassion (*misericordia*) and just punishment (*iustitia*) licenses

[53] 'quia secundum ypocrasis doctrinam repente euacuare calidare uel infrigidare fallax est experimentum et nature penitus inimicus quia natura non patitur repentinas mutaciones. Unde sic paulatim est nature restauracio et ideo sepe perit si in consequenti dieta non fuerit refrenata. Sic homines penitentes paulatim sunt premonendi nec nimis grauendi sed in utilibus edocendi et super uacuis refrenandi. Unde postquam natura a malis est euacuata restaurata et confortata et ad pristinum statum reducta.' Ibid. fol. 84[r].

[54] It was common to portray Christ as the best physician whose mercy is so great that he assimilates all the patients' diseases into his own body. See Robert Holcot, *In librum sapientie regis Salomonis prelectiones ccxiii* (Basel, 1586), *lectio* cxviii, 397, who distinguishes between three levels of medical treatment: the passive *speculatio* which leads to compassion at most, the more active *examinatio* of accidents, and the most efficacious *assimilatio* of the patient's disease to the physician's body as Christ historically applied.

charitable attitudes and activities as well as, in extreme cases, violence and exclusion in the domains of body and of soul. Yet this congruence is not absolute, since the physician of the soul is expected to be more compassionate than just.[55]

The second chapter in *Antidotarius animarum* is entitled 'In What Manner should the Physician Conduct himself Towards the Patient?' (*Qualiter se debeat habere medicus ad egrotum*). Servasanto describes in terms of medicine the preparatory knowledge necessary for effective spiritual cure. The physician of the body must take into consideration the complexion, compositions, and combinations of organs and humours, seasonal dispositions, sex, and age when he prescribes a medical treatment. Galen, who teaches that hot food is detrimental to the complexion of children and youths who are inflamed by innate heat, provides here the scientific foundation for this argument; just the opposite applies to old people.[56]

The need to adapt the treatment to the patient is discussed in the following two chapters. The wise physician should gather information, knowledge, and experience concerning the patient and also the medicines and antidotes he prescribes. He must take into consideration symptoms and accidental qualities (*signa et accidentia*), nature (*natura rerum*), qualities (*qualitates*), complexions (*complectiones*), powers (*virtutes*), weaknesses (*debilitates*), functions (*operationes*), the diversities of diseases (*morborum diversitates*), durabilities (*diuturnitates*), and oppositions (*contrarietates*). The gravity of the illness (*quantitas*) should determine the degree (*gradus*) of the remedy. Hence the medicine must suit the particular patient and disease, and simple disease should be treated with simple medicines, complex with composite. On the spiritual level, knowledge of herbal medicines is equated with the knowledge of spiritual herbs (*spirituales herbe*). Thus the lascivious should be treated with fasting, the avaricious with almsgiving, and the proud with devout and humble prayer. The medical differentiation among medicines that are attractive (*medicina attractiva*), transformatory (*immutativa*), digestive (*digestiva*), laxative (*laxativa*), constringent (*constrictiva*), curative (*curativa*), restorative (*reparativa*), and preservative (*preservativa*) helps Servasanto to describe the ways in which the priest extracts (*attrahere*) sin from the heart's depths;

---

[55] 'Sed notandum quod semper medicus animarum magis debet declinare ad misericordiam quam ad iusticiam quia misericordia superexaltat iudicium'. Servasauto da Faenza, *Antidotarius animarum*, fol. 151[ra].

[56] 'Docet enim Galienus: puerorum ac iuvenum corpora insito sibi calore fervere et noxios asserit his etatibus calidos cibos esse frigidosque valere sicut econtra senibus frigida nocent et calida valent.' Ibid. fol. 150[va].

changes (*immutare*) the moral disposition of the patient; dissolves the abscess of sin by sweet words; frees (*laxare*) the soul from sin through penitence and contrition; constrains (*constringere*) the excessive desires of the proud; and cures and preserves the spiritual health by the *electuarium* (syrup-like medication which dissolves in the mouth) of meditation on and imitation of saints and *perfecti*, and by baths of tears. According to Hippocrates, when it is necessary for the preservation of health, the body has to be cleansed and purged.[57] This should be done by inducing the evacuation of digested rather than raw material. The same is true for spiritual medicine: a digestive medicine must be applied after the patient has spiritually taken the prescribed laxative medicine in the form of worthy penitence. The physician of the soul, like his physical counterpart, should thus recognize the diversity of sin in order to prescribe the appropriate remedy. In prescribing penance the priest should study the penitent and adapt the practice to his personality as well as to his physical and psychological complexion. Since it is biologically more difficult for the choleric person to fast than for the phlegmatic, it is more difficult to fast for the young than for the old. This must be known by the priest when he prescribes fast or prayer.[58] Thus the priest must carefully investigate the temperament of the sinner's soul (*disposiciones cordium*) and prescribe different therapies for the young and the old, for new transgressors or habitual sinners.[59] The variety of sinners' spiritual complexions determines a unique treatment adapted to the individual complexion; for it is harder for a poor person to give one denarius than for a rich person to give a hundred. Similarly, it is much harsher to impose on a farmer a single recitation of *Pater noster* than to impose on a hermit a whole day of prayer.[60]

Both penitent and patient should be prepared to bear the burden of the treatment, like knights who carry the weight of armour, or pilgrims who tackle rough paths, and to follow the advice of the physician or the priest. Servasanto underlines the purgative effects of penance and the penitent's duty to stay on the path of righteousness once he has performed satisfaction.

[57] 'Nam secundum ypocratis doctrinam oportet medicari et mouere digesta non cruda'. Servasanto da Faenza, *Liber de exemplis naturalibus*, MS Paris, BN lat. 3436, fol. 84[r].

[58] 'in tanta penitentia singulorum attendenda est natura quia gravius est ieiunare colerico quam fleumatico ceteris paribus propter maiores calores ipsum interius cibum consumentes et digestionem celerius celebrantes et ideo mox cibum alium appetit. Facilius est ex eadem causa ieiunare seni quam iuveni unde Avicenna dicit quod senes facile ieiunium ferunt; sed pueri difficiliter ferunt facilius enim convenit orare quam ieiunare.' Servasanto da Faenza, *Antidotarius animarum*, fol. 151[rb].

[59] Servasanto da Faenza, *Liber de exemplis naturalibus*, MS Paris, BN lat. 3436, fol. 82[v].

[60] Ibid. fol. 83[r–v].

Like the recurrence of illness in the physical world, the recurrence of sin is an ominous sign.[61] Servasanto introduces citations from medical authorities to his moralizing text, and the level of his medical language is higher than all the preachers cited above. In this respect, his mode of employing the medical model is similar to that of Giovanni. For these particular chapters Servasanto drew on Bartholomaeus Anglicus's chapter on medicine, rearranging it, adding more material, and creating the parallels with the priest.[62]

This general medical imagery seems to have been useful for preachers not only because it was understood by all (since everyone had some real medical experience), but also because it was quite flexible, and applicable to such a variety of religious issues. The same signifier could signify different things, and this left space for the preacher or the religious thinker to imprint his own creative contribution. It could also be conveniently used for upholding the demand of the Church for absolute and universal obedience from the believers. It enabled the preacher to speak intelligibly about every part of the complex structure of the Christian faith, about every function-holder, from Christ to the confessor, and about every mood and attitude of believers towards God and his precepts.

How would the frequent use of metaphors connecting God, Christ, the priest, and spiritual well-being with physicians, the medical profession, and physical health affect the audience and the self-image of the real physician? Without concrete evidence, I can only suggest that the frequent employment of the physician–patient model enhanced the status both of medicine and of the physician. It certainly reflects the preachers' and their audiences' basic medical knowledge, and, perhaps, also a widespread interest in medical matters.

It is remarkable that the literary prominence of the medical model around 1300 did not further iconographic representations of Christ the Physician or the Apothecary. The earliest known representation of Christ as a physician is in a Dutch book printed in 1510. It then becomes popular throughout the following two centuries, particularly in Germany and the Low Countries.[63] The iconographic motif of Christ the Apothecary

---

[61] Servasanto da Faenza, *Antidotarius animarum*, fol. 151^V–152^V.

[62] Bartholomaeus Anglicus, *Venerandi patris Bartholomei Anglici . . . opus de rerum proprietatibus* (Nuremberg, 1519), vii. 69, 'De medicina'. Cf. Pierre Bersuire, *Reductorium morale super totam bibliam*, iv. 28, 108^2–111^1, 'De medico'.

[63] *Lexikon der Christlichen Ikonographie*, i. ed. E. Kirschbaum (Freiburg am Breisgau, 1968), 190–1; *Reallexikon zur deutschen Kunstgeschichte*, iii. ed. O. Schmitt, E. Gall, and L. H. Heydenreich (Stuttgart, 1954), 639–43.

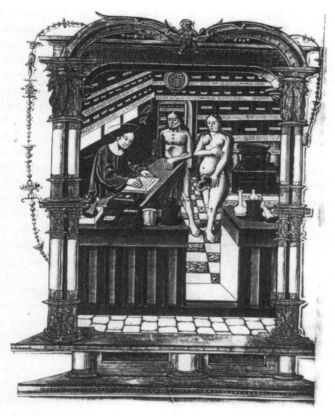

Christ the Apothecary

Bibliothèque Nationale de France (MS Paris, BN, Fr. 1537, fol. 82ᵛ).

becomes common particularly in southern German Baroque art of the sixteenth to eighteenth centuries.[64] The earliest iconographic depiction of Christ the Apothecary appears in a well-executed miniature in a French manuscript produced in Rouen between 1519 and 1528. It portrays Christ as an apothecary in his shop prescribing medicine to Adam and Eve.[65]

[64] *Lexikon der Christlichen Ikonographie*, i. 174; *Reallexikon zur deutschen Kunstgeschichte*, iii. 636–9; W.-H. Hein, *Christus als Apotheker* (Frankfurt am Main, 1974).
[65] MS Paris, BN Fr. 1537, fol. 82ᵛ; *La Médecine médiévale à travers les manuscrits de la Bibliothèque Nationale* (Paris, 1982), 19, 81; Hein, *Christus als Apotheker*, 18–19. The illustration accompanies a poem composed for a competition held by a literary confraternity in Rouen on the Feast of the Immaculate Conception in a manuscript of *c.* 1519–28.

The other four categories of medical similes in Giovanni's *Sde* emanate from the 'medical model' described above. On the foundation of the similarity between medical cure and spiritual care, Giovanni proceeds to more concrete comparisons which he grounds on specific medical information, and the section to come examines this unique feature (also shared by Servasanto and Bersuire). The second category of medical terms is that which appears in the discourse on sin.[66] Giovanni's moralizing approach to disease in general, and in particular the way in which he uses specific medical structure both for the description and for the explanation of spiritual illness, is significant. He makes an effort to describe meticulously the clinical symptoms of each and every disease, relying solely on Avicenna as his source for these pathologies.

The third category is made up of anatomical similes which describe and explain various aspects of orthodox Christian life. If Giovanni relies on Avicenna for his knowledge of pathologies, Constantinus Africanus is his main cited source on anatomy and physiology, though he sometimes mentions Galen, Hippocrates, and Haly as well. He equates the virtue of *caritas* with nerves, flesh, sense of touch, legs, back, the chin, and the heart. He describes grace as bone-marrow, and the reception of the divine word as physical digestion, the sense of hearing or the ears themselves, and the formation of voice. He discusses prayer within the context of breathing, and compares pastoral care to breast-feeding.[67] Each such simile includes a detailed anatomical or physiological description which is then moralized. Of all religious practices, Giovanni decorates penance with the largest number of anatomical similes.[68] Lungs, eyelids, bile, the spleen, and even the four kinds of stomach-ache according to Avicenna's differentiation are used to signify it. One simile compares physical conception to the spiritual conception of the penitent through God.[69]

Other contemporary preachers also made use of medical allusions when speaking about the sacraments. Servasanto depicts grace as a lubricating medicine which strengthens the mental complexion in its devotion,

---

[66] See Ch. 2, pp. 106–11, and Appendix Ib.

[67] See Appendix Ic and Appendix II.

[68] This may be an evolution of the frequent use of 'medical' discourse about penance in earlier penitentials, e.g. Alan de Lille's *Liber poenitentialis*, and Canon Law, e.g. bk.19 ('De poenitentia') in Burchard of Worms's *Libri decretorum*. J. Agrimi and C. Crisciani, *Medicina del corpo e medicina dell'anima: Note sul sapere del medico fino all'inizio del secolo XIII* (Milan, 1978), 46–9.

[69] *Sde*, vi. 54, 338⁴–339¹. Cf. Ch. 2, pp. 65–8.

prevents corruption, revives natural heat, cures sterility, and helps to overcome famine. He also compares it to the medicinal effect of the moon over the quantities of bone-marrow.[70] His discussion of baptism includes a comparison with medicinal baths, and he equates penance with medicinal herbs and extreme unction with medicinal unction. Penance, which appears as a sour-tasting medicine but conceals moist, fruitful, comforting, nourishing, and strengthening powers within it, enables Servasanto to display his knowledge of medicinal herbs, which, though sour-tasting, are effective cures. He thus allows us a glimpse of some common herbal therapies, which appear in the medicinal texts attributed to Dioscorides, and compares certain plants to penance, as follows. The almond tree (*arbor amigdalus*) has an effective cosmetic use; it also mitigates headache and disinfects bruises. Oil produced from it kills intestinal worms, cleans the ears and helps as an antidote for dog-bites. Aloe expels melancholy, strengthens the organs and cleans them from viscous humours, clarifies the eyesight, relieves the spleen of obstruction, defends against dropsy, generates good colour for the body, kills worms, fights mouth-stench, and curbs genital ulcers, while Aristolochia (*aristologia*) expels poisons from the body and removes the stench from corpses. Cassia has a strengthening, purgative, maturative, and particularly palliative effect on bad breath and defects of the heart; thorny caper (*capparis spinosa*) softens the belly, sedates toothache, and kills stomach-worms; and centaury (*centaverea*) sedates stomach-ache, clarifies the eyesight, cures paralysis, and kills stomach-worms. Finally, the leaves of the ash-tree (*fraxinus*) provide antidotes to poisons.[71]

The fourth category is similes in which each of the main groups within the Christian community is likened to a certain organ of the body. This organic view of the Christian community is obviously not new, but Giovanni uses it in a distinctive fashion. He goes beyond the usual depiction of prelates as the head, the princes as the shoulders, or the believers

---

[70] Servasanto da Faenza, *Liber de exemplis naturalibus*, MS Paris, BN nouv. acq. lat. 259, fol. 42va, 45va.

[71] Ibid. MS Paris, BN nouv. acq. lat. 259, fol. 27vb for baptism, 32^{rb-va} for herbal penance, 38^{rb-va} for extreme unction. The *Liber de occultis virtutibus* attributed to Ascolapius [*sic*] is his source for describing in this context various therapies for haemorrhoids. These include sitting on lion's skin and smearing the body with tallow made of lion's kidneys. He attributes to Constantinus three medicines preventing epileptic fits; their ingredients include dog-hair, ground ass-hoofs, and bull's gall-bladder. W. Schneider, *Lexikon zur Arzneimittelgeschichte* (Frankfurt a. M., 1974), 5/3, 130–2 (Amygdalus); 5/1, 70–4 (Aloe); 5/1, 124–9 (Aristolochia); 5/1, 246–52 (Cassia); 5/1, 231–3 (Capparis); 5/1, 258–62 (Centaurea); 5/2, 107–11 (Fraxinus).

as the limbs, and turns every organ into an iconic sign.[72] The saints are compared to the spleen, apostolic people to the symmetry of the ribs, preachers to the eyes, and members of the religious orders to the teeth, which are well-rooted in the flesh yet live outside it.[73] Teachers of the Church are likened to the kidneys, nuns to the thighs, the just and the perfect to the heart and the liver, and the proper treatment of the new converts to the treatment of the newly born.[74] The liver represents the just and perfect men (*iusti et perfecti viri*), since by supplying the stomach (which signifies the common good, *res publica sive bonum commune*) with the necessary heat for digestion, it helps the whole body. The community is thus similarly enriched by the presence of the *perfecti*.

The liver is where secondary digestion takes place. It attracts the juices which have been produced by primary digestion, and turns them into sanguine matter by boiling (*ebulitio*). At this stage of his discussion Giovanni stresses that the form (*forma*) of the blood originates in the heart, as Aristotle argued. The waste produced in this process is emitted by the urine via the kidneys. Sanguine matter is of four kinds: blood itself; choler, which is warm and dry and concentrated in the bile; melancholy, which is cold and dry and concentrated in the spleen; and phlegm which is cold and humid and is concentrated in the lungs. The digestive process in the liver is equated with the compunction of the *perfecti*, which is secondary, coming after penitence, and is directed at venial sins. It produces compunction which arises from contemplating prelapsarian existence in the past, base, sinful existence in the present, the threatening prospects for the future, and potential existence in paradise. These four thoughts correspond to the four kinds of sanguinal matter. The pathologies of the liver include overheating and dramatic loss of heat producing failure of the digestive power and endangering the health of the body; in extreme cases, dropsy may evolve from them. The penitent is also exposed to similar spiritual fluctuations.

The last category is anatomical similes depicting the human mind and intellect. Giovanni equates memory with the stomach,[75] thoughts with

---

[72] *Collected Papers of C. S. Peirce*, ii. ed. C. Hartstorme and P. Weiss (Cambridge, Mass., 1932), 156–60. For a discussion of the political aspects of the use of bodily metaphors and especially of the emergence of the metaphor of the heart, see J. Le Goff, 'Head or Heart: The Political Use of Bodily Metaphors in the Middle-Ages' in M. Feher, R. Naddaff, and N. Tazi (ed.), *Fragments for a History of the Human Body*, iii (New York, 1990), 12–27.

[73] Robert Holcot, *In librum sapientie*, 345–6 (7.26, *lectio* cii, p. 345–6) refers to the *doctores et prelatus* as *dentes ecclesie* and cites Aristotle.

[74] See Appendix Id.

[75] Cf. St Gregory, *Regula pastoralis*, iii. 12, in *PL* 77, 69.

hair, mind with the chest, wisdom with taste, tongue, and saliva, knowledge with the nose, and contemplation with sleep, blood, and eyes.[76] He likens the pleasantness of contemplation (*dulcedo contemplationis*) to blood, and supports his argument by scientific knowledge. He refers to Aristotle's assertion that the origin of blood lies in the heart. Like many other medical tags employed by Giovanni, this one probably originated in Bartholomaeus Anglicus's *De proprietatibus rerum* (iii. 7). But Giovanni also mentions the Galenic theory that it is the liver from which blood originates, and thus undermines his analogy[77] and shows that he has collected the medical information for his *exempla* from various chapters in the encyclopaedia. He harmonizes the apparently contradictory explanations, and salvages his simile by alleging that both explanations are correct and can coexist. The liver is indeed the origin of the blood as far as its matter is concerned (*quo ad materiam*); the heart, where the blood receives its 'bloodiness' (*forma sanguinis*), is the origin of blood as far as its essence is concerned (*quantum ad formam*). The by-product of the production of blood is heat, which he equates with the fire of love (*ardor amoris*) flowing to the soul of the contemplator. Its curative effect (i.e. the pleasantness that it causes) is like the invigorating effect of hot and humid blood on the body. The heat of love, together with the humour of the fear of God (*timor*), create a feeling of utmost delight and render the contemplator spiritually healthy (*sobries et sanus*).

An Interpretation

The high-level medical knowledge of Giovanni, Servasanto, and Bersuire, and the manner in which they employ it in a non-medical context, is the most striking point in the discussion above. Early-thirteenth-century preaching literature is characterized by its use of scriptural *auctoritates*. The average sermon does not usually contain patristic and other

---

[76] See Appendix Ie.

[77] '(secundum Arist.) sedem habet in corde, quia dicit quod cor est principium sanguinis sicut et venarum, ut manifestum esse dicit per anathomiam. Sed secundum Gale. sedes sanguinis est in hepate sicut in suo fonte; quia in calore hepatis est locus secunde decoctionis et inde sanguis per membra dirigitur, ut eorum calore tertio decoquatur. Prima enim decoctio fit in stomacho, secunda in hepate, tertia in omnibus membris.' *Sde* vi. 16, 310[4]–311[1]. Cf. Bartholomaeus Anglicus, *De proprietatibus rerum* 5.39 for the information concerning the disagreement between the Galenic and Aristotelian approaches; Pierre Bersuire, *Reductorium morale* i. 20, 21[2].

ecclesiastical *auctoritates* until the end of the century.[78] Our three figures demonstrate the continuing development in preachers' style, which by the turn of the thirteenth century allows and even encourages the introduction of profane *auctoritates* into the sermon.

The 110 similes from *Sde* VI enumerated in the Appendix are saturated with technical medical knowledge and show Giovanni's familiarity with current medical material. He was not merely a name-dropper. Sixty-three of the similes appear in *Sde* VI without a specific medical attribution; yet, of its 78 chapters, there is hardly one which does not include a reference to one medical authority. The breakdown of the references reveals a distinctive distribution of the authorities. Constantinus Africanus is the most frequently cited source for anatomical and physiological observations, with 31 references, while Avicenna (or an intermediate source which cites him) is Giovanni's main source for diseases, with 28 references. Galen is cited seven times, and, together with the five citations of Hippocrates, we obtain twelve citations in all of the Greek medical authorities. Aristotle is mentioned eight times as a medical source; anonymous *medici* or *physici* are referred to three times. Haly is mentioned twice and Johannitius, Averoes, Al-Ghazali, Isidore (as a medical source; Giovanni makes frequent use of his texts in other contexts), Ambrose, and Varro are mentioned once each. The popularity of Avicenna at that period, particularly in Italy, may well explain his frequent appearance in Giovanni's book. In making so much use of Constantinus Africanus Giovanni was wholly traditional, since the *Pantegni* in particular had a powerful impact on thirteenth-century encyclopaedias. Giovanni is also familiar with the debate among academic physicians about the differences between the Aristotelian and the Galenic approaches to the prime organ(s) and the process of conception. He attempts to harmonize them in order to anchor his similes in firm scientific theory.

Giovanni prides himself on citing only from great thinkers. He makes it clear that he employs this knowledge not in order to turn natural science into faith but in order to extract from it useful and instructive material. He argues that in their moral treatises, theologians and great philosophers have often effectively employed incredible fables. Therefore one certainly should not reject lessons from nature, which are always true.[79]

[78] R. H. Rouse and M. A. Rouse, *Preachers Florilegia and Sermons: Studies on the Manipulus florum of Thomas of Ireland* (Toronto, 1979), 74.

[79] *Sde* Prol., 4[1].

It was this interest in the real, concrete dimension of the simile that made the introduction of medical and other scientific authorities useful, indeed essential: the only way to demonstrate the truth of the example from nature was to base it on recognized scientific authority.

Giovanni could have drawn his medical knowledge directly from medical treatises, from older encyclopaedic sources, or from contemporary concordances.[80] Since it appears that the mendicants were not particularly interested in building up a medical section in their libraries, whether for study or for practice,[81] the question of Giovanni's sources is all the more interesting. A close comparison between the medical matter in *Sde* and Bartholomaeus Anglicus's *De proprietatibus rerum* v–vii[82] reveals similarities sufficiently distinctive to conclude that Giovanni drew many of his Constantinus and Aristotle citations from Bartholomaeus (d. 1272).[83] Constantinus was the most frequently cited medical source in Bartholomaeus, which would explain his predominance in *Sde*. However, Bartholomaeus was not Giovanni's source for Avicenna: most of his disease similes may have been taken directly from Avicenna's *Liber canonis* or from another encyclopaedic collection which I have not located. Giovanni's audience probably did not realize that much of his medical knowledge was second-hand, since he, like other preachers, never cited his precise source. Nor did he mention

[80] There is no sign that Giovanni used the medical concordances of Jean de St Amand (Johannes de Sancto Amando, *c.*1261–*c.*1312) who learnt and taught philosophy and medicine in Paris. Neither did Giovanni use *Liber de natura rerum* of the Flemish Dominican Thomas Cantimpratensis (de Cantimpré) (d. *c.*1276), whose first book was devoted to human anatomy, or Vincent de Beauvais's *Speculum maius* (*Speculum naturale* xxviii and *Speculum doctrinale* xii–xiv).

[81] The borrowing record from the Barcelona Dominican House 1255–77 shows no evidence for the presence of medical books; no medical books are recorded in the 1278 catalogue of Lucca, *c.*1277 Pisa, 1307 Dijon, and 1386 Bologna. K. W. Humphreys, 'The Medical Books of the Mediaeval Friars', *Libri*, 3 (1954), 95–103.

[82] On the medical sources of Bartholomaeus Anglicus, *De proprietatibus rerum*, see M. C. Seymour, *Bartholomaeus Anglicus and His Encyclopaedia* (London, 1992), 23–5, 59–76, 87–96. On Bartholomaeus Anglicus see F. Getz, 'The Faculty of Medicine', in J. I. Catto and R. Evans (ed.), *The History of the University of Oxford*, ii: Late Medieval Oxford (Oxford, 1992), 376–7, and R. French and A. Cunningham, *Before Science: The Invention of the Friars' Natural Philosophy* (Aldershot, 1996), 212–18.

[83] For example: *Sde* vi. 62 uses the simile of the forehead and quotes Constantinus, Aristotle; Bartholomaeus, v. 10 cites the same sources almost literally and adds also Haly. *Sde* vi. 30 employs the simile of bone-marrow and relies on Constantinus and Varro, who are quoted verbatim in Bartholomaeus, v. 58. The story about Orpheus which appears in the voice simile *Sde* vi. 25, 317³ appears in Bartholomaeus, v. 23 with exact reference to the *Viaticum*, etc.

Bartholomaeus in his prologue. Preachers who used such a manual would cite a medical piece of knowledge 'according to Avicenna, Constantinus or Galen' and would not add 'as cited by Bartholomaeus Anglicus'. Without a reference to Bartholomaeus in the prologue, preachers who used the *Sde*, and certainly their audience regarded the medical knowledge exposed to them as originating from a primary source.

This is true also of Pierre Bersuire's *Reductorium morale*.[84] Though acknowledging his indebtedness to Bartholomaeus in the prologue and sporadically throughout the text, he presented his medical authorities as primary sources of the same kind as the Bible and the Fathers. This can be seen in the layout of the text and in its content. Thus in MS Oxford, Bodleian Library, Douce 177, which contains the first ten books of the *Reductorium*, medical authors and titles are rubricated in the same way as the patristic and biblical sources, and the citations are underlined in red. When discussing the duration of the period of formation of the foetus (46 days for males, and longer for females) Bersuire supports the information by saying 'as says Galen in *On the Aphorisms*, Augustine in *On John* and Constantine in *Pantegni*', thus surrounding Augustine by two medical authorities and treating all three as equally important.[85] The extensive citation of medical sources by name does not prove that clerics actually used academic medical texts for religious purposes; nevertheless, it is evident that the preachers who drew on Giovanni's or Bersuire's books made an effort to anchor their arguments in scientific medical knowledge, and that in so doing they inevitably conferred a degree of religious significance on medical authorities.

The works of Giovanni, Servasanto, and Bersuire shed distinctive light on the relationship between medicine and religion in the early fourteenth century. If Arnau reveals how easy and natural it was for a physician to cross into the field of religious discourse, they show that amongst some clerics there was a tendency to annex medicine to the religious debate. In doing so they were not interested in becoming directly involved in medical practice but in promoting the effective presentation of a variety of religious messages. The outcome of this movement was religious language

---

[84] See p. 207 below. I used the 1583 Venice edition of the *Reductorium*. This edition includes the first fourteen books, since it was common to bind separately the two last books (which include the often cited moralized Ovide). On the *Reductorium*, see C. Samaran, 'Pierre Bersuire, prieur de Saint Éloi de Paris', *Histoire littéraire de la France*, 39 (1962), 304–49, and on the four first books which I have used, ibid. 304–25.

[85] 'sicut dicit Galenus super Aphorismos, Augustinus super Iohannem, et Constantinus in Pantegni'. *Reductorium*, iii. 2, 67².

saturated with high-level medical language, which does not thereby automatically indicate that the author had any professional ties with medicine.
Yet this pattern of expressing religious themes helps to explain why some
physicians dared to imitate it and then encroach on the clerical domain: it
legitimized and facilitated spiritual activity among physicians.

Is the pattern revealed by Giovanni and Servasanto a development
specifically associated with the turn of the thirteenth century? Was it a consequence of a growing public interest in medicine at a time when medicine
was recognized as a science and beginning to assert its prestige? To answer
these questions demands comparisons with earlier periods which go beyond
the scope of this book. But in order to locate texts such as Giovanni's *Sde* in
their historical context, I shall offer a few earlier examples of the employment of medical knowledge for religious and moral purposes.

Book vi of Rabanus Maurus's monumental encyclopaedia *De universo*
or *De rerum naturis* attempted to use the physiology of the body to convey religious messages.[86] Rabanus organized his encyclopaedia entirely
within the framework of Christian cosmology, and intended it to be a
clerical tool for scriptural interpretation. Unlike Isidore's encyclopaedia,
which sought to sum up the knowledge of antiquity, Rabanus compiled
the *De universo* to lay the basis for a universal Christian science of biblical studies. For physical and material information it was based on Isidore
of Seville's *Etymologies*, and for mystical insights it was based on the
anonymous allegorical glossary, *Clavis sacre scripture*. Although this
Carolingian text may appear remote in time and irrelevant, it does have
structural and thematic similarities with Giovanni's work which permit
cautious comparison. Like Giovanni, Rabanus starts his book with the
notions of outward and inward man as provided by 2 Corinthians 4: 16,
giving similar philosophical and religious premises for the two books.
Rabanus also gives moral/religious interpretations of every bodily organ
from head to toe. But here the similarity ends. Rabanus begins with the
concrete, the physical, and moves quicky to the mystical. While Giovanni
attempts to anchor every simile in updated medical knowledge, Rabanus
gives etymological explanations, and his mystical interpretation of the
organs of the body is clearly non-scientific. Eyes are called *oculi* because
they are covered by lashes which hide them (*occultare*) and defend them
from accidental harm or damage; they also store a hidden interior light

---

[86] *PL* III, 137–80; F. S. Paxton, 'Curing Bodies—Curing Souls: Hrabanus Maurus,
Medical Education and the Clergy in Ninth-Century Francia', *Journal of the History of
Medicine and Allied Sciences*, 50 (1995), 246–50.

(*occultus lumen*) which explains their essential role in creating understanding. Of all sense organs they are nearest to the soul, because in them
lies the power of judgement (*judicium mentis*). Unlike Giovanni, Rabanus
is not interested in the structure of the eye, but founds his simile on functional analogy. He then discusses the eye as an organ of sight, physical
and interior/spiritual (*visus cordis*), relying solely on scriptural quota-
tions.[87] Unlike Giovanni, he rarely introduces learned medical allusions.[88]
Thus the difference between Giovanni's approach and that of Rabanus is
great, and may be partially explained by the fact that most of the texts
that Giovanni cited through the medium of encyclopaedias were as yet
unknown in the Carolingian period. If this is so, then perhaps the appearance of new encyclopaedias in the middle of the thirteenth century
played an important role in making technical medical knowledge accessible to preachers.

Two twelfth-century moralistic sources seem to be close in certain
particulars to *Sde*, having emerged in a century which witnessed the
revival of humoral characterology in Western natural philosophy and the
free exploitation of comparisons and similes as a preaching technique.[89]
The first is *De medicina anime* by the Augustinian canon Hugues de
Fouilloy (Hugo de Folieto 1100/1110–1172/3).[90] Hugues explains the
macrocosm through the human microcosm by reference to the theory of
elements, the humoral doctrine, temperaments, seasons, and astrology.
He also twice names Hippocrates as his source.[91] In these respects he predates Giovanni, whose text was more developed.

---

[87] Rabanus Maurus, *De universo*, PL 111, 148. The jaws are called 'maxilie per diminu-
tionem a malis sicut paxillus a palo, taxillus a talo'. They therefore signify the teachers of
the Church and the corporeal discipline by which the disobedient are coerced (cols.151–2).
Bone-marrow is called 'Medulle . . . quod modefaciant ossa. Irrigant enim et confortant.'
It signifies internal thoughts (col.164). Every such description is founded on scriptural
verses.

[88] For example, after a very short definition of the pupil and its importance to sight,
Rabanus adds: 'Physici dicunt easdem pupillas quas videmus in oculis, morituros ante
triduum non habere, quibus non visis certa est desperatio'. Ibid. col. 150.

[89] R. Klibansky, E. Panowsky, and F. Saxl, *Saturn and Melancholy: Studies in the History
of Natural Philosophy, Religion and Art* (London, 1964), 102–11; Agrimi and Crisciani,
Medicina del corpo, 40–53; D'Avray, *The Preaching of the Friars*, 225–39.

[90] Hugues de Fouilloy, *De medicina anime*, PL 176: 1183–1202; on Hugues, see in W. B.
Clark, *The Medieval Book of Birds: Hugh of Fouilloy's Aviarium* (Philadelphia, 1992), 5–9;
Agrimi and Crisciani, *Medicina del corpo*, 43–5.

[91] See n. 47 above; *De medicina anime*, PL 176: 1185 ('Dicunt enim physici sanguineos
esse dulces', applying the humoral doctrine to ethical and religious disposition), 1190 (on
the role of the spleen as the hothouse for black choler and as the cause of melancholy), and
1195–8 (the nine Hippocratic signs for health), which appear almost literally in *Sde* x. 74,
485³–487⁴.

The second twelfth-century source is Guillaume de Saint-Thierry's 'On the Nature of Body and Soul' (*De natura corporis et anime*).[92] Guillaume's anthropology is distinctive in giving a separate and important role to the material component of man. If a thorough investigation of the human microcosm within and without reveals its beautiful unity and harmonious order, and if through this knowledge we may partially understand the Creator of all things, then medical knowledge acquires a religious significance. Guillaume stresses that the physiological part of his work relies on the work of philosophers and physicians (*ex parte philosophorum vel phisicorum*).[93] He exploits Constantinus's *Pantegni* throughout the work without specifically naming it. He cites Hippocrates in his discussion of the elements, and he refers directly to Constantinus's *Liber graduum* in his treatment of digestion.[94] Unlike Giovanni, Guillaume discusses the outward man solely in terms of the perfection, unity, and harmony which he discerns in him: for Guillaume it is the body as a whole which has a religious significance, not the individual organs. Yet he is anxious to emphasize that physicians and philosophers who have elevated the outward man have failed to comprehend the true dignity of the inner man made in the image of God. He urges his readers to advance from the body to the soul, to go beyond what philosophers or scientists of the world think or guess about it, and to consider what the Catholic fathers have learned from God.[95] He then devotes the rest of the work to what the body teaches us about the various parts of the soul and their function.

Despite the difficulties of comparing different types of literary genres, a comparison of Rabanus, Hugues, Guillaume, and Giovanni, who shared a common moralizing goal, can yield significant insight into the use of medical language in a religious/moral context. Rabanus shows that using the human body as a source of moral speculation was conventional at least as early as the Carolingian period. Hugues demonstrates the comfortable accommodation of the doctrine of humours within the philosophical and theological discourse of the twelfth century. Guillaume

[92] Guillaume de Saint-Thierry, *De natura corporis et animae*, ed. M. Lemoine (Paris, 1988); B. McGinn (ed.), *Three Treatises on Man: A Cistercian Anthropology* (Kalamazoo, 1977), 101–52 (English trans.); at 1–34 a discussion of Guillaume's medical sources.

[93] Guillaume de Saint-Thierry, *De natura corporis*, 69 (McGinn, 103).

[94] Ibid. 75 (McGinn, 106). Elsewhere when speaking of veins which lead blood to the spleen, of the role of the lungs for the expansion and contraction of the heart, and of the protective membranes for the brain, he is satisfied with anonymous 'medici' or 'physici' as sources. Ibid. 85, 93–5, 105 (McGinn, 110, 113, 117).

[95] Ibid. 123, 127 (McGinn, 123).

actually stresses that his medical knowledge relies on medical authorities. Thus Giovanni and other preachers around 1300 were following a well-trodden path and represent a new pitch of development rather than a new technique. Giovanni and his contemporaries employed a much wider range of medical topics, and introduced more sophisticated examples and citations from recognized medical authorities. Like their predecessors, preachers around 1300 compared the small world (the body) with the greater world (the universe). Both are presided over by a supreme spirit (*spiritus summus*, the soul in the body and God in the universe), both contain inanimate parts (*partes non viventes*, humours and nails for the body, terrestrial or celestial bodies in the universe), parts that are senseless (*partes non sentientes*, hair and bones in the body, plants and vegetating objects in the universe), parts that lack understanding (*partes non intelligentes*—the acting organs, *membra officialia*, in the small world, beasts in the larger), and an intellective power (*virtus intellectiva*). The human heart which supplies the body with sense and motion, and the divinely created firmament which gives life and motion to the world below, are both firstly generated bodies which exert maximal influence and occupy the centre of the cosmos (*corpus generatione primum, et influentia maximum, locum occupans medium*).[96] Yet the preachers were not merely fascinated by the anatomy and physiology of the body as proofs for divine perfection and intelligence. By the end of the thirteenth century, medical knowledge served to illuminate more than the macrocosm/microcosm analogy so popular in the twelfth century; it was applied to particular facets of human life and religion, and became a comprehensive language for conveying religious messages. The human body and the scientific knowledge which deciphered it became key didactic tools for exposing the faithful to the Christian faith and for guiding them into orthodox practice. This development coincided with the growing prestige of medicine as a scientific and academic discipline, though this circumstantial connection between the two cultural processes still needs to be substantiated.

This diachronic view demands a synchronic one as well. Is Giovanni's 'stock metaphorique' common to other preachers of his time? The examples I have cited from Servasanto da Faenza and other preachers suggest that it was. Yet are we facing here what is primarily a local, mendicant phenomenon confined to urban, Tuscan communities where there was a

---

[96] Servasanto da Faenza, *Antidotarius animarum*, fol. 20^r–22^v. Aristotle supported by Isidore and Rabanus are cited as the scientific sources for this description.

lay public with intellectual interests? My argument that these medical tropes illustrate a development taking off in the twelfth century, on a rising curve in the later thirteenth and early fourteenth centuries, may be supported by reference to a later example and from a slightly different geographical and denominational setting. Pierre Bersuire (Berchorius, Bercheure, d. 1362),[97] a Benedictine monk active during the pontificates of John XXII, Benedict XII, and Clement VI, produced two major compilations in the 1320s and 1330s; the *Reductorium morale*, probably composed between 1325 and 1337, and the *Repertorium morale*, probably composed between 1335 and 1342. The *Repertorium* includes several thousand words extracted from the Bible, organized alphabetically and interpreted morally. The *Reductorium* displays (among many other things) medical knowledge in a theological context. Like all the authors hitherto considered, Bersuire observes nature and attempts to unravel its true meaning for the benefit of all the faithful.[98] Thus, since nature promotes faith, medical science, along with other disciplines, acquires a moral and religious significance. The first four books of the *Reductorium* are saturated with medical references (see Appendix II), and their inner structure is meticulously arranged along thematic lines. The first book moralizes on general medical terms and concepts such as humours, complexions, and qualities; the second, on the organs of the body from the head to the legs; the third, on the seven non-natural things essential for good health; and the fourth on diseases.

Bersuire's encyclopaedia, compiled a generation after that of Giovanni, provides us with another example of moralized *exempla* containing high-level medical language. His work contains all the elements discussed in relation to Giovanni's *Sde*, thereby suggesting that the pattern of expression revealed in *Sde* was not a particularly Italian or mendicant phenomenon. Nevertheless, though the style of moralizing is similar to Giovanni's, the medical analogies are more detailed and bear specific reference to the

---

[97] On Bersuire see *DS* 12/2, 1508–10; Samaran, 'Pierre Bersuire', 259–450; J.-Th. Welter, *L'Exemplum dans la littérature religieuse et didactique du Moyen Âge* (Paris, 1927), 345–9; J. Engels, 'Berchoriana', *Vivarium*, 2 (1964), 62–124. Bersuire has an entry in Wickersheimer's *Dictionnaire biographique des médecins en France au Moyen Âge* (Geneva, 1936), 617, though there is no evidence for his affiliation to the medical profession.

[98] '[E]go videns quod omnis natura gaudet bonum sibi concessum aliis communicare et bonorum suorum participem invenire, non solum mihi laborare volui sed ad utilitatem omnium fidelium labores meos ordinare contendi.' He describes this work as nothing but 'quedam morales reductiones quedamque proprietatum moralizationes et quedam exemplares applicationes quibus scilicet conditiones virtutum et vitiorum possint ostendi et quibus exemplis et figuris mediantibus possint illa que ad fidem et mores pertinent manu duci.' *Reductorium*, Prol., 1$^{1-2}$.

medical authorities. Unlike Giovanni, Bersuire specifies in the prologue that he is very much indebted to Bartholomaeus Anglicus as the primary source for his scientific knowledge, and indeed, both the structure of the *Reductorium* and the individual medical citations are taken directly from Bartholomaeus's *De proprietatibus rerum*.[99] Bersuire occasionally refers to the *Magister de proprietatibus rerum*, and apologizes that for the sake of brevity he has omitted many medical details concerning the topic under discussion.[100] Unlike Giovanni, Bersuire often provides precise references to his medical sources, scarcely mentions Avicenna when speaking about diseases, and discusses cures, not just symptoms.

None of the authors mentioned in this section ever referred to contemporary physicians in their analogies; but on one occasion Bersuire cites Arnau de Vilanova, active around 50 years before himself. Bersuire identifies melancholics with those who hold false, deceptive, and vain beliefs. One of the medical authorities he introduces when describing the peculiar behaviour of the melancholic is 'Magister Arnaldus de Villa Nova'. According to Bersuire, Arnau treated a melancholic patient who did not eat because he thought he was already dead (and the dead do not eat). Arnau dressed himself in black, pretended to be dead, and invited the patient to go with him to the cemetery, where other friends dressed in black and pretending to be dead stood eating lavishly. He invited the patient to join the feast and thus cured him (perhaps not of the depression but of the syndrome of self-starvation). The story is indeed taken from Arnau's *De parte operativa*, though it has acquired some dramatic elements which are absent in Arnau's original text.[101]

Bersuire's analogical use of medical material is similar to Giovanni's, but it provides the user with a larger choice of signified objects for every signifier. A bodily organ or a disease can signify several things, some of which may be diametrically opposed to each other. Choler, for example, denotes zeal and the severity of justice. However, it may also denote the

---

[99] Samaran, 'Pierre Bersuire', 316; for the other authorities he uses see ibid. 320–2.

[100] *Reductorium*, iii. 2, 87².

[101] 'De alio vero qui tempore magistri arnaldi de villa nova, mortuum se credebat nolloque modo comedere volebat asserens quod mortui comedere non debebant. Idem tamen magister assumpta veste nigra mortuum se finxit et sub illo colore ipsum infirmum ad cimiterium duxit, ubi alios socios nigro vestitos splendide comedentes stare disposuerat, ipsosque mortuos comedere, asseruit, et sic eorum exemplo ipsum infirmum caute ad comedendum invitavit et ita eum sanavit.' *Reductorium*, i. 23, 25² (cf. MS Oxford, Bod. Lib., Douce 177, fol. 28ᵛ). Cf. Arnau de Vilanova, *De parte operativa*, fol. 128ᵛᵇ: 'Nam si mortuum seipsum imaginetur et inde cibos abhorreat alius siccus mortuus associetur et se propter mortuum asserens eum concomitans cibos tamen in eius presentia comedens.'

heat of anger, lust, avarice, and envy.[102] Thus preachers could use their discretion in choosing analogies. Bersuire apparently used examples from nature to express harsh criticism of the clergy (prelates, confessors, and preachers).[103] The medical model thus enabled him explicitly to draw out notions which otherwise he could not openly utter. The upward curve in the use of higher medical language which started in the patristic period and moved through Rabanus and the twelfth-century texts did not stop with Giovanni. Bersuire shows that the development of medical discourse in the religious context progressed even further, becoming more detailed and sophisticated and betraying a growing inclination to buttress the analogy by specific medical sources.

My treatment of sermon literature has necessarily been incomplete. The preaching sources I have used essentially provide accessory material which could be fitted into a sermon. *Sde*, *Reductorium*, and Servasanto's *Summa* and *Antidotarius* are encyclopaedias that introduce medical tropes in a deliberate and self-conscious way, giving us a less balanced idea of the overall structure and pattern of thought of the speaker and his audience than the actual sermons.[104] To amend this bias it will be necessary to check the sermons themselves more carefully, and to examine the use of similes in actual preaching. Medical knowledge based on explicitly cited authorities did enter Giovanni's sermons.[105] More such examples should be investigated, and possible differences between various kinds of sermons (whether vernacular or Latin, whether academic and targeting the clergy or directed at the laity and targeting specific social groups), should be taken into consideration.[106]

Throughout this section I have alluded to the possible influence of medical similes on the public perception and the self-image of the physician. I interpreted the borrowing of medical concepts and subject matter

---

[102] *Reductorium*, i. 22, 24^1; ii. 21, 42^1–43^1, which deals with the throat and offers a variety of moral interpretations preceded by: 'Si vis dicere . . .; sed si vis . . .' or 'potes intelligi . . . vel dic . . .'

[103] In *Reductorium*, ii. 31, 49^1–50^1, blood instead of milk in the breast signifies the carnality which characterizes many of the clergy. In *Reductorium*, iv. 1, 87 the loss of hair which is part of a skin condition called *eruginosa squamositas* signifies clerics who lapse as a result of the bad examples (fumes) of prelates (head). In *Reductorium* iv. 9, 91^2–93^1, paralysis is caused by a failure of nerves, which signify prelates; when they abuse their function the other organs of the Christian body lose their motion.

[104] D'Avray, *The Preaching of the Friars*, 82.

[105] See 'The Vocabulary of Disease' in Ch. 2, pp. 109–11.

[106] See, e.g. N. Bériou and F. O. Touati, *Voluntate dei leprosus: les lépreux entre conversion et exclusion aux XIIème et XIIIème siècles* (Spoleto, 1991) who show how the study of *ad status* sermons can highlight changing social attitudes towards lepers.

as creating an atmosphere conducive to the participation of physicians in religious debate. I also argued that it could confer on human physicians an element of religious authority. Now some broader conclusions concerning the audience may be essayed.

First, the texts I have used in this section suggest an audience keen to acquire deep, scientific, and subtle explanations from their preachers. Second, the manuals of Giovanni, Servasanto, and Bersuire suggest that medical knowledge was widely diffused throughout society.[107] Temperaments, the humours, the humoral imbalance theory of pathology, and the basic therapeutic devices were all common intellectual currency by then. Since physicians judged the health of patients by the patients' own account of their illness, inevitably the two parties began to share a common vocabulary. Third, the writings I have discussed show that religious discourse may also have helped to popularize academic medical terms. Sermons were one of the major means of mass communication, and they introduced Scripture and the heritage of Christian thought to the unlearned or unlettered. The use of scientific *auctoritates* in sermons to lend weight to the preacher's conclusions helped to introduce the profane sciences to the masses also. Dominican friars played an important role in diffusing Aristotle and the 'new learning' in the Italian towns to a lay urban audience well versed in various modes of civic rhetoric;[108] similarly, Giovanni, Servasanto, and Bersuire conveyed their medical knowledge to large audiences which encompassed both the clergy and the laity. In the prologue to *Sde* Giovanni explains that, by the aid of *exempla*, spiritual and refined things are revealed to the senses, since all our knowledge originates from sense perception (*omnis nostra scientia oritur ab sensu*). This is the way to expose the people (*vulgus* and *simplices*) to such sophisticated knowledge.[109] The passage from

[107] For a similar conclusion concerning Renaisssance society, see J. Henry, 'Doctors and Healers: Popular Culture and the Medical Profession', in *Science, Culture and Popular Belief in Renaissance Europe*, ed. S. Pumfrey, P. L. Rossi, and M. Slawinski (Manchester, 1991), 191–221. For the widespread use of medical imagery in late-fourteenth-century and fifteenth-century English sermons see Rawcliffe, *Medicine and Society*, 17–21, 216–18.

[108] D. L. D'Avray, 'Sermons on the Dead before 1350', *Studi Medievali*, 31 (1990), 215–16; C. Delcorno, 'La predicazione volgare in Italia (sec. XIII–XIV). Teoria, produzione, ricezione', *Revue Mabillon*, 65 (1993), 83–107.

[109] 'non eos tantum apud curiosos auditores faciet gratiosos quos mira nature opera vel humane inventionis studia narrata et patefacta delectant, sed etiam apud vulgus et simplices fructuosos et acceptos constituet, dum per exempla ad sensum spritualia et subtilia declarabunt.' *Sde*, prol., 3[3]. At the beginning of his *Sermones de sanctis* he similarly says: 'quasdam predicationes conscribere magis congruas ad predicandum in populo quam forte ad sermonicandum in clero.' MS Florence, Bibl. Naz., Conv. Soppr. J. I 41, fol. 1[ra] (cited in Delcorno, 'La predicazione volgare', 86 n. 13).

the sensible to the spiritual, from the concrete to the abstract, was a constant feature of medieval religious thinking. To this phenomenon Giovanni, Servasanto, and Bersuire contribute their unique style which is based on a literary borrowing of scientific material, whether directly from the original text or by way of summaries and encyclopaedias. All this blurred the apparent dichotomy between metaphorical and logical reasoning. The result was both to medicinalize religious discourse and to turn medicine, even in its scientific form, into a branch of theology.

Focusing on Giovanni's or Bersuire's use of medical subject matter and authorities should not blind us to the large areas of other scientific knowledge they were using. Had I used *Sde* i, I might have concluded that Giovanni 'astrologizes' his religious discourse, *Sde* ii that he 'mineralizes' it, or *Sde* iii to v that he 'zoologizes' or 'biologizes' it. So is there anything unique about the medical similes? *Sde* generally regards physical nature as a source of divine truths and messages. When it comes to questions of faith and morals, Christ remains the main inward model (*intrinsecus exemplar*); however, nature as the outward model (*exemplar extrinsecus*) is almost as effective. The principle that 'the act of seeing is equivalent to the instruction of the soul' (*oculorum visio est mentis eruditio*) was fundamental to Giovanni's thinking, and did not privilege the body or medicine over the other arts.[110] In this respect Giovanni, Bersuire, Sevasanto, and Arnau were alike in regarding natural phenomena as symbolizing and reflecting each other and the divine, and their incorporation into the religious domain becomes desirable and even essential. Since comprehending nature amounts to comprehending God and his precepts, analogy based on resemblance (*similitudo*) of all natural objects and phenomena becomes a vehicle by which to construct a legitimate discussion of divine matters. Thus in *Sde* i, Ptolemy is the main cited source but a whole variety of other, mainly classical sources is employed; while in *Sde* ii Dioscorides, and in *Sde* iii to v and vii Aristotle, are the main cited scientific sources. The use of medical sources and subject-matter in a spiritual context is thus in itself not unique, and should be interpreted as part of the general change in attitude towards nature. It is also part of a growing philosophical sophistication which characterizes the writings of mendicant preachers towards the end of the thirteenth century.

Though I cannot prove that there was anything unique in Giovanni's

---

[110] *Sde*, Prol., 3^{2-3}. *Geistliche Aspekte mittelalterlicher Naturlehre*, ed. B. K. Vollmann (Wiesbaden, 1993).

employment of medical knowledge, I would like to make three observations which suggest that this may have been the case. First, in all the other non-medical books of *Sde*, Giovanni hardly attempts to demonstrate his knowledge of recent developments in the particular science. Most of his sources are classical, and the few new texts he uses (mainly translations of Arabic sources) merely serve to underline their general absence. Only in *Sde* viii, dealing with law, does Giovanni seem conversant with new medieval sources, especially Hostiensis. The preference he accords to the two advanced academic disciplines seems to be intentional. Similes from other fields of knowledge are usually confined in *Sde* to an anecdotal level. When dealing with medicine he tries to introduce sound and sometimes very dry observations.

Second, no other field of scientific knowledge provides so coherent and comprehensive a model of description and explanation as medicine. The medical subject-matter of the body, the medical practitioner, the patient, and the curing process acquire moral and religious significance. The other sources of scientific figurative language did not rely on the powerful and ancient congruence between God or Christ and the expert practitioner in that particular science. In medicine, this resulted in a complex reciprocal sign/signified relationship which endowed the real physician with a quasi-religious aura and gave his science its peculiar role in religious discourse. And third, the sermons I have discussed in this section suggest that medical imagery was a more powerful source of figurative language than other types of images. While the Bible and Christian theology always remain the substructure in the sermons, the auxiliary role of medical imagery is unique.

Giovanni, Servasanto, and Bersuire use a much higher-level medical language than Arnau. The particular characteristic of their approach is the use of relatively high-quality medical similes adorned with frequent and accurate citations from medical authorities. They all seem to have made a sincere attempt to convey a picture which would agree with current scientific knowledge. As a 'control' for my study of Arnau, these three authors shed new light on physicians who were inclined to theologize; for, when high-level medical language becomes a commonplace in religious discourse, the entrance of physicians into the clerical realm becomes understandable and even natural. Furthermore, the preachers' writings show that high-level medical language was common currency and cannot automatically be related to the medical background of the author. Arnau's 'medical language' differed from that of the preachers in some aspects. He was overwhelmingly loyal to medicine as the main source of his figurative language, and neither relied on encyclopaedias nor gave a moral interpretation to his medical examples. His densely used anatomical and pathological images were intercalated spontaneously into his spiritual writing, constituting an exterior expression of the medical way in which he approached spiritual problems as a physician who cures the spiritual disease of the Christian body.

It will be necessary to consult other sources for further evidence of more spontaneous and unforced use of medical imagery in order to validate the broader hypothesis of a growing use of medical subject-matter in religious discourse in this period. The three authors I have discussed, however, provide us with a powerful example of the fusion between religion and medicine at the turn of the thirteenth century. The medical model, as one of several 'calculi of thought' in preaching manuals of the period, provides ample evidence for the combination of abstract and concrete modes of thought in the genre of preaching literature. Medieval medical knowledge as a cultural agent seems to have possessed a reality of its own, and to have informed or shaped the human experience as much as it was informed or shaped by it.

5

Medicine and Religion:
Between Competition and Cooperation

So far I have shown how the medical profession contributed to, and sometimes initiated, religious speculation in two learned physicians, and, more
generally, how it provided the clergy with a vocabulary for discussing a
variety of moral and theological issues. But is this account compatible with
the notion that a long-lasting tension and antagonism between physicians
and clerics first became detectable in the early Christian period?[1] Do the
medical writings ascribed to Arnau prove potential or actual friction with
parallel clerical attitudes and practice? After a brief description of clerical
attitudes to physicians and human cure in the early Christian period
(stressing in particular the critical aspects of these attitudes), I shall outline the major foci of potential tension between clerics and physicians in
the thirteenth century, and examine their expression in Arnau's texts.
Every subsection in this chapter justifies an independent study. Rather
than exhaustively analysing each topic, I intend to use Arnau's medical
and spiritual texts, as well as some of the apocryphal ones to chart the
main paths which further research could follow.

The Historical Context

It is illuminating to start this brief historical introduction to the alleged
tensions between physicians and clerics with an anachronistic digression.

---

[1] Of the vast literature on the religious aspects of ancient medicine I have used V.
Nutton, 'Murders and Miracles: Lay Attitudes towards Medicine in Classical Antiquity',
in *Patients and Practitioners*, ed. R. Porter (Cambridge, 1985), 23–53, and 'From Galen to
Alexander: Aspects of Medicine and Medical Practice in Late Antiquity', *Dumbarton Oaks
Paper*, 38 (1984), 1–14 (esp. 5–8); L. G. Westernik, 'Philosophy and Medicine in the Late
Antiquity', *Janus*, 51 (1964), 169–77; D. W. Amundsen, *Medicine, Society and Faith in the
Ancient and Medieval Worlds* (Baltimore and London, 1996), *passim* and esp. 1–29, 127–57,
175–221; D. W. Amundsen and G. B. Ferngren, 'Medicine and Religion: Early Christianity
through the Middle Ages', in M. E. Marty and K. L. Vaux (ed.), *Health/Medicine and the
Faith Traditions: An Inquiry into Religion and Medicine* (Philadelphia, 1982), 93–131; G. B.
Ferngren, 'Early Christianity as a Religion of Healing', *Bulletin of the History of Medicine*,
66 (1992), 1–15; S. R. Ell, 'Concepts of Disease and the Physician in the Early Middle
Ages', *Janus*, 65 (1978), 153–65; F. Kudlien, 'Der Arzt des Körpers und der Arzt der
Seele', *Clio Medica*, 3 (1968), 1–21.

In November 1858 John Henry Newman addressed the students of medicine at the recently founded Catholic University of Ireland.[2] Newman's lecture communicates a strong sense of competition between medicine and theology, between medical truth and superior religious truth, between the physician's orders and the priest's precepts, between the material and hence limited scope of medicine and the elevated, moral, and spiritual essence of religion. The mind and soul have legitimate sovereignty over the body, and in consequence the sciences relating to them take precedence over those sciences relating to the body, Newman tells the students in Dublin. As the soldier must yield to the statesman when they collide, so must the physician to the priest. When the indefinitely higher law of morals and religion comes to some different conclusion from the medical truth, religion must prevail, determines Newman, and he presents two examples for such a case. The first describes the Sister of Charity, who, for the sake of her soul, would not obey the law of self-preservation as regards her body, thus causing her medical adviser great irritation and disgust. The second example depicts a struggle between the priest and the physician attending a dying person. The priest wishes to perform his sacramental duty lest the patient die without due preparation; the physician says that the thought of religion will imperil the patient's recovery. In both cases, which reflect the two traditional loci of clerical suspicion towards physicians (Extreme Unction and medical therapy which is incompatible with a religious way of life), Newman confidently upholds the priest's right and duty to have the ultimate decision. Newman's fear of the immanent collision between medical men and priests reflects his struggle against the dangerous effects of secularism and the materialism accompanying it, on the Christian Catholic way of living. For him, bringing the Faculty of Medicine under the shadow of the Catholic Church is thus highly expedient and desirable. Are such notions of competition and collision between medicine and theology relevant to the European reality around 1300?

Though at first a religion of caring rather than curing, the Christian religion evolved into one of healing during the fourth century. It was not necessarily opposed to secular healing, but it presupposed an alternative medicine on which a true Christian might rely. God, the source both of healing substances and their application, gave these to men to relieve them from their ills. A man who recognized the true nature of his illness

[2] John Henry Cardinal Newman, 'Christianity and Medical Science: An Address to the Students of Medicine', in *The Idea of a University* (New York, 1968), 380–91.

(namely his sins) would first turn to Christ the *Medicus*, and beg for his cure. Christianity took over from pagan healing cults not only their function but also their language, their imagery, even their sites.[3] There was no rejection of Hippocratic and Galenic theories; but they were totally subordinated to God's will and the divine plan. Christ was the saviour on earth, the Real Physician to both soul and body who brought healing (*salus*) through salvation, and whose help was available to all believers at no financial cost.

From classical culture and philosophy Christian thinkers adopted the analogy of the body and the soul, the notion of a similarity between the training of the body and the discipline of the soul, and the consideration of medicine as a counterpart of ethics. The first known analogy between Christ and the physician appeared in *c*.110 with Ignatius of Antioch, who also spoke of Christ as an antidote to sins. This analogy gradually became more common during the second century on the basis of a strong competition with the cult of Asclepius, and the Stoic tradition which stressed the healing function of the philosopher as a physician to souls.[4]

The early apologists of Christianity laid stress on the effectiveness of Christian cures, and their message of hope to the sick was a major factor in the eventual triumph of Christianity over other cults. All patristic sources who discussed medical issues shared the notion that the use of medicine was not intrinsically inappropriate for Christians; but they placed significant limitations on Christians' recourse to human medical care. Divine omnipotence could cure through medicine or without it.[5] The existence of a specifically Christian method of healing and the explanation of disease as rooted in sin exacerbated a tension, already visible in the Jewish tradition, which appeared in different discussions among the early Fathers who took two approaches to secular healing within a Christian society. The boundaries separating the two approaches were diffuse, and thinkers sometimes used both of them.

The first, enunciated by Clement of Alexandria, Basil of Caesarea, and John Chrysostom, for example, proclaimed medicine to be laudable,

---

[3] K. H. Rengstorf, *Die Anfänge der Auseinandersetzung zwischen Christusglaube und Asklepiosfrömmigkeit* (Münster, 1953).

[4] G. Fichtner, 'Christus als Arzt. Ursprünge und Wirkungen eines Motivs', *Frühmittelalterliche Studien*, 16 (1982), 7; L. Edelstein, 'The Relation of Ancient Philosophy to Medicine', *Bulletin of the History of Medicine*, 26 (1952), 310 ff.

[5] D. W. Amundsen, 'Body, Soul and Physician', in *Medicine, Society, and Faith*, 6–7.

and espoused an obligation to care for the body. Medicine was a gift from God, and thus essential and beneficial to mankind. However, because they accepted the link between sickness and sin, and shared the view that the soul was of infinitely greater value than the body, even some adherents of this approach were ambivalent towards human medicine. For Jerome, health, though desirable, was a relative good. The health of the unrighteous was a gift of the devil. On the other hand, the sickness of the just was a cause for rejoicing, in that the spirit was made stronger and more perfect in the weakness of the flesh.[6] These clerics regarded disease as a testing time through which man might earn special rewards. They thus tended to seek moral rationalizations for illness and to submit medical phenomena totally to the omnipotent will of God. But how does a physician fit into a world in which God allows Christians to endure physical ills because such ailments heal the swelling of pride, test and prove patience, punish and eradicate sins, remind Christians of their mortality, and cause them to rely on God? A clear answer was not offered, but medicine and religion were interwoven in a manner which ruled out the independent activity of physicians. The emergence in late antiquity of a peculiarly Christian image of the body which was endowed with intrinsic, inalienable qualities vindicated medicine, especially *vis-à-vis* dualist tendencies which abhorred the body. The body became a sacrosanct temple, created by God, who allotted to it an important role in his divine plan at the price of medicine's submission to the control of religious authorities.[7]

The second approach was adopted by other Church Fathers who were hostile to classical culture and regarded physical medicine as incompatible with Christianity in its highest form.[8] Although few were as violent as Tatian (*fl.* 160–180), who regarded the use of drugs as apostasy,[9] members of this group argued that the medicine of the physicians was suitable for the average, ordinary Christian; but for those of higher religious capabilities (like ascetics and hermits), prayer, devotion, and faith alone sufficed. This approach stressed the moral and religious benefits of disease and allowed Cyprian, for example, to advise his African flock to welcome the plague of 252 as a proof of God's love and

---

[6] Jerome, *Epist.*, 39. 2, *CSEL* 54, 295–8; Augustine, *Epist.* 38. 1, *CSEL* 34, 64–5; D. W. Amundsen, 'Suicide and Early Christian Values', in *Medicine, Society, and Faith*, 84–5.

[7] P. R. L. Brown, *The Body and Society: Men, Women and Sexual Renunciation in Early Christianity* (London and Boston, 1987), 437–9.

[8] Origen, *Contra Celsum*, ed. H. Chadwick (Cambridge, 1980), 8. 60: 498.

[9] D. W. Amundsen, 'Tatian's "Rejection" of Medicine in the Second Century', in *Medicine, Society and Faith*, 158–74.

mercy.[10] The activity of God and the passivity of the Christian in death portrayed in these writings left no room for suicide,[11] but at the same time potentially limited the role of human medicine to cope with disease.

Occasionally this approach portrayed recourse to earthly medicine as a sign of faithlessness. Gregory of Tours, for example, describes a cleric suffering from cataract and eventually losing his eyesight. When the treatment of physicians is of no avail, he goes to the shrine of St Martin where he undergoes a treatment of fasts and flagellation. Apparently this treatment is more effective than the conventional one, for the archdeacon partially regains his eyesight and returns home. Yet there, on the advice of a Jewish physician, he undergoes further treatment, this time by cupping-glass. The result of the bleeding is catastrophic: he again loses his eyesight, and now the shrine of St Martin cannot improve this condition, for the faithless and ungrateful archdeacon is deemed unworthy of this celestial medicine. The lesson of the story is clear: if you benefit from divine medicine you should not require earthly medicine. Divine medicine starts when earthly medicine fails. For Gregory, asking for medical advice was sinful (that the physician was Jewish probably made it worse), for it signified a lack of faith and ingratitude towards the Lord.[12] The story reinforces the view that competition for healing power was rife in early medieval Europe where a great range of therapeutic paths was offered to the sick. Physicians and magicians, pagans and Jews, secular or regular priests, Christian holy men and women, the living and the dead were all competing for the same clients as suppliers of health care. Valerie Flint has examined the social competition for the role of the healer in early medieval society, and has shown that early medieval physicians and saints occasionally made common cause against non-Christian practices of medical magic.[13] In the

---

[10] Cyprian, *De mortalitate* 15, *CCSL* IIIa, 24. Tertullian, *De anima*, ed. J. H. Waszink (Amsterdam, 1947), 30. 4: 42, delighted in plague as one of God's cures for overpopulation. He was far from rejecting medicine and suggested that nature should be the primary source of knowledge in all questions of life (ibid. 27. 4: 38), expressed his support of physicians in their struggle against disease (ibid. 43. 8), and energetically rejected the Platonic notion of the body as a prison for the soul (ibid. 53. 5: 72).

[11] Amundsen, 'Suicide and Early Christian Values', in *Medicine, Society and Faith*, 86–90.

[12] Gregory of Tours, *Libri historiarum X*, v. 6 in *Monumenta Germaniae Historica, Scriptores rerum Merovingicarum* I/1, ed. B. Kursch (Hannover, 1951), 203. For a balanced overview of Gregory's attitudes to medicine see E. James, 'A Sense of Wonder: Gregory of Tours, Medicine and Science', in M. A. Meyer (ed.), *The Culture of Christendom: Essays in Medieval History in Commemoration of Denis L. T. Bethell* (London and Rio Grande, 1993), 45–60.

[13] V. I. J. Flint, 'The Early Medieval 'Medicus', the Saint—and the Enchanter', *Social History of Medicine*, 2 (1989), 127–45 and *The Rise of Magic in Early Medieval Europe* (Oxford, 1991), 301–28.

struggle against the non-Christian witch doctor and enchanter, two chan-nels proved particularly effective: monastic medicine (which involved medical learning, Christian healing powers of the priest and liturgy,[14] and organization and control of healing shrines) and deliberately Christianized magical compromises encouraged by the Church and its representatives.

Critical attitudes towards human medicine reappeared throughout future centuries, and were shared by prominent thinkers; yet they never entered the mainstream, and were generally confined to hermits, certain monastic communities, and mystics. Illness was thus prominent in women's spirituality. Many mystics saw physical anguish as an opportu-nity for their own salvation and that of others. Some even prayed for dis-ease as a gift from God or as a sign of divine love and care.[15]

Bernard of Clairvaux is an example of the survival of the second approach into the high middle ages. He strongly objected to the use of sec-ular medicine by monks. He was prepared to tolerate the use of common herbs, but criticized those who sought bodily medicine for committing acts inappropriate to their religious profession.[16] Such attitudes may explain the relative absence of medical books from lists associated with monastic infirm-aries. On the other hand, records of the infirmarer (*infirmarius*) suggest that, within monasteries, skilled medicine was supplied to the monks with-out obstacles, and refute the idea that monks were generally hostile towards medicine.[17] Bernard of Clairvaux did not represent the majority of monks.

Because such rejection still persisted in the thirteenth century, cleri-cal authors had specifically to endorse the use of medicine by monks. For example, Hugues de Saint-Cher's commentary on Ecclesiasticus 38: 1, 'him also God has established in his profession', determined that medi-cine had been established for our benefit (*utilitas*), and added: 'and here is a proof that members of religious Orders may consult physicians'.[18]

[14] F. S. Paxton, 'Liturgy and Healing in an Early Medieval Saint's Cult: The Mass *in honore sancti Sigismundi* for the Cure of Fevers', *Traditio*, 49 (1994), 23–43.

[15] C. Walker Bynum, *Fragmentation and Redemption: Essays on Gender and the Human Body in Medieval Religion* (New York, 1991), 189, and 'The Female Body and Religious Practice in the Later Middle Ages', in *Fragments for a History of the Human Body*, ed. M. Feher, R. Naddaff, and N. Tazi (New York, 1990), i, 167.

[16] Bernard of Clairvaux, *Epistolae*, ed. J. Leclercq and H. Rochais, in *Opera*, vii (Rome, 1974), epist. 345, 287.

[17] B. Harvey, *Living and Dying in England 1100–1540: The Monastic Experience*, (Oxford, 1993), ch. 3, esp. 81–111; K. Park, *Doctors and Medicine in Early Renaissance Florence* (Princeton, 1985), 99–101; D. Nebbiani-Dalla Guarda, 'Les livres de l'infirmerie dans les monastères médiévaux', *Revue Mabillon*, 66 (1994), 57–81.

[18] 'Et est hic argumentum quod medicis licet uti religiosis', in *Pars prima (–sexta) huius operis continens textum Biblie, cum postilla Hugonis*, iii (Paris, 1533), fol. ccxvii^v. Cf. Nicholas de Gorran's (OP. d. 1295) commentary, MS Paris, BN lat. 486^a, fol. 109va.

The apparent contradiction between Isaiah, who advised King Hezekiah to lay plaster of figs upon his boil (Isaiah 38: 21), and St Agatha, who proudly told Peter that she had never treated her body with carnal medicine, was solved by Hugues, who emphatically determined that 'the privileges of the few do not constitute a general law' (*privilegia paucorum non faciunt legem communem*).

In addition to a disagreement over the interpretation of diseases and the way they could be cured, other clerics deemed physicians liable to produce theological errors and to transgress the boundaries of their discipline. Among the devastating criticisms of physicians by John of Salisbury in *Policraticus* and *Metalogicon*[19] was a reprimand for deviating from the rules of their profession through the frailty of their faith. For while they attributed excessive authority to nature, they commonly assailed its Creator by opposing the faith.[20] John had heard many physicians disputing in an unorthodox way about the soul's virtues and properties, about the body's growth, corruption, and even resurrection, and about creation. He was perplexed, amazed, and even bemused by self-admiring physicians who erred through lack of faith, and who could never agree upon any cure for a malady. 'When I listen to them (*medici theorici*), they seem to be capable of raising the dead and pretend to be no less powerful than Asclepius or Mercury.'[21] After acknowledging that not all physicians deserve rebuke, since at least with respect to practitioners (*medici practici*) their activity is necessary and we all might fall into their hands because of our sins, and quoting Ecclesiasticus 38: 4, which calls for medicine not to be abhorred, he concluded his discussion by sarcastically blaming physicians for pretending to be God. This link between the medical profession and religious errors shows that some clerics were suspicious of academic physicians' orthodoxy and in particular disapproved of the speculative part of medicine.

The cases of Arnau and Galvano suggest that the ease with which they moved to the clerical domain was common among physicians. The *Glossa*

---

[19] John of Salisbury, *Ioannis Saresberiensis Policraticus I–IV*, ed. K. S. B. Keats-Rohan (*CCCM* 118; Turnhout, 1993), ii. 29, 169–71, and *Ioannis Saresberiensis Metalogicon*, ed. J. B. Hall (*CCCM* 98; Turnhout, 1991), i. 4, 18–19. He criticized the avarice of physicians, their incompetence, excessive quest for reward and glory, superficiality, diversity in opinion, intellectual stiffness, ignorance, presumption, and ostentatious pride.

[20] 'At phisici dum nature nimium auctoritatis attribuunt, in auctorem nature adversando fidei plerumque impingunt.' *Policraticus*, 170.

[21] Ibid.

Ordinaria[22] to Psalms 87: 11 [88: 10] ('Wilt thou shew wonders to the dead? shall [physicians] arise and praise thee?') provides us with a unique reference to this question. The marginal gloss quotes Augustine, who referred to the corrupt translation from the Hebrew that caused the original giants ('refa'im', *gigantes*) to be interchanged with physicians (rof'im, *medici*), and adds, paraphrasing Augustine:

If therefore the text means they are proud giants (that is the sages of this world), then rightly are they called physicians who promise through their art the health of souls and against whom it is said: 'Salvation belongeth unto the Lord' (Psalms, 3: 9 [3: 8]). If [the text means] they are good giants (namely, large and strong), then these are physicians who can cure the living by their ministry but cannot raise the dead. For only grace restores them to life and faith, hence: 'No man can come to me, except the Father which hath sent me draw him.' (John, 6: 44)[23]

Hence there are two kinds of physicians: those good physicians, who do not transgress the limited professional boundaries which are determined by the living bodies, and those proud ones who claim to perform the task of curing souls as well as bodies.

Nicholas of Lyra explains why the interlinear gloss 'almost not' (*quasi non*) was added above the verb 'praise' (*confitebuntur*) in Psalm 87: 11. It was done to stress the opposition towards physicians who pretended to raise the dead 'because their art does not extend to this domain' (*quia non se extendit ad hoc ars ipsorum*). Hugues de Saint-Cher (OP. d. 1263) makes a clearer distinction between evil and good physicians. The profane sages (*sapientes huius seculi*) are the evil physicians who cause people to sin and promise them impunity and long life; they are 'inflated by pride' (*alti in superbia*). The good physicians are the good prelates and preachers who are 'raised up by knowledge' (*alti in scientia*) and can direct and cure the living yet do not raise the dead, since only divine grace can bring that about.[24]

[22] On the *Glossa Ordinaria*, see B. Smalley's article in *TRE* 13, 452–7 and M. T. Gibson's introduction to the Facsimile Reprint of the *Editio Princeps* of Strasbourg, 1480/81 (Turnhout, 1992), pp. vii–xi.

[23] 'Si ergo superbi gigantes dicuntur, id est sapientes seculi, bene dicuntur medici qui per artes suas promittunt salutem animarum, contra quos dicitur *Domini est salus*. Si boni gigantes, gigantes—id est magni et fortes, et ipsi medici qui viventes curare ministerio possunt sed non mortuos excitare. Sola enim gratia reviviscunt ad fidem, unde: *Nemo poterit venire ad me nisi pater traxerit eum.*' *Glossa Ordinaria* on Ps. 87: 11, in *Biblia sacra, cum glossa ordinaria*, iii. 1112–13 ('Nunquid mortuis facies mirabilia; aut medici suscitabunt et confitebuntur tibi'); cf. Augustine, *Enarr. in Ps.*, CCSL 39, 1215.

[24] *Glossa Ordinaria* on Ps. 87: 11, in *Biblia sacra, cum glossa ordinaria*, iii. 1111–12. Hugues de Saint-Cher, *Postilla*, ii. 2, fol. ccvi^vb. Cf. Jacopo da Voragine, *Sermones aurei ac pulcherrimi variis scripturarum doctrinis referti de sanctis per anni totius circulum concurrentibus* (Cologne, 1478), 161 where this verse starts a discussion of the medical aid offered by Cosmas and Damian, who rightly attributed their success to God.

Bonaventura used Luke 8: 43 (the haemorrhaging woman) to contrast the omnipotence of God with the failure of human medicine. But he also explained his perception of the role of medicine in the universe. The art of medicine is not autonomous, and its efficacy will always depend on the supreme power (God) and nature. He asserted that:

The art of the physicians is laudable when it follows the celestial power and basic nature. . . . Yet the action of the physician will become blameworthy when he disregards nature or does not give preference to divine power as is said of Asa.[25]

By determining that one ought to praise and honour the physician only on condition that he does not contravene nature and does not put his own power before the divine, Bonaventura implied that some physicians refused to submit to the superior authority of God, and he expressed his suspicion of their religious reliability.

Though most suppliers of medical services around 1300 probably fell into the category of the 'good giants', the exegetes cited above reveal deep-seated fears of physicians who annex the clerical domain of the human soul and offer to cure it. It is plausible to assume that these views reflect the real image of some physicians during the thirteenth century and the existence of a real tension between clerics and physicians.

The 'Clerical' Approach to Disease

Is it possible to speak of a specific 'clerical approach' towards disease and medicine in the late thirteenth century? Did clerics view disease differently from physicians? The examples I have picked from John of Salisbury, the *Glossa Ordinaria*, and Bonaventura's exegesis suggest that ambivalent attitudes towards medicine and physicians did persist among clerics in the twelfth and thirteenth centuries. Yet they do not suffice for any generalization. Thomas Aquinas denied medicine the status of a theoretical science (*scientia speculativa*) and relegated it to the status of a practical science (*scientia operativa*).[26] His attitude reflects a real suspicion

---

[25] 'medicorum ars est *laudabilis* quando sequitur supernam potentiam et naturam substratam. . . . Sed tunc erit *vituperabilis* operatio medici, quando negligit vel considerare naturam vel non anteponit divinam potentiam, sicut dicitur de Asa.' Bonaventura, *Commentarius in Evangelium Lucae*, in *Opera Omnia*, vii (Quaracchi, 1895), 210[a]–211[a] at 211[a]. See his commentary to Luke 4: 23, ibid. 101[a], and to Luke 5: 31, ibid. 131[b].

[26] Thomas Aquinas, *Super Boetium De trinitate*, Q. 5.1, in *Opera Omnia*, 50 (Rome and Paris, 1992), 140: 251–93; also in A. Maurer, *St. Thomas Aquinas: The Division and Methods of the Sciences* (Toronto, 1986), 19–22. Cf. Robert Kilwardby (*c*.1215–79), *De ortu scientiarum*, ed. A. G. Judy (Oxford and Toronto, 1976), 10. 57, 39. 363, pp. 27–8, 129, who, following Hugh of St Victor's division, relegated medicine to the status of mechanical art. On Hugh's low estimation of *medicina* see Bylebyl, 'The Medical Meaning of *Physica*', 30.

towards the theoretical aspects of medicine, and should be regarded as an attempt to maintain a clear separation between medicine and philosophy and theology in the academic context. Yet it teaches us nothing about his actual perception of disease and attitude to the physician. Moreover, similar tendencies to restrict medicine to an art occasionally appear in the writings of academic physicians like Arnau.[27]

The value of a reconstruction of past attitudes depends on the selection of sources. When no direct evidence exists for the question under consideration, the researcher must base his interpretation on a cautious analysis of indirect sources which should be sufficiently representative to enable a qualified generalization. How would an early-fourteenth-century literate person interested in describing the 'clerical attitude to medicine and the physician' approach the problem? He could consult one of the encyclopaedias available at that time. He could turn to the Bible and its commentators, and deduce what clerics thought of medicine from the way they interpreted biblical 'medical' narratives. He could also collect relevant information from sermons delivered on various occasions. An encyclopaedia, biblical commentary, and preaching material are the sources I have used in order to outline the 'clerical approach to medicine' around 1300, texts which were widely used and sufficiently representative to form the basis of generalizations.

What kind of image would emerge to our medieval reader from the influential encyclopaedia of Vincent de Beauvais? In a chapter entitled, 'How Should one Apply the Physician's Advice?' (*Qualiter consilio medici sit utendum*), Vincent introduces nine authorities on the issue.[28] The first four authorities he cites are favourable towards medical cure and the physician, the fifth is neutral, and the last four are critical either of human cure or of the human physician. Isidore reminds the readers of Isaiah (3: 21) and Paul (1 Timothy 5: 23) who suggested medical treatment to Hezekiah and Timothy; hence medicine must not be despised.[29]

---

[27] Cf. 'The Divine Source of Medical Knowledge', Ch. 3, p. 117.

[28] Vincent de Beauvais, *Speculum naturale*, xxxi. 99 (Venice, 1591), 406[ra].

[29] *Isidori Hispalensis episcopi etymologiarum sive originum libri xx*, ed. W. M. Lindsay (Oxford, 1911), iv. 9.1. See also iv. 13 where he explains why medicine is not included among the other liberal arts. Whereas each art embraces only one subject, medicine embraces them all, and thus makes it imperative for a physician to know them all. He concludes his discussion in 13.5 saying, 'Hence it is that medicine is called a second philosophy, for each discipline claims the whole of man for itself. Just as by philosophy the soul, so also by medicine the body is cured.' This passage is quoted fully in Vincent de Beauvais, *Speculum doctrinale* xiii. 2, 217[r]–218[v]. For an English translation of Isidore, see W. D. Sharpe, 'Isidore of Seville: The Medical Writings', *Transactions of the American Philosophical Society*, 54/2 (1964), 1–75.

Augustine's rule instructs the canons to accept medical council without muttering and preaches total submission to the physician's advice in times of disease.[30] Jerome's commentary on Habakkuk 1: 2–3 depicts the physician as rightfully overruling the patient's will.[31] The fifth authority is Seneca, who in two letters to Lucilius and in the tragedy *Oedipus* glorified patience yet did not actively praise disease. By expressing Oedipus's loathing of being cured by foul medicine, Seneca prepares the ground for the last four authorities, who are suspicious of the physicians' activities.[32] The sixth authority is a fragment of Bernard of Clairvaux's Homily 30 on *Song of Songs* (c.1138–40) which depicts a dichotomic relationship between Christ's and Galen's disciples and communicates hostility to physicians.

Bernard determines (and Vincent quotes him in full) that those who observe the dietary rules (*observantes ciborum*) neglect the moral rules. What Hippocrates teaches—ways to preserve life, *animas salvas facere*— Christ and his disciples reject. The physician represented by Hippocrates and Galen is thus a reversed image of the faithful Christian; he is the ally of the Epicureans[33] and the incarnation of the corrupt world and of those who prefer bodily pleasure (*voluptas*) to good morals. Bernard emphatically demands that the faithful choose between the two. He ridicules the attempt to cure with the aid of herbal medicines and on the basis of the theory of complexion, and says: 'I am a monk not a physician; one should not think about complexion but about profession of vows' (*nec de complexione judicandum, sed de professione*). Rhetorically, he asks whether he should expose his monks to the judgement of Galen, Hippocrates, and those who emerge from the Epicurean school. And, proudly, he declares himself as the disciple of Christ who abhorred and despised everything that Epicurus and Hippocrates preached.[34] This attitude to the medical

[30] Augustine, *Regula* 9, in *PL* 32: 1383.

[31] Jerome, *Super Abacuc* I. 2–3, *CCSL* 76 (a), 582.

[32] 'non sum tam demens ut egrotare cupiam, sed si egrotandum fuerit, nihil effiminate faciam. Non enim pati tormenta optabile est sed pati fortiter. *Idem* in edippo: Abi [sic] ergo turpis est medicina, sanari piget.' Vincent de Beauvais, *Speculum naturale*, xxxi. 99, 406ra. Cf. Seneca, *Ad Lucilium epistulae morales*, ii (London and Cambridge, Mass., 1952), 67.4 and 67.6, pp. 36, 38, and *Oedipus*, ed. B. W. Häuptli (Frauenfeld, 1984), 517.

[33] Cf. A. Murray, 'The Epicureans', in P. Boitani and A. Torti (ed.), *Intellectuals and Writers in Fourteenth-Century Europe* (Tübingen and Cambridge, 1986), 138–63; at 159 Murray mentions a *medicus* who has launched Boniface VIII into denial of resurrection and immortality of the soul; on Pietro d'Abano, another Epicurean physician, see ibid. 161–2.

[34] Cf. *S. Bernardi opera* i: *Sermones super Cantica Canticorum*, ed J. Leclercq, C. H. Talbot, and H. M. Rochais (Rome, 1957), sermon 30.10, 210–18, at 217. 'Num Hippocratis seu Galieni sententiam, aut certe de schola Epicuri, debui proponere vobis? Christi sum discipulus, Christi discipulis loquor. . . . Epicurus atque Hippocras, corporis alter voluptatem, alter bonam habitudinem prefert; meus Magister utriusque rei contemptum predicat.' On the intellectual

sources does not prevent Bernard from employing the usual metaphors of Christ as a medicine or a physician elsewhere, or talking of phlebotomy of the soul and making parallels between the bodily and the spiritual healing process. Yet, by selecting only Bernard's critical views, Vincent hides from the reader the monastic context of the homily and consequently introduces Bernard's view as a general proposition.

Then follows, as the seventh authority, a long citation from canon 22 of Lateran IV. Together with the previous authority, it stresses the superiority of spiritual cure.[35] The eighth authority in Vincent's article is Sidonius Apollinaris (d. *c.*486). He advises avoiding the counsel of incompetent physicians who frequently disagree with each other.[36] Hildebert of Lavardin (d. 1133 as Archbishop of Tours) concludes the critical part of the chapter by lamenting excessive care for the body and the neglect of the soul. While people rush to the physician of the flesh, they must know that cure will be slow without proper care for the soul.

Vincent devotes a substantial amount of space to those critical of medicine and the physicians, though this does not necessarily mean that he was in favour of the critical approach. He followed the *sic et non* method, but his discussion did not end with a harmonizing synthesis which would eliminate the contradictions. Consequently, our reader would certainly receive an ambivalent message from Vincent. Criticism of the physician's avarice or incompetence was wholly compatible with a favourable attitude towards human medical cure. However, Bernard's suspicious attitude was incompatible with the praises found in the citations from Isidore and Augustine. Chapter 97 in *Speculum naturale* deals with the various causes for disease and clearly reflects this ambivalent message, this time with respect to the causes of disease.[37] Vincent devotes the larger part of his discussion to Isidore's and Haly's beliefs that disease is a wholly natural phenomenon; but he introduces Jerome's commentary on Matthew 9: 6 (the cure of the paralytic) and his *Contra Iovianum* ii, which

circumstances of this homily, see W. Hiss, *Die Anthropologie Bernhards von Clairvaux* (Berlin, 1964), 121 n. 137. For other comparable ideas of Bernard, who claimed that medicine sought to increase bodily vigour beyond what health requires, and who tried to detach charity from medicine by equating medicine to the care of the body and charity to the care of the soul, see Bernard, Abbot of Clairvaux, *The Steps of Humility*, tr. G. B. Birch (Cambridge Mass., 1942), 58–60.

[35] For canon 22, see above, 'Patterns of Relationship between Religion and Medicine', Ch. 1, pp. 9–10, and Vincent de Beauvais, *Speculum doctrinale*, xii. 2, 100[vb] (*De institutione medici*) which repeats canon 22.

[36] Sidonius Apollinaris, *Epistulae* ii. 12, in *PL* 58, 490.

[37] Vincent de Beauvais, *Speculum naturale*, xxxi. 97, 405[vb].

stress the moral causes for physical diseases and the need to cleanse the soul from sin in order to avoid or eliminate disease.[38]

Most clerics did not reject the notion of natural causes for disease. However, they added to the explanation of physical disease a spiritual nuance which introduced God and the moral behaviour of the patient as additional causes of all pathologies. I shall call this hereafter the 'clerical approach to medicine and the physicians'.[39] This approach linked health (*sanitas*) with spiritual salvation (*salus*). It included the assertion that diseases may be triggered by a moral cause and the claim that they have a moral/religious significance. Physical disease purges the soul; it curbs pride, fortifies the other virtues and provides a means of identifying oneself with Christ (especially from the thirteenth century onwards); it is an occasion for repentance and, as such, an expression of God's care and an opportunity to increase one's merit (Job's argument); it may be a due punishment for sin, a means of correcting the sinner, or an expression of divine anger. Epidemics may be signs of the approaching end of the world. It also included the recognition of the superior role of God in restitution of health and the importance of spiritual cure for physical health. Hence, in discussing disease, clerics tended to emphasize the overwhelming importance of confession for spiritual and physical health.

What would our imaginary medieval person hear from his priest or from the preachers when they spoke of disease? I have chosen John Bromyard's popular *Summa predicantium* as an illustration of the 'clerical approach' to disease in the first third of the fourteenth century because it includes most of the arguments typical of this approach.[40] The *Summa* was an expansion of a previous work by Bromyard entitled *Opus trivium*. It is more than double the size of the *Opus* and has a similar layout, containing articles arranged in alphabetical order (*Abiectio–Xtus*), numbered, subdivided, and furnished with cross-references. This encyclopaedia for preachers treated the capital sins and cardinal virtues as well as theological topics such as angels and free will, and topics suitable for moral discussion such

[38] Jerome, *In Matth.* 9.6, in *PL* 26, 55.

[39] I. Noye, 'Maladie', *DS* 10, 137–52; H. Schipperges, 'Krankheit' (pt. iv–v), *TRE* 19/5, 686–94; J. Agrimi and C. Crisciani, *Medicina del corpo e medicina dell'anima: Note sul sapere del medico fino all'inizio del secolo XIII* (Milan, 1978), 5–24, and *Malato, medico e medicina nel medioevo* (Turin, 1980), 26–33.

[40] Joannes de Bromyard, *Summa predicantium* (Nuremberg, 1518), fols. clviii^{rb}–clx^{ra}. For its dating, see L. E. Boyle, 'The Date of the *Summa praedicantium* of John Bromyard', *Speculum*, 48 (1973), 533–7. P. Binkley, 'John Bromyard and the Hereford Dominicans', in *Centres of Learning: Learning and Location in Pre-Modern Europe and the Near East*, ed. J. W. Drijrers and A. A. MacDonald (Leiden, 1995), 254–64.

as war, cities, and merchants. The marginally numbered paragraphs and the detailed indices also facilitate reference. The reader was expected to select the material he needed and fill it out with thoughts of his own; and sections of text could be extracted from the *Summa* and inserted virtually unchanged into a sermon. Bromyard, who died in *c.*1352, may have completed his Latin sermon encyclopaedia shortly after the summer of 1348. He was licensed to hear confessions in the diocese of Hereford in early 1326, and started working on the *Summa* shortly thereafter. By 1330 he had completed the article on *Iudicium Dei*,[41] so it is plausible to assume that he completed the article on illness (*Infirmitas*) prior to that date.

The article on illness, which aims to help people cope with corporeal disease, is divided into nine sections. From the beginning, it is clear that though Bromyard does not completely abandon the 'Giovanni-style' mirror-image relationship between physical and spiritual disease, this approach plays a minor role in his explanation. Instead, he describes a pattern of cause and effect. Disease is first and foremost a moral phenomenon which has accidental physical manifestations. Sinners suffer disease, and justly so. Bromyard looks on physical disease as a beneficial phenomenon controlled by the moral behaviour of the patient; thus, a prerequisite for physical cure is the healing of the spiritual flaw. Confession should both precede physical convalescence and also continue after good health has been restored, lest disease return. Bromyard thus permits the preacher to use disease as a means of claiming control over believers, even after the cure.[42]

If God sends disease and does nothing without due reason, it is appropriate to investigate his intention in inflicting diseases on people. His first intention is to expel sin from the human soul. Bromyard tells of an abbot who refused to cure a sick fornicator, knowing that 'a serious illness turns the soul sober' (*infirmitas gravis sobriam facit animam*, Ecclesiasticus 31: 2). Second, it is through disease that the castle of the soul is opened; God in his mercy urges the sick person to resume communication with him through his ministers. Third, God, like a teacher who sometimes has to scourge the children, flogs humans with diseases so that they will again have regard for 'the book of conscience'. And fourth, disease stimulates lazy people into performing good deeds. When ill they suddenly start to give alms, thus fulfilling Paul's words, 'When I

---

[41] Boyle, 'The Date', 535.

[42] *Summa predicantium*, fol. clviii[vb]. See in the article entitled *Tribulatio*, fol. ccclxxiiii[r], on illness as an instrument for the Church to exert its control, widen its influence, and guide lost souls who are urged to seek God.

am weak then I am strong' and 'for strength is made perfect in weakness (*in infirmitate*) (2 Corinthians 12: 9–10).

All this leads Bromyard to declare that illnesses are signs of divine care and of great love towards mankind. They are a sign of divine mercy, because through them the eternal punishments we deserve for sins we have committed are commuted to temporal infirmities. Lazarus is a proof that those whom God loves he smites (John 11: 3 'Lord, behold, he whom thou lovest is sick'). An *exemplum* follows about a hermit who once was not afflicted by an annual illness. The hermit bewailed having been cast into oblivion, and 'God sent him good fevers' (*bonas febres*).[43]

In this scheme there seems to be no place for the physician; there may not be any place for temporal curing activity at all, and the only medicine relevant to the disease is the spiritual one. Therefore, when quoting from Ecclesiasticus 38, Bromyard drops the first part of the chapter (which could hardly not be linked to the corporeal physician) and cites verse 9 only ('My son, when you are ill, do not delay but pray to God, for it is he who heals'). In this context, the message is unequivocal: prayer is the only Christian reaction to disease, and it will be answered because disease by definition brings man nearer to divine providence.

Bromyard also contends that diseases purge us of sins and make the righteous shine in their moral superiority. Disease is a haven from this life, where health (*sanitas*) does not last; it is a door to eternal salvation (*salus eterna*). What seems to be a fatal disease, therefore, is really a cure for the soul.[44] Six more *exempla* of 'diseased condition' as a desirable state follow, summed up by the contention that since disease is similar to Christ's passion it offers the opportunity to acquire Christ's virtue.

The practical implication of this approach is the need for patience, as Seneca preached. God is responsible for the disease, but is also the supreme physician who does not err in the medicines he prescribes. The uniqueness of divine medicine is that it is given by a physician who loves the patient as deeply as a father loves his son; this physician knows how to cure, and requires nothing from the patient but that he will not fall ill again. The implied critique directed at physicians then becomes fully explicit, when Bromyard elaborates on a list of obstacles which prevent a

---

[43] *Tribulatio,* fol. clix^r; cf. Matt. 8: 15. *Fasciculus morum,* 136–40, describes physical disease as 'vinculum Christi per quod quos amat castigat'.

[44] Cf. Dominicus Cavalca de Vico Pisano (OP, d. 1340), *Medicina del cuore* (Rome, 1754), 147–56, and Robert Holcot, *In librum sapientie regis Salomonis prelectiones ccxiii* (Basel, 1586), *lectio* xciii, 313–15.

patient from following the therapy prescribed by physicians.[45] The human physician is everything that the supreme physician is not. His weaknesses, uncertainty, ignorance, avarice, betrayal of the patient's trust, lack of proper human relationship, and damaging malpractice undermine the patient's confidence in him and the efficacy of the whole treatment. On the other hand, God knows the causes of the disease and the safe and certain way of cure, and he does everything without charging a fee.

Bromyard then deals with visiting the sick and the physician's duty to call the priest before he starts treatment (according to canon 22 of Lateran IV). He quotes a gloss of Hostiensis castigating failure to do so as mortal sin, and thus presents the visit of the priest as more important than the visit by the physician. Christ, who overcame sin and cured bodies, taught mankind first to seek the medicine of the soul by extracting sin from it. Patients should seek cure from Christ, the supreme physician, and as they patiently suffer for the health of their bodies they must be prepared, for the health of their souls, patiently to endure disease.[46]

Bromyard's treatise ends with a discussion of death and prayers for the dying. Thus, in *Summa predicantium*, disease and its cure have been fully and utterly appropriated by religion. There is no reference to secular medical sources or to natural reasoning. The place allotted to physicians in the curing process is almost negligible, and the text is shot through with contempt towards them.

Yet how typical was Bromyard's approach to disease amongst his fellow Dominicans and clerics in general? Giovanni, at least, did not share Bromyard's approach, for in a funeral sermon to a physician he openly declared that 'in distribution of remedies, medicine derives its efficacy not from God alone but also from physicians'.[47] Nevertheless, Bromyard's views were shared by some patients of the surgeon Henri de Mondeville, a contemporary of Arnau who had studied and perhaps taught medicine and surgery at Montpellier before establishing himself at Paris. Henri tells of simple patients (described as *vulgus*) who, believing

---

[45] *Summa predicantium*, fol. clix[va].

[46] 'ut prius medicinam querant anime quod prius ferrum de vulnere, id est peccatum de anima extrahant, confitendo quod medicinam a summo medico querant christo, et tantum ei debet in membris suis pro salute anime quantum daret pro salute corporis et quod pro salute corporis multa sustineret ita illam patienter sustineat infirmitatem pro salute anime.' *Summa predicantium*, fol. clix[vb].

[47] 'non solum a Deo medicina, sed medicis efficaciam habeat in distributione medicine'. Giovanni da San Gimignano, *Conciones funebres* (Paris, 1611), 724.

that medical knowledge is infused directly from God and the saints as a divine gift, and that God is the author of every illness and the only source of health, reject learned surgery all together. They shun all medicine and turn to religious treatment performed by divine surgeons (*divini cyrurgici*) such as hermits, anchorites, and old harlots (*antique meretrices et metatrices*). Holy water and incantations are the means by which these religious lure (*alliciunt*) the patients into receiving 'divine' treatment. Other patients are such ardent believers that they are practically indifferent to ill health and refuse to be cured by human hand. Henri describes there how a surgeon preparing medicines accidentally broke the mortar. The *populus* interpreted it as a divine miracle suggesting that he should not have attempted to treat a disease which must only be cured by divine surgeons.[48] We do not know if these patients were clerics or pious laymen. But we can conclude that a Bromyard-like approach to disease was not merely a rhetorical invention in the beginning of the fourteenth century.

The Role of Scripture in the Medieval Perception of Medicine and the Physician

From preachers like Bromyard, our late-medieval explorer would gather that the Bible and its commentaries could be used to emphasize the moral significance of disease and the superior importance of spiritual over corporeal health. He could then go directly to the glossed Bible, as I have done, and supplement this with Hugues de Saint Cher's *Postils* and Nicholas of Lyra's commentary. In general, the commentators give a spiritual explanation to any biblical phrase or story with a medical theme; the cause of disease is always moral, and cure follows a spiritual conversion.[49] They repeatedly communicate a notion of the superiority of the True Physician (*Verus Medicus*) over the mere healer (*curator*), since the first heals all diseases of soul and body. The speed of cures obtained by

---

[48] *Die Chirurgie des Heinrich von Mondeville*, ed. J. L. Pagel (Berlin, 1892), Tract. II, Not. introduct. 2, 68; E. Nicaise (tr.), *Chirurgie de Maître Henri de Mondeville* (Paris, 1893), 101–2, 182–3; M. R. McVaugh, *Medicine before the Plague: Practitioners and their Patients in the Crown of Aragon 1285–1345* (Cambridge, 1993), 172; M. C. Pouchelle, *The Body and Surgery in the Middle Ages* (Cambridge, 1990), 43–4.

[49] See e.g. *Glossa Ordinaria* on Job 5: 17–18, in *Biblia sacra, cum glossa ordinaria*, iii. 83–4. The various healing stories of Christ, Asa (2 Chr. 16: 12–13) and Hezekiah (Isa. 38: 1–6) were ideal stories to initiate such debate; *Glossa Ordinaria* to 2 Cor. 12: 9–10 hails the state of sickness and gives Nicholas of Lyra an opportunity to elaborate on the theology of disease. See also *Glossa Ordinaria* on Exod. 15: 26, 'ego enim Dominus sanator tuus' (i. 629–30) and on Jer. 17: 14 (iv. 711).

divine intervention in comparison to their slowness by human or natural channels is further evidence of this superiority.[50]

In what follows I shall mainly discuss the interpretations of Ecclesiasticus 38: 1–8,[51] which discuss the respect due to physicians, and which Bromyard avoided (intentionally, I suggested) in his article on disease. A literal reading of these verses suggests that the text referred to human physicians. How did the commentators explain this plea to honour the physician and not to despise God-given medicine?

Whereas all commentators agree that verses 9–15 speak of the spiritual cure of disease caused by sin and hence of the spiritual physician, their interpretations of verses 1–8 differ. The first approach is that which appears in the interlinear and marginal glosses in the *Glossa Ordinaria*.[52] These glosses are largely an edited version of patristic and Carolingian exegesis, compiled in the mid-twelfth century at the latest. They communicate to the reader an ambivalent message, since every phrase discusses both aspects of medicine and both kinds of physician. The writers of the commentaries and the editors of the *Glossa* seem to have been dissatisfied with a purely literal reading of the text. Looking for a way to suppress the literal meaning which was most favourable to human medicine, they chose the option of interchangeability between literal and spiritual reading while stressing the overall superiority of spiritual over physical health. Every 'physician' (*medicus*) and 'medicine' (*medicina*) appearing in the text is both spiritual and corporeal; every reference to *salus* denotes both spiritual and physical health. If my reading is correct, the confused medieval reader would immediately understand that the authors were making an orchestrated effort to play down the call for exceptional respect for physicians, and hence were somewhat critical of human physicians. However, parallel to the functional separation and the explicit preference of spiritual over human physicians, our medieval reader could conclude that by closely juxtaposing spiritual and corporeal physicians, the commentaries create extreme similarity between corporeal and spiritual physicians and hence raise the status of the corporeal physician. This clearly appears in the marginal gloss to the opening words in Ecclesiasticus 38: 1: 'Honour the physician' (*Honora medicum*):

---

[50] *Glossa Ordinaria* on Luke 4: 38 and on Matt. 8: 14. The feverish people were relieved only gradually of the weakness that is caused by the disease. Simon's mother-in-law was cured at once.

[51] Cf. above, 'Patterns of Relationship between Religion and Medicine', Ch. 1, p. 3.

[52] *Glossa Ordinaria* on Ecclus. 38: 1–15, in *Biblia sacra, cum glossa ordinaria*, iii. 2161–4.

He wants us to be prudent in all things, because God's works are very good. Hence we ought not to spurn those things that the Creator has made for our benefit. There are corporeal physicians and there are spiritual physicians. Corporeal physicians cure bodies; spiritual physicians cure souls. Therefore both kinds should be honoured but one should prefer the spiritual ones.[53]

It was Rabanus Maurus in his Ecclesiasticus commentary (written between 835 and 840) who made the distinction between corporeal and spiritual physicians and medicine. He also determined that the health of the soul is superior to the health of the body. Thus, Ben Sira's praise for the physician and medicine could be read as praise for clerics and the methods they use to cure sick souls. Nevertheless, the gloss does not discard the possible literal interpretation which also explains the first eight verses of Ecclesiasticus 38 as praise for the physician and the art of medicine. This interchangeable approach recurs throughout the text of the gloss. The interlinear gloss to 38: 3 ('The knowledge of the physician', *Disciplina medici*) adds 'corporeal or spiritual' (*corporalis vel spiritualis*); to 38: 7 ('Curing through these', *In his curans*) the marginal gloss adds: 'Physicians oppose diverse diseases by diverse means—food and drink, plasters and unguents—so that the remedies will suit the disease. Spiritual physicians act similarly' (*Contra diversas infirmitates, diversa opponunt medici, cibos scilicet et potus, emplastra, et unguenta; ut morbis conveniant medicamenta. Similiter faciunt medici spirituales*). The subject of the last part of 38: 7 ('his work continues without cease', *non consummabuntur opera eius*) is understood as 'the true physician' (*verus medicus*) and the 'works' (*opera*) are interpreted as 'remedies' (*medicamenta*); the peace in 38: 8 ('The peace of God on the surface of the earth') is specified as the time when death is eliminated in victory. From verse 9 onwards the text is interpreted constantly as denoting the spiritual healing of infirmity caused by sin.

The second approach is that which appears in Hugues de Saint-Cher's *Postils*. Hugues openly declares that the whole chapter deals with spiritual medicine, avoids much reference to physical medicine when dis-

---

[53] 'Discretos vult nos esse in omnibus, quia opera Dei bona sunt valde, unde non debemus ea spernere, que constat creatorem ad utilitatem nostram fecisse. Sunt corporales medici sunt et spirituales. Corporales medici corpora, spirituales curant animas. Utrique ergo honorandi, sed spirituales preferendi.' *Glossa Ordinaria* on Ecclus. 38: 1, in *Biblia sacra, cum glossa ordinaria*, iii. 2161. Its source is Rabanus Maurus, *Comm. in Ecclus.*, PL 109, 1030–3. On Rabanus's interpretation of Ecclus. 38, see Paxton, 'Curing Bodies—Curing Soul', 241–4. Rabanus likens the physical physician who heals with herbs to the spiritual physician who cures souls with God's precepts.

cussing Ecclesiasticus 38, and devotes most of its interpretation to Christ, the spiritual physician. Hugues opens his commentary thus: 'This chapter is totally about spiritual medicine that cures sins and is the reason why the physician should be honoured.' Literally, *honora medicum* is directed at both physical and spiritual physicians. Mystically, however, one should honour the True Physician of the souls through due worship.[54] He similarly explains the other verses of that chapter.

In his commentary on Ecclesiasticus, Nicholas de Gorran (OP. d. 1295) takes a middle line between Rabanus and Hugues de Saint-Cher.[55] Like Rabanus's commentary, his explanations for verses 1–8 include the qualifications 'of the body or the soul' (*corporis vel anime*) or 'corporeal as well as spiritual' (*corporalis quam spiritualis*); but a mystical interpretation attributing every utterance to Christ dominates his commentary. That medicine is a divine gift (*donatio*, 38: 2) does not alter Gorran's view of it. It is God who determines the efficacy of the treatment, and therefore the sick should seek God and trust his powers. Gorran, who omits the physician in this context, buttresses his view with the story about Asa who did not seek God but rather put all his trust in the art of medicine. In general, it is to God and not to the physician that men owe obedience, gratitude, and trust. The human physician is at best a secondary actor. Gorran's apparent relegation of medicine to a back seat did not imply a rejection of human cure. He argues that, since every cure is a result of divine grace, medical art is a spiritual art (*ars spiritualis*) which cannot be sold, and therefore those physicians sin who sell their work.

The third nuance in the exegetes' approach to medicine returns to a more literal reading of the text, as the commentary of Nicholas of Lyra suggests. Nicholas felt unease at the confusion between the physical and the spiritual elements in the interpretation of Ecclesiasticus 38. He obviously sensed that, according to a literal reading, the human physician was at the core of the text (or, at least, of its first eight verses). This prompted him to start his commentary by answering the question of why the discussion about the honour due to the physical physician precedes that about the honour due to the spiritual. He declares that one should proceed in explanation from the sensible things, which are easily noted, to those which are grasped only spiritually, and therefore from the physician to the prelate. Nicholas explicitly acknowledges God's role as the

---

[54] 'In hoc capitulo agitur per totum de medicina spiritualis qua peccata curantur propter quam medicus est honorandus.' Hugues de Saint-Cher, *Postilla Hugonis*, iii, fols. ccx-vii[rb]–ccxviii[rb].

[55] MS Paris, BN lat. 486[2], fol. 109[va].

prime originator of the medical art by which he relieves humans from the agony of disease. But, according to him, the first eight verses are dedicated to the human physician, whilst the spiritual physician, identified as the priest (*sacerdos*), appears only in verse 9. This he deduces from verse 14 ('and they too beseech the Lord to direct their peace', *ipsi vero Dominum deprecabuntur ut dirigat requiem eorum*) and says, 'hence it is evident that here the text does not speak of corporeal physicians who do not cure ill people through prayer, but of priests'.[56] The priest's role is to bring divine peace (*requies*) by praying and by performing the sacraments, and he should be honoured for it. Nicholas does not deviate from the basic notion of the superiority of spiritual medicine over physical. At the end of his commentary to verse 9 he says, 'The first reason for honouring the spiritual physician is the health of the soul which is more valuable than the health of the body; consequently one should honour the prelate more than the corporeal physician.'[57] He uses identical vocabulary when describing the activities of both physicians; but it looks as if he is trying to stabilize the boundaries between the two faces of medicine which complement each other to produce a complete cure: the human physician supplies natural medicines, the spiritual physician cures the soul through prayers. By developing this interpretative nuance (the nearest of all to a literal reading) Nicholas of Lyra (1270–1340), who wrote in a period marked by a real boost in the status of medical science and of the physician, accords with the prevalent tendency to establish clear disciplinary boundaries among the sciences in general and between medicine and theology in particular.

None of the commentators from Rabanus to Nicholas of Lyra explicitly rejected the work of the physician or the herbal remedies created by God for the restoration of physical health. Their main concern was not with the health of the body but with the cure of the soul. Nevertheless, a medieval reader could infer from them some clerical attitudes towards corporeal medicine. Our medieval explorer would have to be learned indeed to be able directly to consult the glossed Bible. Had he done so, he would face the three interpretative nuances which diverted from a simple reading of the text. Whichever he preferred, he would be

---

[56] 'ex hoc apparet, quod non loquitur hic de medicis corporis, qui non curant infirmos per orationes, sed de sacerdotibus'. *Glossa Ordinaria* on Ecclus. 38: 14 in *Biblia sacra, cum glossa ordinaria*, iii. 2164.

[57] 'Prima causa honorandi medicum spiritualem est sanitas anime, que melior est corporis sanitate, et per consequens prelatus magis honorandus est quam medicus corporalis'. *Glossa Ordinaria* on Ecclus. 38: 9, in *Biblia sacra, cum glossa ordinaria*, iii. 2163.

impressed by the superiority of spiritual over physical health and would detect the hidden message that physicians deserved no overwhelming respect. Even if he were not sufficiently learned to look directly at the commentaries, he could be exposed to these messages elsewhere. Verses from Ecclesiasticus 38: 1–15—a paragraph from a fairly obscure book which has never been part of the Hebrew canon—were particularly popular amongst preachers who preached on the days commemorating Luke, Cosmas and Damian, and Sylvester. It was through this vehicle of sermons that the 'religious approach' to medicine and the physician was reiterated faithfully to the believers. Thus, in the sermons under consideration, the call to honour the physician was interpreted as pointing at the spiritual physician; the preachers only referred to the physician of the body when they wished to underline the differences between the two. For example, in two sermons dedicated to St Sylvester, Jacopo da Voragine discusses Ecclesiasticus 38: 2 'From God is every cure' (*A deo est omnis medela*). The divine cure is baptism in this context, and Jacopo explains its efficacy for bodily and spiritual health. Ecclesiasticus 38: 1, 'honour the physician for he is essential to you' (*honora medicum propter necessitatem*), enabled Jacopo to elaborate on the spiritual and physical needs (*necessitates*) which made him essential for his clients. The required honour was given to Sylvester, who was the personification of the real physician.[58]

To assess the impact of Ecclesiasticus 38 it is necessary to examine how it was used and understood by the physicians. This will show whether there was any 'medical way' to read these verses. It is my hypothesis that physicians could use the text and its commentaries as a license to engage spiritual matters. Though it is impossible to determine with certainty whether Arnau had access to a glossed Bible which included the Ecclesiasticus commentaries now found in the printed *Glossa Ordinaria*, it is plausible to assume that he did. From the inventory of his books, we know that he had access to some form of biblical commentary;[59] furthermore, on several occasions he explicitly referred to the common gloss (*glossa communis*).[60]

---

[58] Jacopo da Voragine, *Sermones de sanctis* (Cologne, 1478), no. 25–6.

[59] R. Chabás, 'Inventario de los libros, ropas y demás efectos de Arnaldo de Villanueva', *Revista de Archivos, Bibliotecas e Museos*, 9 (1903), nrs. 58, 61, 66 (glossed Song of Songs and Proverbs), 98 (*Postille super xii prophetiis*), 141, 143, 146, 148, 149, 171, 239, 240, 256 (*Primo ii postille super Matheum et Lucam super Actus et super Apocalipsim*), 262 (*Postilla super Matheum*), 268, 271 (*textus cum glossis super epistolis Pauli*), and 274 (*Psalterium glossatum*).

[60] *Antidotum*, MS Vat. lat. 3824, fol. 245va–b. Martinus de Atheca refers to Arnau's Daniel commentary in *Tractatus de tempore adventus Antichristi*, in J. Perarnau, 'El text primitiu del *De mysterio cymbalorum ecclesiae* d'Arnau de Vilanova', *ATCA* 7/8 (1988/9), 147–53. Cf. *Glossa Ordinaria* on Dan. 12: 11 in *Biblia sacra, cum glossa ordinaria*, iv. 1771.

Ecclesiasticus 38 provides Arnau with a key argument and a powerful tool against those who maintained the apparent dissonance between the medical profession and spiritual activity. Ecclesiasticus 38 discusses both the spiritual and the physical physicians, according to Arnau. However, he sees the medical dimension of Christ's activity as the justification for expanding the subject of these verses from Christ and the spiritual physicians to all other physicians. Those who deny Arnau the right to express himself in theology because he is a physician and not a theologian are blaspheming God, who specifically presented Christ to mankind as a medicine and as a physician, and ordered humanity to honour this physician. Since spiritual medicine is the subject of Ecclesiasticus 38 and the reason why man must honour both the spiritual and human physician, denying human physicians spiritual activity (as his opponents do) violates the spirit of the text.[61] Elsewhere, in order to justify his spiritual activity, he (or one of his associates) cites the medical dimension of Christ's activities conveyed in Ecclesiasticus 38 as the precedent for physicians who deal with theology.[62] Thus, the spiritual interpretation of Ecclesiasticus 38 enables him confidently to demand a recognition of the physicians' right and duty to join the spiritual/theological debate and to maintain the divine source of medical knowledge, and allows him to maintain his conviction that the honour that the physician deserves emenates from both his spiritual and physical missions.

Yet Arnau also found the literal interpretation of Ecclesiasticus 38 useful for his arguments. Scripture orders that the physician be honoured because of his spiritual and physical activities. Those who offer to honour him as a physician and reject him as a theologian are violating the spirit of the text.[63] As we have seen, Arnau and Galvano employ Ecclesiasticus 38 as a pivot of their belief that medical knowledge proceeds directly from God and that the physician is a chosen divine agent.[64] They were not alone in emphasizing an interpretation which the biblical commentators usually did not share. Henri de Mondeville also explicitly interpreted the chapter as applying to the surgeon when he said:

---

[61] *Apologia de versutiis et perversitatibus pseudotheologorum et religiosorum*, in MS Vat. lat. 3824, fol. 147va.

[62] *Tractatus quidam*, in MS Rome, Archivio Generale dei Carmelitani III Varia I, fol. 63ra (also in M. Batllori, 'Dos nous escrits espirituals d'Arnau de Vilanova, *AST* 28 (1955), 63).

[63] *Interpretatio de visionibus in somniis*, in M. Menéndez y Pelayo, *Historia de los heterodoxos españoles*, iii (Buenos Aires, 1951), p. lxxi. Cf. Ch. 3, n. 113.

[64] See above, Ch. 3, n. 29 for the literal use of Ecclus. 38 in *Liber de vinis* and n. 73 for Galvano's literal use of Ecclus. 38.

When Ecclesiastes [*sic*] 38 says: 'Honour the physician for he is essential to you', he manifestly intimates (*manifeste insinuens*) that he alone does not cure diseases as some people believe (otherwise he would not have ordered that we honour surgeons or physicians for it would not be necessary). And when he adds, '[f]or He makes the earth yield healing herbs' (Ecclesiasticus 38: 4), it is evident (*patet*) that he did not intend [to speak about] the physician of the soul because it is not from earth that he had created the medicine of the soul.[65]

Even churchmen sometimes interpreted Ecclesiasticus 38 literally, as did Giovanni da San Gimignano in a funeral sermon for physicians. According to Giovanni, verse 11 ('Give the physician his place', *Da locum medico*) refers to the human physician, because he plays an essential role in dispensing charity. Thus, though God can cure by words alone, the physician's activity is essential.[66] The first written statutes of the medical school at Montpellier, produced in 1220 by Cardinal Conrad with the explicit agreement of the bishops of Maguelonne, Agde, Lyons, and Avignon, start with a rhetorical declaration which directly quotes Ecclesiasticus 38: 4 as binding testimony of the need to venerate the science of medicine.[67]

Exegetical scholarship as a learned art was directly accessible only to a literate minority. Nevertheless, its content reached a broader audience, mainly through sermons. In Chapter 4 I discussed the use of the 'medical model' in preaching literature. The metaphorical comparison between Christ, preachers or priests, and physicians largely communicated a favourable image of physicians. However, biblical stories depicting actual acts of healing provided a different image which stressed the moral flaws of physicians and the shortcomings of human medicine. The story of Hezekiah (Isaiah 38: 1–6) who, struck by a corporeal disease, cried to God in prayer and thereby prolonged his life, was frequently used by preachers to discuss the relationship between spiritual and physical

---

[65] Henri de Mondeville, *Die Chirurgie*, Tract. II, Notab. introd. 25.11, pp. 133, 135; Nicaise, *Chirurgie*, 199, 202; Pouchelle, *The Body and Surgery*, 44. This he declares after stating that the only manual work explicitly attributed to Christ in Scripture was *officium cyrurgici*. He concludes: 'ubi opus cyrurgicum pre aliis approbatur'.

[66] Giovanni da San Gimignano, *Conciones funebres*, 721–8 (centred on Jer. 8: 22, 'medicus non est ibi'). About this collection, see E. Winkler, 'Scholastische Leichenpredigten: die *Sermones funebres* des Johannes von St. Geminiano', in *Kirche, Theologie, Frömmigkeit* (Berlin, 1965), 177–86; D. L. D'Avray, *Death and the Prince: Memorial Preaching before 1350* (Oxford, 1995), 44–6.

[67] 'Nimirum hanc scientiam sapientis sententia persuadet venerari testans, quia Altissimus creavit de terra medicinam et vir prudens non abhorrebit illam'. *Cart. Mont.*, 180/2.

health, and to stress the efficacy of prayer.[68] Bertrand de la Tour held that, whereas all the other physicians were satisfied by gifts and money (and thus betrayed their greed), the celestial physician was satisfied solely by prayer.[69] Another biblical story popular with preachers was Luke 8: 43 and Mark 5: 26, which relate the story of the woman who had the issue of blood for twelve years. The inability of the physicians to heal the woman and the deterioration of her condition led preachers to present the physicians as representing passions of the flesh (*carnales affectus*), which do not revive and heal but kill and damn the patients. In no other profession is there such a concentration of evil people, hence the woman rightly consulted Christ, the only source of true cure.[70] Similarly the good king Asa, who in old age was stricken by pride and avarice (1 Kings 15: 23), devoted himself to the medical art, which is 'the diligence, sagacious knowledge and experience of carnal desires', rather than to God.[71]

The contamination of the physician's image by this type of interpretation was exacerbated even further when *exempla* portraying physicians as agents of the devil were introduced to the sermons, other preaching material, and hagiographic literature. John Bromyard, for example, describes the devil touching the sinner's heart as a physician taking the patient's pulse in the wrist with three fingers. Both deceive the patients by comforting them without grounds. He also depicts sloth as the medicine of the devil; the infernal physicians (*medici inferni*) appear in the *exemplum* as those who provide the monk with the medical reason for not waking up on time for Matins.[72] Caesarius of Heisterbach asserts that the origin of the physician's knowledge is from the demon.[73] The *Dialogus Miraculorum* tells of a priest who was

---

[68] *Glossa Ordinaria* on Isa. 38: 1, in *Biblia sacra, cum glossa ordinaria*, iv. 335–42 at 335–6.

[69] 'Omnes enim alii medici placantur muneribus et pecuniis ait Chrys. super Mat. Medicus autem celestis qui libentius sanitatem spiritualem quam corporalem efficit sola oratione placatur.' Bertrand de la Tour, *Sermones quadragesimales epistolares* (Strasbourg, 1501/2), fol. xiiii[ra].

[70] L.-J. Bataillon, 'Les images dans les sermons du xiiie siècle', *Freiburger Zeitschrift für Philosophie und Theologie*, 37/3 (1990), 357–8 (a sermon of Gérard de Mailly, who explains the woman's rational supplication).

[71] 'industria, sagaci scientia et experientia carnalium affectuum . . . non ergo est in medicis confidendum.' Antonio da Padova, *Sermones dominicales et festivi ad fidem codicum recogniti*, ed. B. Costa, L. Frasson, and I. Luisetto (Padua, 1979), ii. 441.

[72] Bromyard, *Summa predicantium*, *Misericordia*, ix. fol. ccxiii[rb–va]; *Accidia*, v. fol. vi[rb].

[73] *Die Wundergeschichten des Caesarius von Heisterbach*, iii. ed. A. Hilka (Bonn, 1937), 52.

overwhelmed by a desire for a certain woman. As he was suffering 'it was said to him by a physician—or rather by the devil through a physician' (*dictum ei a medico—immo per medicum a diabolo*) that in order to convalesce he must fornicate with that woman. Having regard for this life and not for the future, he liaised with the woman and this brought about his quick death.[74] This image is connected with the fear that medical therapy involves practices which are incompatible with Christian ethics. Alpais of Cudot saw the devil appearing in a vision as a doctor; for her, the very offer of a cure was a temptation.[75] And the Franciscan Guibert de Tournai, in the first of three sermons directed at lepers (*Ad leprosos et abiectos*), describes the devil as a physician who suggests to those wishing to lead a frugal life that this undermines the complexion and hence is a cause of disease. In the name of defending the complexion, they then reject spiritual therapies such as vigils and fasts.[76] The use of the term *medicus* as referring to the devil also appears in Biblical commentary. In *Glossa Ordinaria* on Luke 8: 43 the *medici* whose help the woman with the flow of blood vainly seeks are interpreted in the marginal gloss thus: 'Physicians—demons who as if looking after human beings, demand that they worship them [the physicians/demons] instead of God.'[77]

Other preachers criticized what they saw as materialism in belief among their audience. Turning to physicians in illness was one of the expressions of this objectionable materialism.[78] Complaints against the excessive care of the body at the expense of spiritual health sometimes appeared in sermons, suggesting competition between priests and physicians. With reproach Giovanni da San Gimignano describes how the ill immediately obey even the most unpleasant demands of the physician, and never neglect anything which has any bearing upon their health, whereas nobody listens to the most skilful and wisest of all physicians—

---

[74] *Dialogus Miraculorum*, ed. J. Strange (Brussels, 1851), Dist. IV. 101, 271. See also F. C. Tubach, *Index exemplorum: A Handbook of Medieval Religious Tales* (FF Communications, 204; Helsinki, 1969), 128/1561.

[75] N. G. Siraisi, *Medieval and Early Renaissance Medicine* (Chicago and London, 1990), 14.

[76] 'Et factus est dyabolus phisicus disputans de complexionibus, et si perseveremus in bono proposito minatur mortem imminentem.' N. Bériou and F.-O. Touati, *Voluntate dei leprosus: les lépreux entre conversion et exclusion au XIIème et XIIIème siècles* (Spoleto, 1991), 130: 25–8.

[77] 'Medici, demones, qui quasi consulentes hominibus, pro Deo se coli exigunt.' *Glossa Ordinaria* on Luke 8: 43, in *Biblia sacra, cum glossa ordinaria*, v. 817.

[78] A. Murray, 'Religion among the Poor in Thirteenth-Century France: The Testimony of Humbert de Romans', *Traditio*, 30 (1974), 319, n. 198.

Christ.[79] Giovanni does not criticize excessive care of the body, but demands a similar concern for the word of God.

The inverse use of the medical model (spiritual physicians are what human physicians are not), and the employment of spiritual allegory criticizing human medicine and physicians, reflect real attitudes in some devout circles. These attitudes were communicated to the broad public. Hence the Bible provided a framework for a wide range of attitudes towards secular medicine and its officers, and was used to stress the absolute superiority of the True Physician over the human physician. Preachers also sometimes used it to criticize the human physician and the cure he offered, although it was used as well (by Arnau and by some clerics) to enhance the status of the human physician and corporeal medicine as fully congruent with the spiritual physician and his medicine.

Ambivalence and suspicion were two of the characteristics of clerical attitude towards physicians. This was certainly not the only possible clerical approach to medicine and the physicians, yet neither was it a negligible one. How justifiable were these attitudes in the light of Arnau's medical writings and those ascribed to him? In what follows I shall discuss three questions which theoretically could justify clerical caution and even suspicion of physicians. First, how compatible was the 'clerical approach' to disease with that of the physicians who ignored its moral and religious significance? Second, does the therapy prescribed by Arnau and his fellow practitioners support the image of physicians endangering Christian morals? And third, were physicians reliable in fulfilling their religious duties to ensure the spiritual health of their patients?

The Aetiology of the Physicians

Does Arnau adopt in any form the 'clerical approach' to disease? His definition of disease precludes any direct supernatural causes. Except for one formulaic description at the beginning of *De venenis*, in which God

---

[79] 'Maxime deplorandum est, quod homines tanto studio corpus curent, anime vero salutem parvi aut nihil faciant. Precipit aliquid medicus etiam difficile agendum, pro corporis sanitate recuperanda, confestim illius dicto egroti obtemperant, nihilque pretermittitur eorum que saluti corporis conducere videntur. At Christus sapientissimus Doctor et peritissimus animarum nostrarum medicus et restaurator, verbis suis quotidie remedia ad salutem animarum necessaria proponit, docet, ostendit, nemo tamen aures attentas prebet.' This is from a sermon about the necessity of death by Giovanni da San Gimignano, *Conciones funebres*, 245. Cf. Ramon Llull, *Liber de virtutibus et peccatis sive ars maior praedicationis*, CCCM 76, 207: 99–104.

affectionately sends diseases as part of his salvatory scheme,[80] nowhere in his medical treatises does Arnau accept that disease is a corrective benefit imposed by God on the human being, possibly as a result of his sins. For Arnau, physical affliction (*morbus vel lapsus*) is one of the 'things against nature' (*res contra naturam*) and must be treated as such. In calling the physician servant (*minister*) or partner of nature (*socius nature*),[81] Arnau allocates to nature a major role in determining the order of the physical and the spiritual aspects of the universe. The physician may have the power to present natural phenomena as if they were miracles,[82] but practical investigation (*investigacio realis*) is the key to finding the correct pattern of practice (*recta forma operandi*) in any medical condition and to acquiring concrete, manifest, and certain knowledge.[83] In his theoretical discussion of disease in *Speculum medicine*, Arnau distinguishes between disease and its causes and accidents, discusses the two phases of failing health (*lapsus*), enumerates the various types of diseases (regional, epidemic, regiminal, contagious, and hereditary), differentiates between simple and composite diseases, and ignores any reference to divine involvement in the process which leads to disease or cures it. Human medicinal intervention and manual practice (*medicari et manualiter operari*) is the only means for cure.[84] His aetiology is thus strictly natural, firmly in keeping with the Hippocratic legacy and common to other academic physicians.[85]

For Arnau the relationship of the physician, the art of medicine, and good health is logically likened to the relationship of the farmer, agriculture, and the product of the land. In each case the human is only a secondary agent and not the first cause. The product—health—thus cannot be regarded as absolutely produced by human skill (*absolute artificialis*); it is the result of a natural process. The foundation of the body is natural *per se*; but *per accidens* it is artificial.[86] The physician is not

---

[80] 'Creator ominum deus in secula benedictus percutiens pie ac sanans emisit ex thesauro uberrimo ineffabilissime clementie sue naufragio humane salvationis lapsus corporales et spirituales.' *De venenis*, in Arnau de Vilanova, *Opera* (Lyons, 1520), fol. 216vb.

[81] Giovanni da San Gimignano, *Conciones funebres*, 721 calls the physician *Dei minister et nature*. This might reflect Giovanni's recognition of his elevated, quasi-religious status. It also may hint at his wish to submit the physician to God and not only to nature.

[82] *Liber de vinis*, in Arnau de Vilanova, *Opera*, fol. 263ra.

[83] *Contra calculum*, ibid. fol. 305vb; *Doctrina Galieni de interioribus*, in *AVOMO*, xv. 306–7.

[84] *Speculum medicine*, in Arnau de Vilanova, *Opera*, fols. 27ra–32rb.

[85] See Bernard de Gordon's explanations for epilepsy, depressive mania, and nightmares, in L. E. Demaitre, *Doctor Bernard de Gordon: Professor and Practitioner* (Toronto, 1980), 159–61.

[86] 'Nam corpus eius principium per se naturale est, per accidens vero artificiale'. *De parte operativa*, in Arnau de Vilanova, *Opera*, fol. 123ra.

supposed to occupy himself with altering nature, which according to Galen is the producer of everything (*omnium operatrix*). As manager of the non-natural things (*administrator rerum non naturalium*), he is utterly subordinate to nature, and at most can claim to be nature's aid (*auxilium*).[87]

Yet at the same time both disease and medicine are for Arnau parts of the divine order of the world. He clearly reveals this in the opening chapters of the treatise *Contra calculum*, which may have been written in 1301 shortly after he cured Boniface VIII of kidney stones.[88] Here he says that medicine is a science created by divine providence for the benefit of mankind to counteract the ailments resulting from Adam's sin. Original sin is a criminal attempt to supply a medical cure for created things, disregarding divine order. He implicitly compares Adam and Eve to physicians who try to supply medicine without God's consent: in his opinion, a faithful physician is required to practise his art in full accordance with divine will. Like Avicenna, Arnau stresses that medicine cannot absolve anyone from death, but can merely postpone man's death until the moment nature has ordained for it; he thinks it wrong, therefore, to hope for eternal health.[89] In Part II of *De Cautelis medicorum*[90] he warns the physician against promising health, because 'then he would eliminate a divine function and unjustly harm God'.[91] In *De humido radicali* he defines and discusses death as a purely biological process naturally caused by the impotence of the life-giving heat to restore the radical moisture, which has been lost. The process is natural; it can be regulated by the physician, but not prevented. The active role of God is limited to exclusive knowledge concerning the precise duration of the efficacious

---

[87] *Contra calculum*, ibid. fol. 305rb; *De simplicibus*, ibid. fol. 233va. Galen's demiurge-God was never willing or able to do things that are impossible by natural standards. See G. Keil, 'Galen's Religious Belief', in *Galen: Problems and Prospects*, ed. V. Nutton (London, 1981), 117–30.

[88] *Contra calculum*, fols. 305va–306ra; J. A. Paniagua, *El Maestro Arnau de Vilanova médico* (Valencia, 1969), 64.

[89] *Liber canonis*, i. *c. de necessitate mortis eius*. Cf. Avicenna, *Liber canonis*, i. fen 3, 1, 53ra.

[90] Part II of the treatise—regarded by H. E. Sigerist, 'Bedside Manners in the Middle Ages: The Treatise *De cautelis medicorum* Attributed to Arnold of Villanova', in *Henry E. Sigerist on the History of Medicine*, ed. F. Martí-Ibáñez (New York, 1960), 133 as not authentic—is repeated almost literally at the concluding paragraph in Arnau's *Repetitio super can. Vita brevis*, in Arnau de Vilanova, *Opera*, fol. 281rb, and may well be treated as an authentic text of Arnau.

[91] 'tunc extirparet divinum officium et facit Deo iniuriam'. *De cautelis medicorum*, ibid. fol. 216rb.

activity of natural heat.[92] For Arnau, it is the remote sin of Adam which renders medicine necessary; ordinary sin apparently has no effect on health, and the moral and religious attitudes of the patient are irrelevant to the healing process. As far as medical causation is concerned, God exists as the prime cause of maladies, as an omniscient being, as the creator of medicine, as the summit of acuity, or the prime intellect; but he is so remote that he becomes almost irrelevant to the healing of most diseases. The physician, inscribed as God's helper, performs the actual cure by regulating the substance of things non-natural according to due quantity, quality, and time.[93] This is an approach to disease quite different from the 'clerical' one.

In one of Arnau's later spiritual treatises he argues that longevity is not a matter of any mundane privilege or grace such as youth, physical strength, complexion, health, lineage, or power. No one, whether young or old, ordinary person or king, knows when he will die. Death is determined solely by divine will, which is influenced by the behaviour of the individual. The physician is powerless in this respect.[94] The spirit of this opinion complies with the clerical approach to disease, and contradicts, in part, the foundation of his medical writings, which ignored the link between moral behaviour and state of health. This could indicate the growing ambivalence towards corporeal medicine which engulfed Arnau towards the latter and more pious stage of his career. But it is more likely that he simply wanted to satisfy the spiritual taste of the Beguin community that commissioned the treatise.

In his spiritual texts, Arnau, who is loyal to the rule 'God and nature make nothing in vain',[95] recognizes nature's role as a prime principle for organizing life, explaining the universe, and ordering the moral and spiritual aspects in it. Such a view, which accords with the major role which he allotted to nature in the medical domain, uncomfortably coexisted, in

---

[92] 'Huius autem durationis mensuram solus ille cognoscit et terminum eius previdet cui patet proportio caloris vivifici ad humidum in restaurando et informando ex omnibus convenientissime concurrentibus ad naturam viventis corporis . . . et hoc in quolibet corpore que inquam, cognoscere secundum veritatem precisam solius credimus esse Dei.' *De humido radicali*, II. iv, ibid. fol. 42rb.

[93] 'Oportet ergo ponere unum intellectum primum, qui omnia agnoscat, sicut Deum. Medicus autem ministrando nature substantiam rerum non naturalium scilicet moderate secundum debitam quantitatem et etiam qualitatem et tempus, adiutor eius inscribitur, egro vero inimicus'. *Contra calculum*, fol. 305vb. Cf. Pouchelle, *The Body and Surgery*, 37–44, 45, and 226 n. 22 for Henri de Mondeville, who also distanced himself from God.

[94] *Per ciò che molti* in R. Manselli, 'La religiosità d'Arnaldo da Villanova', *Bullettino dell'Istituto Storico Italiano per il Medio Evo e Archivio Muratoriano*, 63 (1951), 98.

[95] *Tractatus de tempore adventus Antichristi*, 155: 900–1.

Arnau's case, with a growing belief that sense-perception is subsidiary to intellectual understanding.[96] When it comes to the human being as a distinct and certainly the most elevated of all animal species, Arnau introduces two categories—human nature and natural reason—which determine human behaviour and distinguish it from other animals. He defines human nature as the natural inclination that distinguishes mankind from the rest of the animals and accords with the role of the human species to perform 'deeds demanded by the faith, obligation under the law, justice and prudence, liberality and piety, friendship, and all civic virtues'.[97] Natural reason, as one of human nature's major characteristics, should rule every person unless he is mad, melancholic, or utterly bestial.[98]

Human nature is full of faults and weaknesses (*infirmitates humane nature*) which are particularly evident in the human body. Nevertheless, when contrasted with the excellence of divine majesty, faulty human nature can provide an important insight to the measure or degree of God's love towards humans.[99] Despite its shortcomings, Arnau is prepared to regard human nature as a possible and even a desired guideline to human behaviour. A comparison with the world of animals provides decisive proof of the extent of the benefit that God has bestowed upon the human species. Seeing (*visio*) a toad and comparing oneself with it will lead everyone to the true knowledge of God, his liberality and the benefits of creation.[100] The world of animals is thus a major instrument for theological inference.

The concept of the human species as elevated above all animals and portraying the natural (and hence desirable) order of things offers clear criteria for assessing human behaviour. Thus, if asked how bodily as well as spiritual health may be acquired, the answer should be: If you wish to possess bodily health, preserve a balanced complexion; and if you wish to

---

[96] *De prudentia catholicorum scolarium* in Graziano di Santa Teresa, 'Il *Tractatus de prudentia catholicorum scolarium* di Arnaldo da Villanova', in *Miscellanea André Combes*, ii (Rome and Paris, 1967), 446–7.

[97] 'opera fidei sive legalitatis et iustitie ac prudentie, liberalitatis ac pietatis et amicitie et omnis honestatis civilis'. *Allocutio Christini* in J. Perarnau, 'L'*Allocutio Christini* . . . d'Arnau de Vilanova', *ATCA* 11 (1992), 101: 291–3.

[98] *De helemosina et sacrificio* in J. Perarnau, 'Dos tratados 'espirituales' de Arnau de Vilanova en traducción castellana medieval: *Dyalogus de elementis catholice fidei y De helemosina et sacrificio*', *Anthologica Annua*, 22–3 (1975–6), 622.

[99] *Allocutio Christini*, 87.

[100] *Allocutio Christini*, 80–2: 29–53 and 85: 56–9. On the toad as a symbol of either death or the pain of divine punishment and as an agent of evil see M. E. Robbins, 'The Truculent Toad in the Middle Ages', in *Animals in the Middle Ages*, ed. N. C. Flores (New York and London, 1996), 25–47.

attend the health of the soul, preserve your noble qualities which nobody can do unless he performs only those things which fit his high or higher nature.[101]

The well-being of the body and the soul go hand in hand, and the physician who defines himself as the servant of nature (*minister nature*) employs nature not only for medical treatments but also for explaining abstract religious ideas. To explain the desired behaviour that makes men nobler, Arnau ventures into the well-ordered world of animals. Nature provides every species with a certain natural rank (*gradus*) by which its behaviour is judged. If the behaviour conforms to this rank the creature is noble (*nobilis*); it will be judged vile and inferior (*vilis*) if it performs actions which conform to the norms of lower species. It will be judged as nobler (*nobilior*) if it does what is expected of a species of a higher degree. Greyhounds which hunt mice exemplify vile conduct which contradicts their nature. If they hunt hares or rabbits they are noble (*nobiles*). They will be nobler (*nobiliores*) if they hunt wild beasts. Similarly, the hunting behaviour of falcons exemplifies the categories according to which human behaviour should be judged. Greyhounds and falcons (usually describing the brutish dimension of human behaviour) become a model which should be imitated by humans. If people perform actions which conform only to the norms of human nature, they should be judged noble (*nobiles*). The nobler (*nobiliores*) among the humans are those who indulge in angelic forms of activity such as contemplating God, his truths, and dignities, and praising him. The conclusion of the discussion is therefore that 'the lover of God must perform those deeds which conform to his high rank so far as it fits his species. This becomes evident from a comparison with other animals.'[102] Hence when Arnau calls the corrupt rich *desnaturats*, he accuses them of deviating from the nature of their species and lacking the natural qualities which should distinguish it.[103]

Nature also determines the boundaries of the therapy the physician can offer, since 'nothing should be done that nature does not allow'.[104] Thus, physicians should prefer natural means such as physical exercise,

---

[101] 'Si vis salutem corporis possidere, serva temperamentum. Et si vis salutem anime consequi, serva nobilitatem. Quam nemo servare potest, nisi solum operetur illa que tantum conveniunt gradui sue altitudinis aut sublimioris nature.' *Allocutio Christini*, 99–100: 264–7.

[102] 'amator Dei debet illa opera exercere que gradui sue altitudinis conveniunt quantum ad speciem et hoc in comparatione ad alia animalia'. Ibid. 102: 298–300; 101: 281–8 (for a comparison between human and animal behaviour). Cf. *Raonament d'Avinyó* in Arnau de Vilanova, *Obres Catalanes*, i. ed. M. Batllori (Barcelona, 1947), 187, 190.

[103] Ibid. 191.

[104] 'nihil est agendum quod natura non faceret'. *De simplicibus*, fol. 242vb.

baths, and diet in order to overcome disease.[105] The result of such an approach towards disease was to deprive supernatural forces (miracles or active divine intervention) of any significant role in the curing process, except for some rare cases. Arnau treated even epilepsy—an illness with significant religious connotations both for diagnosis and for cure—overwhelmingly as a natural phenomenon. Only in extreme cases of epilepsy would he appeal to divine help. Such was the case when an epileptic fit struck the patient in his sleep, accompanied by tremor. Arnau described it as incurable by mortal physicians.[106] Similar attitudes are expressed by the author of *De epilepsia*, attributed to Arnau. For him it is not the wrath of God or a demonic influence that causes epileptic fits, but natural causes, though he is aware that he is treating a disease that was cured by Christ. Facing a rare species of analepsy, he determines that when an unfortunate patient is reduced to a state of total immobility but still retains his sense-perception, the skill and experience of physicians cannot suffice for a cure in any way unless by the aid of the supreme physician, Jesus Christ, who healed epilepsy free of charge. However, he immediately beseeches Jesus to bestow on him his light, and then proceeds to offer advice on other species of the disease.[107]

Magic played a minor role in the therapies Arnau offered. He used a magical seal to cure Boniface VIII of his kidney disease, and specifically mentioned a hermetic lion-seal which, when in contact with the loins, immediately mitigated the pain caused by kidney stones.[108] He was prepared to concede the existence of demons, but at the same time he forcibly determined that the deceptions of magicians, the delusions of enchanters, and the shaking of sorcerers had no efficacy in medical therapy.[109]

---

[105] *De simplicibus*, ibid.; *Contra calculum*, fol. 305vb.

[106] 'medicinam aut curam non recipit mortalium medicorum.' *Afforismi*, in Arnau de Vilanova, *Opera*, fol. 121ra.

[107] 'languori infelici eius nullo modo medicorum peritia subvenire sufficit nisi summo medico Iesu Cristo opitulante, qui peregre proficiscens, morbum lunaticum gratis curavit . . . Ipsum ergo lumen Iesu verum obsecro, quatenus misericorditer me doceat.' *De epilepsia*, ibid. fol. 313^{va-b}.

[108] On this episode see H. Finke, *Aus den Tagen Bonifaz VIII* (Münster, 1902), 200–26 and esp. 205–6. *De Sigillis*, in Arnau de Vilanova, *Opera*, fol. 302ra. Arnau did not mention the magical path in the monograph he dedicated to kidney stones (*Contra calculum*). Cf. *Speculum medicine* fol. 7ra and the seventh lion-seal in *De sigillis*, fol. 302ra. On the doubtful origin of *De sigilis*, see Paniagua, *El Maestro*, 74–5 and McVaugh, *Medicine before the Plague*, 163–5.

[109] 'et magorum prestigia et incantatorum delusiones et maleficiorum vexationes ac etiam festinantes impressiones non aliter efficaciam habent, licet demones subministrent'. *De parte operativa*, fol. 127ra.

Similarly, the author of *De epilepsia* was strongly opposed to the application of any kind of what he called superstitious method.[110] Exactly like Arnau, he distinguishes between legitimate methods, which are based on the natural properties and manifestly good effect of the curing object, and superstitious methods, which might include divine symbols, Sunday prayers, and tying amulets to the diseased organ. For him, as for Arnau, the healing effect was derived from the material substance of the healing object, its quantity and physical composition. He therefore rejected any kind of enchanters, diviners, and soothsayers, as well as augury or any occult doctrine which Holy Scripture and the canons of the Church had not sanctioned.

Bernard de Gordon also attacked the use of magic in medical contexts, but several times he suggested the use of quack remedies and magical cures. Though his preference was for rational treatment, he only adopted magical cures as a last resort when all natural treatments were ineffective (for example, in the case of epilepsy).[111]

Arnau upheld the view that medicines might be affected by astral constellations and supplemented by various stones and minerals containing effective natural healing powers. Arnau, who may have been the author of *De iudiciis astronomie* ('On the prognostications of astronomy'), shared with most academic physicians the notion that superior constellations (such as the stars or natural properties of certain minerals) had a distinctive influence over the lower things (*res inferiores*) which included every kind of human action (*humanis operatio*). Skilled physicians had to acquire and use sufficient understanding of the powers of the universe (*virtutes orbis et materie*). As for the use of natural healing objects, as long as they were exploited for cures in a way consonant with their particular nature and natural properties (*virtus specifica*), their use was allowed and even recommended.

The medical texts wrongly attributed to Arnau contain a few examples of appeals to divine help. Their scarcity even in these texts suggests that his avoidance of supernatural curing methods was not unique. Thus *Breviarium practice* declares that when a lethargic person develops certain clinical signs (such as tremor of the members and discolouring of the

---

[110] *De epilepsia*, fol. 315^{va-b}. Cf. Augustine, *De doctrina christiana libros quattuor*, ed. H. S. Vogel, Florilegium Patristicum, 24 (Bonn, 1930), II. xx. 30–1 and xix. 45, pp. 33–4, 41–2. *Breviarium practice*, in Arnau de Vilanova, *Opera*, fol. 189ra also rejects the use of spells to ease the pains of women in childbirth, saying, 'Que alia incantatoria habentur, vere fideles fugiant.'

[111] Demaitre, *Doctor Bernard*, 157–9; McVaugh, *Medicine before the Plague*, 164–5.

urine) 'we should entrust him to the holy spirit and transfer him to the priests and run away from him'.[112] When phrenesis has been diagnosed the prudent physician is advised not to treat it but to relinquish it to the soothsayers (*prognostici*) since it is not the physician's role to resuscitate.[113] Semitertian fever (*Hemitritaeus*) can be healed by divine hand rather than by human intervention;[114] and the author of *Breviarium* also describes how he went to a priest who removed from his hands more than a hundred warts by touch, marking the sign of the cross on them and reciting the *Pater noster*.[115]

Sterility, impotence, and any other conditions which prevent intercourse or conception constituted another set of medical problems which could not be easily solved by natural means. In this area, healing methods involving divine aid were most often advocated. But even here physicians seem to have looked on this only as a last resort. The pseudo-Arnau's 'Remedies against Evil Effects of Magic' (*Remedia contra maleficia*) at first glance gives the impression that there is no place for conventional medicine when coition is hampered by black magic.[116] In such cases only divine help will do; as its author says, 'Put your hope in God and he will confer upon you his mercy.' However, diagnosis of the condition should be by the usual means of careful observation and investigation. As to prevention, a physician should understand the various kinds of magic to counteract its effects. Direct priestly intervention may be confined to the case of magic worked through a spell composed of sacred letters or words (*character*), which should, when found, be brought to the priest. The *Breviarium* analyses the various causes of sterility and admits that when a woman is afflicted by it from the beginning of her life or because she has reached the age of 50 or 60, only a divine miracle will be able to ensure conception. The story from the apocryphal History of Hanna, about the 60-year-old Elizabeth who miraculously gave birth to John the Baptist, is related as an example.[117]

Divine intervention is limited to the minimum in *Tractatus de sterilitate*, attributed to Arnau. When the author deals with female sterility

---

[112] 'ipsum Sancto Spiritui commendemus, et tradamus ipsum sacerdotibus, et ab eo fugiamus.' *Breviarium practice*, fol. 199ra. A prayer over the healing potion offered to a patient bitten by a snake is at fol. 192va.   [113] Ibid. fol. 198ra.

[114] Ibid. fol. 200va.   [115] Ibid. fol. 186ra.

[116] *Remedia contra maleficia*, in Arnau de Vilanova, *Opera*, fol. 215va–b; Paniagua, *El Maestro*, 73–4.

[117] *Breviarium practice*, fol. 187rb. *Liber de vinis*, fol. 265va mentions wine which protects the pregnant woman, reduces the risk of miscarriage, and defends the embryo 'cum adiutorio dei'.

there is no mention of problems which are outside the scope of his medical skills. Men who suffer from *approximeron* (that is, lack of erection and emission) may be the victims of black magic. In this case the cure is in the hands of God. Those who utter the spell must revoke it, though there are medical books, adds the author, which suggest some practical advice to counteract the spell. Quicksilver in a box made of hazelnut may be attached to the neck, or mugwort (*arthemisia*) hung throughout the house of the afflicted couple. When sterility is due to a basic physical flaw such as damage to the flow of the spermatic humour from the brain to the kidney and the genital organs, that defect may only be cured by God, through a miracle.[118] But, on the whole, there are only a few incidents in the medical corpus attributed to Arnau where miracles or active divine intervention are offered as a possible means for curing a disease.

Arnau's spiritual writings reveal a different approach to aetiology. As a devout Christian, he could not and did not explicitly dismiss appeals to God for health. But he seldom mentions this. In *De prudentia catholicorum scolarium*, a didactic manual for scholars probably written before 1297, he parallels the search for knowledge with the search for health. He exhorts the *scholares catholici* to make the effort to reach true wisdom and to live according to it. The first part of the treatise deals with the manner of acquiring that wisdom; the second with how to shun deviance, defend orthodoxy, and resist error. According to Arnau, there is a divine origin to each and every type of wisdom (*sapientia*). Seekers after knowledge should approach God, for he alone can create *ex nihilo* the power of discernment, and also expand and clarify man's existing powers of understanding. The first stage in the process of acquiring knowledge is therefore to have a good desire (*bonum optatum*) to know the truth for the glory of God. Here Arnau introduces a medical analogy, comparing the intellectual process of acquiring truth through God with the process of acquiring health through direct divine aid.[119] Disease and cure constitute an opportunity for a religious experience and for a dialogue with God. Since both true knowledge and good health are divine goods, and since neither the sick person nor the aspirer after true knowledge can acquire their objectives solely by the use of their own powers, the analogy is useful. Knowledge will come as a result of a correct will, as it does for those who pray for health and do not mind how it is brought about (*modo*

---

[118] *Tractatus de sterilitate*, ii. 3, ii. 6, in Arnau de Vilanova, Raymund de Moleris and Jordan de Turre (attr.), *Tractatus de sterilitate,* ed. E. Montero Cartelle (Valladolid, 1993), 126, 136.

[119] *Tractatus de prudentia catholicorum scolarium*, 436–7.

sanandi). Arnau then lists eight ways through which God may exert his healing influence on a physically ill person: by words, by the sole power of the patient's will, or by applying a specific medicine, such as clay, to the eyes of the blind (John 9: 6). God can also heal by sending the ill to physicians such as priests.[120] Cure can be brought by a messenger, as it was in the case of Elisha; it can be brought by touch; it can be sudden or slow, in response to request or not. All these ways manifest the divine origin of health and the pattern of the physician/patient relationship. A person searching for knowledge, as if in a state of bad health, should approach God because he should leave to God things which transcend his own powers. However, he should do so only after having used his own intellectual faculties to their utmost limits.

This is the one example in all Arnau's writings of God's direct intervention in healing. We have already seen how Arnau, Galen's disciple, employs in his spiritual writings metaphors which reflect Aristotelian rather than Galenic physiological theories. There, as here, he does not hesitate to employ in his spiritual writings theories which he would not use in his medical works. This represents an interesting way of being 'theologically medical', and it offers a comfortable manner of mitigating the different emphases of physicians and clerics when they discussed diseases and their cures.

In his medical texts Arnau ignored, though he did not explicitly reject, divine intervention in causing disease or curing it. Nor did he discuss the moral significance of disease. I have found no evidence that this caused tension between him and the clerics. This may hint at an informal division of labour when discussing diseases. When the biological and medical aspects of disease were the issue, the natural approach determined the language and the content of the discussion; in such a context, clerics would subscribe to Arnau's explanation of aetiology and therapy. In a spiritual and religious context the 'clerical approach' to disease would introduce God into the curing process, give moral significance to disease, and stress the priority of spiritual over physical health. In such a context even academic physicians like Arnau might employ the clerical approach.

Visiting the Sick and the Dying

Arnau mentions two occasions when physicians and clerics are likely to meet—visiting the sick, and comforting the dying. On these occasions

[120] 'Quosdam vero ad medicos, ut ad sacerdotes mitendo.' Ibid. 436; cf. Matt. 8: 4 and Luke 5: 14, in which Jesus advises the leper 'ostende te sacerdoti'.

physicians and priests serve the same client at the same time. They are cus-
tomarily offered the place of honour at the dinner table in the client's house
(an offer the physician ought to reject, according to the author of *De cautelis
medicorum*).[121] Each one provides his treatment, and maximum cooperation
between the two is needed. On each of these occasions Arnau has something
critical to say of the clerics. In *Confessio Ylerdensis*, delivered in 1303 to the
Archbishop of Tarragona in Lleida, he says of the pseudo-religious that
they visit the sick out of cupidity and not charity.[122] Visiting the sick
becomes, for Arnau, a test of the visitor's religiousness. As a physician he
was unimpressed by the priests (especially mendicants) whom he met at
bedsides, and was repelled by clerical visitors motivated by gain. He regarded as 'tavern goliards' false regular clergy (*religiosi*) who tried to obtain wine
and expensive food. Because they needed laymen to maintain their corrupt
way of life, they tried to attract them by sermons, confessions, provision of
Mass, or visiting them in their homes in sickness and in health.[123]

The priest and the physician also meet at times of impending death.[124]
The priestly remedy aims to open the door to salvation, and Arnau is critical of this. He says that a man who throughout his life has done the
opposite of what Christian love prescribes cannot suddenly renounce the
object of his past desires (temporal goods). The heart cannot suddenly
abandon what it has become accustomed to love. Natural reason cannot
ensure real contrition on the death-bed, because natural reason determines that people will always follow their habits rather than embark on a
new path. Arnau brands the hope for last-minute contrition as mad and
corrupt, especially in the case of rich people who throughout their life
lacked *caritas*. Real contrition can only be achieved either through a miracle which softens the patient's heart or through the grace of God, if the
long torment forces the diseased person to a true change of heart and
abandonment of temporal desires. However, usually death does not provide an opportunity for real contrition.[125] Consequently Arnau explicitly
rejects promises of salvation for gravely ill or dying people, and declares
that those who preach thus are false teachers, because they tacitly incite

---

[121] 'Cum autem ad prandium te invitaverit non te oportunum ingeras; nec in mensa primum locum occupes, licet sacerdoti et medico soleat primus locus servari.' *De cautelis
medicorum*, fol. 216rb.

[122] MS Vat. lat. 3824, fol. 175vb.

[123] *Raonament d'Avinyó*, 197.

[124] M.-C. Pouchelle, 'La prise en charge de la mort: médecine, médicins et chirurgiens
devant les problèmes liés à la mort à la fin du Moyen Âge (XIIIe–XVe siècles)', *Archives
européennes de sociologie*, 17 2 (1976), 249–78 at 249–57.

[125] *Raonament d'Avinyó*, 201; *Per ciò che molti*, 96–7.

the faithful to persevere in their corrupt modes of life in this world, and fail to prepare them for the real contrition necessary for salvation. In order to explain his attitude, Arnau compares such deceptive preachers to false physicians who are primarily concerned with the means to enhance their own glory rather than with the well-being of their patients. Thus, when they know that the climax of the sickness is approaching, they mislead the patient and his attendants by admonishing him not to lose hope when he suffers fits of sweat. They give such advice knowing that the outcome of the treatment depends solely on the grace of the Lord. If the patient dies, the physician can always claim that, had he suffered the fits of sweating with patience, he would have been cured. But the physician has neither cured him nor showed him the way to suffer.[126]

The rejection of the promise of salvation through last-moment contrition was an idea shared by various spiritual groups at that time, including the Beguins;[127] the appearance of this idea in Arnau's text, therefore, does not necessarily link it to his medical background. Nevertheless, the similarity between his critique of physicians who promise their patients certain cure and his rejection of preachers' promises of guaranteed salvation is striking, providing further evidence for the known difficulties of enforcing canon 22 of Lateran IV. From 1240 the statutes of Montpellier include an explicit requirement not to counsel any severely ill patient before he has been to the priest. The statutes of 1340 contain a direct quotation of canon 22 of Lateran IV, which perhaps hints at a real difficulty in enforcing this practice. The frequent reiteration of canon 22 throughout the fourteenth century in the Crown of Aragon suggests that other physicians were either lax or critical when it came to its implementation.[128] Item 6 in the *furs* of Valencia from 1329 obliged every medical practitioner, whether physician or surgeon, annually to swear before the newly elected justiciar that he would not start treating a seriously ill or wounded patient if the patient had not first made confession. Only when a delay would be dangerous could this stipulation be deferred to the second visit.[129] Confessors' manuals (*Summe confessorum* or *Summe de casibus*

---

[126] *Raonament d'Avinyó*, 201–2.

[127] See Batllori's remarks in Arnau de Vilanova, *Obres Catalanes*, i. 200 n. 35.

[128] *Cart. Mont.*, 188/5. 'Item, jurent quod nullum recipient laborantem acuta, nisi prius se ostenderit sacerdoti, si possibile sit'; for the 1340 statutes see ibid. 344/10. For the evidence concerning the Crown of Aragon see McVaugh, *Medicine before the Plague*, 171 n. 13.

[129] L. García-Ballester, M. R. McVaugh and A. Rubio-Vela, 'Medical Licensing and Learning in Fourteenth-Century Valencia', *Transactions of the American Philosophical Society*, 79/6 (1989), 60. This demand could also reflect the need actively to acknowledge the authority and legitimacy of the newly elected official.

conscientie) of the late thirteenth and the fourteenth centuries blame physicians' misconduct rather than the patients' dislike of confession for this state of affairs. Some are laconic and cite abbreviated parts of Canon 22; others quote it verbatim and even add some commentaries, and all reflect a reality in which it was difficult to enforce canon 22 of Lateran IV.[130]

In his discourse on the first Hippocratic aphorism, Arnau takes his students step by step through their first encounter with a patient, and nowhere does he mention the need for a confession or the involvement of a priest in any stage of the cure.[131] He also utterly ignores, in his medical and spiritual writings, the belief in the physical effect of confession and extreme unction commonly expressed in biblical exegesis and confessors' manuals. According to this belief, the sacrament of extreme unction affects the person, that is, body and soul together. Though the primary effect of anointing the sick is the cure of spiritual infirmity (venial sin, according to Bonaventura and Scotus, and the remains of sin, *reliquie peccati*, according to the Thomists), it can accidentally bring physical relief, since by strengthening the soul which rules the body it has secondary, physical effects. Grace conferred by this sacrament causes both remission of sins and the conditional alleviation of bodily infirmity.[132] The impact of anointing the sick person on his physical health is unqualified in the *Glossa Ordinaria*,[133] although in the late thirteenth century some reservations were expressed. *Astesana*, for example, cited the opinion of Richard

---

[130] Ramon de Penyafort, *Summa S^{ti} raymundi de Peniafort Barcinonensis . . . De poenitentia et matrimonio cum glossis Iannis de Friburgo* (Rome, 1603), iii.23, 457–8; Johannes von Freiburg, *Summa confessorum* (Augsburg, 1476), iii. Tit. 34, q. lxix, and *Confessionale*, in MS Oxford, Bodl. Lib., Laud Misc. 278, fol. 361ra.

[131] *Repetitio super can. vita brevis*, fol. 275–84^V. McVaugh, *Medicine before the Plague*, 171 n. 13, and 'Bedside Manners in the Middle Ages', *Bulletin of the History of Medicine*, 71 (1997), 217.

[132] B. Poschmann, *Penance and the Anointing of the Sick*, tr. F. Courtney (Freiburg and London, 1964), 234–57, esp. 242–9, 252–7; Z. Alszegly, 'L'effetto corporale dell'Estrema Unzione', *Gregorianum*, 38 (1957), 385–405 at 385–91. For the historical process which by the 9th century transformed anointing the sick from solely a means to restore bodily health to a powerful symbol of spiritual transformation and a means to the eternal cure of the soul, see F. S. Paxton, 'Anointing the Sick and the Dying in Christian Antiquity and the Early Medieval West', in *Health, Disease and Healing in Medieval Culture*, ed. S. D. Campbell, B. B. Hall, and D. N. Klausner (Toronto, 1992), 93–102.

[133] See *Glossa Ordinaria* on James 5: 14–15, in *Biblia sacra, cum glossa ordinaria*, vi. 1302–4 on which the sacrament of extreme unction is based. 'When we are sick,' says Peter Damian, 'languishing on the verge of death by the fever of mortal sins, the spirit of piety helps us and reminds us that we are but dust. It is the unction by which health (*sanitas*) is restored, sin is rejected and awe towards the Lord achieved.' He concludes by asking a rhetorical question: 'Videsne qualiter sacerdotalis manus infirmantis corpus alleviet, et illecebrosam sensuum motionem sacratissima mitiget unctione?' Ibid. fol. 1302. Cf. *PL* 144, 899B.

of Middleton (OFM, d. 1302), who stresses that the physical effect of extreme unction does not automatically remove the disease and its impact on physical disease is only secondary. Its effect may be supernatural (and hence no visible signs will appear); however, the resulting joyfulness of the interior soul may ameliorate the disposition of the body.[134] This accords with the varying opinions of ecclesiastical thinkers on the physical effect of confession or extreme unction. There was a growing tendency among scholastic thinkers to stress the absolute primacy of the spiritual efficacy of this sacrament and to play down (though not to rule out) its bodily effect.

Henri de Mondeville attests to a competitive climate between the surgeon and the priest in times of acute danger to the patient.[135] He describes a hypothetical dilemma (*dubium*) of a severely wounded person who is afflicted with an uncontrolled and highly dangerous haemorrhage and is simultaneously visited by a priest and a surgeon. Who should exercise his professional duties first? The surgeon claims priority, since if the haemorrhage is not stopped immediately, the patient may die before he has confessed. If he succeeds in stopping the haemorrhage the patient may be cured, or at least, his life will be sufficiently prolonged to enable him to perform properly his final confession. However, the priest also claims priority, because even under such circumstances the patient's soul is much more endangered than his body, and hence it is logical first to hasten to save that part which is more at risk. Henri's solution to the dilemma is revealing. He acknowledges the fundamental contradiction between religion and the art of surgery in this case (*aliter secundum artem aliter secundum fidem*). The preferable option is that priest and surgeon act simultaneously. Since this is forbidden by law, however (*non permittetur in lege*—presumably canon law) Henri reluctantly yields to the religious precept.

Arnau's attitude to non-Christian medical aid is another example of the intertwining between medical practice and religious considerations. He repeatedly annoyed clerics by referring to an issue which should have united clerics and physicians, the former for religious/spiritual reasons,

---

[134] *Astesana*, v. 41, 4; cf. Richard of Middleton, *Super quatuor libros sententiarum* (Brescia, 1591), Lib. IV dist. 24, art. 1, q.vi, 357–8 ('Utrum effectus huius sacramenti sit infirmitatis corporalis alleviatio'). Bonaventura, *In IV Sent.* Dist. 23 Art.1, in *Opera Omnia*, iv. 588–90 was his source for that notion, which similarly appears also in William of Pagula, *Oculus sacerdotis*, MS Oxford, Bodl. Lib., Rawl. A. 361, fol. 129[vb].

[135] *Die Chirurgie*, Tract. II, Doct. I.1, Declarat. pr. ad part. 2, 165–6; Nicaise, *Chirurgie*, 247; Pouchelle, *The Body and Surgery*, 46–8.

the latter in order to defend their professional interests. In June 1304 Arnau wrote a letter to the new Pope, Benedict XI, in which he called upon him to amend all his predecessor's defects, and which included Arnau's version of the events of 1300, discussing for the first time his attitude towards receiving medical aid from non-Christian medical practitioners. In the context of an attack on the sins of clerics in general and of the regular clergy, whom he accused of doing the opposite of what they preached, he included the following accusation, which he frequently repeated in later treatises:

And those who should have been accustomed, according to the canons of the Church published by public preaching, to abhor those who introduce Jews and infidels to the cure of their bodies, now ordinarily and daily want only those as healers of their bodily diseases, thus explicitly and publicly treating the saviour with contumely.[136]

The choice of a physician thus becomes, for Arnau, an act of faith.

In *Interpretatio de visionibus in somniis* Arnau attacks the behaviour of the regular clergy, describing it as sick and corrupted. He says that the daily practice in both monasteries and nunneries is not to let physicians through their doors unless they are Jews. He expresses his astonishment at this practice, which is contrary to what they preach and contrary to canon law.[137] He labels calling for the aid of Jewish physicians an abominable, monstrous act of blasphemy, and another example of the uncharitable behaviour of false religious people. The obsessive search for corporeal salvation which is at the core of this behaviour marks a deviation from true faith.[138]

It has been often claimed that the opposition to accepting medical counsel from non-Christian practitioners derived from professional competition within the community of medical practitioners. The ecclesiastical

---

[136] 'Et qui consueuerunt secundum canones ecclesie predicatione publica detestari eos qui iudeos et infideles ad curam sui corporis introducunt iam ordinarie quaque die solum eos habere uolunt suarum egritudinum corporalium curatores in expressam et publicam contumeliam saluatoris.' *De morte Bonifatii*, MS Vat. lat. 3824, fol. 210va. Cf. *Confessió de Barcelona* in Arnau de Vilanova, *Obres Catalanes*, i. 122; *Tractatus quidam*, MS Rome, Archivio Generale dei Carmelitani, III Varia 1, fol. 66va, which denounces those *religiosi* who 'plus credunt iudeo promittenti salutem corporis per artem medicine quam Christo . . . plus sperant de peritia iudei quam de benignitate et uirtute Christi.'

[137] *Interpretatio de visionibus in somniis*, p. lvi; cf. J. Shatzmiller, *Jews, Medicine and Medieval Society* (Berkeley, 1994), 95, 192 n. 60.

[138] *Epistola ad priorissam de caritate*, in Manselli, 'La religiosità', 65; *Tractatus quidam*, MS Rome, Archivio Generale dei Carmelitani, III, Varia 1, fols. 66va–67rb (also in Batllori, 'Dos nous escrits', 68–9).

legislation which prohibited Christians in the Crown of Aragon from receiving medicines and medical care from Jewish practitioners as early as 1243 in the Council of Tarragona[139] was interpreted as bowing to pressure from Christian physicians.[140] Arnau's opposition seems also to have been motivated by religious concern: there was something inherently wrong in calling on non-Christian physicians, and the fault was moral and religious. Thus, in Arnau's view, medical practice, unlike medical knowledge, was not religiously neutral.

In 1310, after having failed to convince James II of the need duly to punish Jews who supplied medical aid to Christians and Christians who sought the care of Jewish physicians, Arnau wrote a draft of constitution for Frederick III's Sicily which demonstrates his attempt to apply the prohibition in practice. There, in a section devoted to the Jews and following an item prohibiting them from holding public office, he says: 'We cannot have faith in those who do not have any faith, nor can those who betrayed their Lord be faithful to others.'[141] Consequently, he forbids the Jews to supply any kind of medical aid to Christians (from merely giving advice to production of medicines and trading in them) because by definition they cannot be reliable physicians (*medici fideles*). Having betrayed the Lord, they cannot be trusted as physicians or apothecaries; as haters of Christians they may cause damage and injury rather than cure. Jews who ignore this prohibition face an imprisonment period of a year, whilst the punishment for a Christian who violates this law is three months' imprisonment, and what he has given to the Jew for his service should be

---

[139] J. M. Pons i Guri, 'Constitucions Conciliars Tarraconenses (1229–1330)', in J. M. Pons i Guri (ed.), *Recull d'estudis d'història jurídica Catalana*, ii (Barcelona, 1989), 272: 'Item quod tam clerici quam layci in percipiendis medicinis et consimilibus prohibitam et dampnatam iudeorum familiaritatem evitent'; McVaugh, *Medicine before the Plague*, 59–60, 98–103.

[140] L. García-Ballester, 'Changes in the *Regimina sanitatis*: The Role of the Jewish Physicians', in *Health, Disease and Healing*, ed. Campbell, Hall, and Klausner, 126–7.

[141] 'In his confidere non possumus, qui fidem non habent, nec alijs poterunt esse fideles, qui eorum dominum prodiderunt et propterea providimus et iubemus ut nullus Iudeorum, qui, cum de illius spectaremur consilio sive cura, forte nobis cum nos odio habeant et procurent imperpendibiliter dispendia vel nociva, medendi artem in Christianos audeat exercere vel medicinas pro christianis conficere aut medicinas eisdem christianis vendere vel eciam ministrare.' *Codice Diplomatico dei Giudei de Sicilia*, i. ed. B. and G. Lagumina (Palermo, 1884), 34–5; H. Finke, *Acta Aragonensia* (Leipzig, 1908), ii. 698. *Capitula Regni Sicilie*, i. ed. F. Testa (Palermo, 1741), cap. lxx, 80; Shatzmiller, *Jews, Medicine and Medieval Society*, 189 n. 47. Similar advice appears in Arnau's *Informació espiritual*, in Arnau de Vilanova, *Obres Catalanes*, i. 235 and in *Tractatus quidam* in MS Rome, Archivio Generale dei Carmelitani, III Varia 1, fol. 66vb.

transferred to the Crown, which will donate it to the poor. Arnau does not explicitly mention fear of poison as the ostensible reason for opposing Jewish medicines, though he may be hinting at this fear. He does not specifically refer to a worry that Jewish practitioners might prevent dying Christians from receiving the last sacraments.[142] But his hostility towards Christians who are receiving medical care from Jewish physicians is part of a general ambivalence and sometimes aversion (frequently expressed in regional Church legislation) towards this habit.[143]

Arnau's attitude here shows how unhappy he was with the contemporary Aragonese situation. There, despite having no access to university studies, Jewish physicians, practitioners, and surgeons were actively and disproportionately practising and attending Christian patients of all social strata. King James II and his successor Alphonse III, as well as members of the urban middle and upper classes, frequently consulted Jewish physicians. In Barcelona between 1300 and 1340 the proportion of Jewish physicians to the Jewish population was perhaps five times larger than the proportion of Christian physicians to the Christian population.[144] Opposition to Christians receiving medical aid from Jews had been in the air since the 1240s; but local Church authorities only began to enforce the ban in the 1330s, when Jewish physicians in Barcelona were required to appeal to the bishop for permission to practise under supervision.[145] In the same decade the Council of Avignon (1337) was to include the argument that Jewish medical practitioners should be forbidden from treating Christian patients, because in such a situation 'the servile status of the Jews is inflated and elevated beyond its boundaries'.[146]

Similar arguments against reliance on Jewish physicians are found in *Tractatus quidam*, attributed to Arnau. In a revealing declaration about

[142] For evidence that this worry indeed occupied Christian minds in the fourteenth century see Shatzmiller, *Jews, Medicine and Medieval Society*, 90–3.

[143] L. García-Ballester, *Historia social de la medicina en la España de los siglos xiii al xvi* (Madrid, 1976), 50–3; P. Diepgen, *Studien zur Geschichte der Beziehungen zwischen Theologie und Medizin in Mittelalter: Die Theologie und der ärztliche Stand* (Berlin, 1922), 20–2; S. Grayzel, *The Church and the Jews in the XIIIth Century* (New York, 1966), 74 n. 147; Shatzmiller, *Jews, Medicine and Medieval Society*, 85–90.

[144] McVaugh, *Medicine before the Plague*, passim. and esp. 55–64. García-Ballester, 'Changes in the *Regimina sanitatis*', 127; García-Ballester, McVaugh, and Rubio-Vela, 'Medical Licensing', *passim* and especially 25–9, tables at 34–5 and documents no. 4, 6, 8, 18, 24, 28, 30; L. García-Ballester, L. Ferre, and E. Feliu, 'Jewish Appreciation of Fourteenth-Century Scholastic Medicine', *Osiris*, 2nd ser., 6 (1990), 85–117.

[145] McVaugh, *Medicine before the Plague*, 98–103.

[146] Mansi, *Sacrorum conciliorum nova et amplissima collectio* 25, 1105; Shatzmiller, *Jews, Medicine and Medieval Society*, 98–9.

his view of the physician's jurisdiction over his patient, Arnau (or one of
his disciples) determines that since the condition of disease demands the
full obedience of the patient to God and to the physician, consulting a
Jewish physician may result in subjecting oneself to the Jew. But giving
the Jew such a position of power is inconceivable.[147] Although a Jew may
be hired for moulding vessels, carpentry, weaving, or performing any
similar manual art, it is forbidden to contact Jewish physicians, since
Jews do not know and cannot follow the Christian rule according to
which the physician should be an intermediary between God and the
patient (*mediator inter deum et egrum*). Paraphrasing Ecclesiasticus 38:
12–14 and James 5: 14–15, which discuss the priest's role in the curing
process and stress the efficacy of prayer, he confidently asserts that,
since a Jew is not a priest of the Church and is not capable of obtaining
the divine grace of health for the patient, those Christians who call on
Jewish physicians scorn both God and the Christian faith.[148] The author
of *Tractatus quidam* denounces these clerics who ask for the help of
Jewish physicians on account of the dangerous example they present to
the believers. By doing so they publicly praise the mortal enemies of
Christ (*inimici mortales Christi*) and hence expose the faithful to the danger of apostasy. This discussion is based on the assumption that medicine is an intrinsic part of Christian culture. Its source is divine grace,
and its very efficacy depends on fulfilling the role allotted to it by the
Church.

Three points must be stressed here. First, nowhere does Arnau's
antipathy towards Jews in general and Jewish medical practitioners in
particular amount to the virulent anti-Jewish attitudes expressed, for
example, in Bernard de Gordon's medical discussion concerning Jews,
who allegedly suffer from bleeding haemorrhoids.[149] Second, some
medieval Jews also upbraided their fellow brethren for recourse to
Christian medical expertise.[150] And third, what emerges from this section
is that, for Arnau, medical practice was not religiously neutral.

---

[147] 'Unde quamuis liceat Christiano uocare iudeum ad uasa fingenda uel fabricanda uel
pannos texendos aut ligna dolanda uel similia officia in quibus non accipit imperium in personas, sed tantum in res que fiunt materia sue artis, tamen si uerus filius est ecclesie cristi
non licet ei in iudeum assumere in ministerium per quod potest imperare personas.' MS
Rome, Archivio Generale dei Carmelitani, III Varia I, fol. 66[vb]–67[ra].
[148] 'Cum ergo iudeus nec sit ecclesie presbiter nec idoneus ad obtinendum egro gratiam
sanitatis a deo, constat quod cristianus qui iudeum ad sui medicationem uocat ambo predicta spernit.' Ibid. fol. 67[ra].
[149] Demaitre, *Doctor Bernard*, 9–10.
[150] Shatzmiller, *Jews, Medicine and Medieval Society*, 121–3.

Medical Practice and Religious Considerations

Thirteenth-century *exempla* often denounce the demonic characteristic of physicians who prescribe therapies incompatible with a monastic lifestyle and lure pious Christians to a life of sin. These fears were not mere literary inventions. At the beginning of the thirteenth century Gilles de Corbeil (*c.*1140–*c.*1224), a court physician of Philip August and a canon of Notre Dame in Paris, wrote his *Hierapigna ad purgandos prelatos.*[151] In this approximately 6,000-line poem, presented as an antidote against the leprosy of the mind and the contagion of sin, Gilles appears as a spokesman for those clerics who were not prepared to renounce the carnal world altogether. He lambasts the attempt of Cardinal Guala, the papal legate, to impose complete chastity on clerics.[152] According to Gilles, this intolerable onus (*onus importabile*) is incompatible with nature, because it necessarily must encourage sodomy. When he accepts prostitution as a necessary evil for those who cannot master their desires, it seems that Gilles the physician rather than Gilles the priest is speaking.

Do Arnau's medical works contain therapies which were incompatible with Christian moral teaching? The few pieces of evidence I have collected suggest that Arnau, like most other physicians, accommodated the prescribed therapy, *regimen,* and judgement to the religious behaviour of his clients. In *Regimen sanitatis ad regem Aragonum,* written between 1305 and 1308 for James II, Arnau deals, among other things, with the appropriate times for meals. He stresses that the natural clock, namely the appetite, should generally determine eating habits. The popular habit of eating at fixed times is the custom of the *vulgus* and emanates from a false understanding by ignorant people. The only occasion on which the natural clock should be ignored despite hunger is when the precepts of the Church or monastic devotion demand it.[153] Thus, sometimes the instructions of religion override medical practice. Arnau also advises the king on

---

[151] C. Vieillard, *Gilles de Corbeil* (Paris, 1909), 74–95, 276–86; G. Rath, 'Gilles de Corbeil as Critic of his Age', *Bulletin of the History of Medicine*, 38 (1964), 133–8; E. Wickersheimer, *Dictionnaire biographique des médecins en France au Moyen Âge* (Geneva, 1936), 196–7; D. Jacquart, *Supplément* to Wickersheimer, *Dictionnaire . . .* (Geneva, 1979), 90–1.

[152] On the debate over clerical celibacy around 1200, see J. W. Baldwin, *The Language of Sex: Five Voices from Northern France around 1200* (Chicago and London, 1994), 61–3.

[153] 'Sumendus est igitur cibus appetente natura, nec diu eciam post esuriem debet sumpcio eius tardari, nisi quia sancte constituciones ecclesie vel honesta occupacio aut religiosa devocio quandoque suggerunt ipsam esuriem tolerare.' *Regimen sanitatis ad regem Aragonum, AVOMO,* x. 1, 429.

how to behave after the meal. He recommends both physical and spiritual rest, and suggests that the king sit and listen to anything which does not lie heavily on the mind, such as stories concerning kings and saints or melodious music.[154] Saints' stories thus have a medical as well as a religious value.

Arnau's contemporary, Bernard de Gordon, provides more examples of the accommodation of medical practice to Christian life. He discusses prayer as an effective soporific for the insomniac patient for whom all other remedies have failed, and recommends fast and scourging against concupiscence. He rebukes Avicenna's suggestion that it was good to get drunk once a month as a complete purge. No Catholic should knowingly get drunk, he says, and asserts that this therapy is totally against God and reason.[155]

The Provençal version of the Life of St Dauphine, who maintained her virginity while married to St Auzias, describes the event in Marseilles (1304) when, owing to pressure by the family concerned about their presumed sterility, the young childless couple consulted Master Arnau.[156] Dauphine feared that the medical examination would expose in public their secret of conjugal virginity. To prevent this from happening Dauphine and Auzias asked the Franciscan Friar Johan Jolia to brief Arnau on the true reasons for their childlessness. When the two arrived in Marseilles, Arnau received them and, filled with sympathy, he promised them full support. During the fifteen days in Marseilles he prescribed a daily diet based on meat and also interrogated them in public about their sleeping habits.[157] In private, Arnau and the pious couple discussed spiritual things. Deeply impressed by their innocence and purity, Arnau became even more devout. To a gathering of expert physicians who assembled to discuss the case in Marseilles, he declared that the couple was unable to procreate until the age of 25 due to four obstacles (*defaihimens e empedimens*) in the woman and three in the man. He thus conspired with Auzias and Dauphine to deceive their family and the medical community, which bowed to his authority. The text is a translation of a Latin original now lost. The Latin *Life of St Dauphine* was written after her death in 1360, and the present text is from the last years of the fourteenth

[154] *AVOMO*, x. 1, 434.

[155] Demaitre, *Doctor Bernard*, 26, 120–1.

[156] J. Cambell, *Vies Occitanes de Saint Auzias et de Sainte Dauphine* (Rome, 1963), 160–3; *Acta Sanctorum*, Sept. VII, 539–55 (life of St Auzias). A. Vauchez, *The Laity in the Middle Ages: Religious Beliefs and Devotional Practices* (Notre Dame and London, 1993), 201–2.

[157] On the importance of regulated sleep for efficient coitus, see *Regimen Sanitatis*, *AVOMO*, x. 1, 435. On the importance of meat consumption for the production of seed, see *Tractatus de sterilitate*, ii. 8, 142.

century. Chronologically and geographically, the event accords with Arnau's known biography; he was in Marseilles in 1304. Whether or not this was a historical event, it portrays well Arnau's image as a physician who shows sensitivity to religious motivations in his medical practice.

Nevertheless, clerics and canon lawyers did not always trust physicians to submit medical judgement to religious considerations. They frequently accused physicians of offering therapies which undermined Christian morals, and directed their suspicion at particular therapies and at the failure of physicians to fulfil their religious duties according to canon 22 of Lateran IV.[158] They entreated physicians always to give preference to the well-being of the soul, and to subject the medical art utterly to theology and to ethics. Physicians were regularly ordered never to prescribe a therapy which would hamper the spiritual salvation of the patient (particularly a member of the regular clergy), lest they misuse their art and harm God, themselves, and their patient.

It is not clear how widely accepted among clerics at the turn of the thirteenth century was the notion that medical therapy might endanger the soul. A single reference suggests the opposite, namely that medical theory (Galen) was employed even by clerics to support sexual continence. In a chapter praising conjugal virginity (*De continentia conjugali*), Servasanto da Faenza also compares continence to sapphire (which represses fever, strengthens the heart, has a sedative effect over fear, restrains sweat and bleeding, expels poisons, preserves the eyesight, mitigates headache, and cures every bruise); both prolong life. He quotes Galen in support of the contention that even a moderate discharge of semen would debilitate the body forty times more than the equivalent loss of blood. Therefore, those who indulge in excessive coition lose their natural complexion, become pallid, and age quickly.[159] He then backs it with two *exempla* from the world of the beasts which shows that coitus weakens the body of bulls, whilst infrequent copulation, as with elephants, causes longevity. The name of the Galenic source is not given, and the author may have just added Galen's name as an artificial scientific

<hr>

[158] Antonino di Firenze, *Confessionale* (Antwerp, 1513), p. lxxxxi^r–v (OP, 1389–1459); Jean Gerson, 'De non esu carnium', in *Oeuvres complètes*, ed. P. Glorieux (Paris, 1962), iii. 93–4.

[159] 'Unde Galienus dicit quod plus debilitat modica seminis emissio quam si quadragies tantum efunderet de sanguine unde et quis multum coeunt colorem perdunt siue pallidi fiunt et cito senescunt.' Servasanto da Faenza, *Liber de exemplis naturalibus*, MS Paris, BN lat. 3436, fol. 140^v. Cf. J. A. Brundage, *Law, Sex and Christian Society in Medieval Europe* (Chicago and London, 1987), 425 for Bonaventura, who similarly was convinced that frequent intercourse was dangerous to health and that every sex act helped to shorten one's life.

authority, since mainstream medical thinkers followed Galen's views according to which moderate sex under favourable conditions was conducive to healthful living for men and women alike. On this particular issue, Soranus of Ephesus (fl. c.100) who had concluded that perpetual virginity was the most healthful of states, would have been a more useful source to rely on; although his advocacy of virginity, which was transmitted in the fifth century to the Latin West by the abbreviated summaries of Muscio and Caelius Aurelianus, had little influence on the medical schools of the twelfth and thirteenth centuries. The prevalent rationale in support of chastity, therefore, could not have been drawn from current medical theory.[160] Servasanto's introduction of Galen in this context is significant, for it shows again that Bernard of Clairvaux's critical approach to Galen was not universal, and that some clerics were adamant to bolster their arguments by recognized medical authorities even at the price of attributing to them spurious views.

When it came to the discussion of the physiology of desire and sexual theory physicians exploited the same range of Latin vocabulary as did the theologians, and were fully aware of the opinions of their theological colleagues in the schools. Yet to the biblical account of sexual desire and its theological elaboration they offered a medical alternative that relied on morally and religiously neutral terms of physiology and psychology.[161] This is manifested in Arnau's discussion of coitus. His treatise on conception tersely describes and analyses impediments to conception without hinting at any moral or religious significance in coitus. Dry, technical discussion of coitus as a natural phenomenon appears in his *Regimen sanitatis ad regem Aragonum*.[162] The longer treatise devoted to coitus and attributed to Arnau in some printed editions from the Renaissance is similarly devoid of any religious references, apart from the formulaic opening, which mentions the Creator who devised coitus to ensure the survival of the animal race (*genus animalium*), and which thus situates coitus as a natural phenomenon common to all animals, including humans. The treatise which largely proceeds from Constantinus Africanus's *Liber de coitu* includes a long list of medicinal therapies to augment sexual desire.[163]

---

[160] J. Cadden, *Meanings of Sex Difference in the Middle Ages: Medicine, Science, and Culture* (Cambridge, 1993), 29, 273–5; Baldwin, *The Language of Sex*, 184–8.

[161] Ibid. 127–8.

[162] *Liber de conceptione*, in Arnau de Vilanova, *Opera*, fol. 213vb–214ra; *Regimen sanitatis ad regem Aragonum*, in *AVOMO*, x.1, 435.

[163] *Liber de coitu*, in Arnau de Vilanova, *Opera*, fol. 272vb–274va; Paniagua, *El Maestro*, 59–60.

Yet religious considerations occasionally do creep into Arnau's med-ical writing when he discusses matters exclusive to monks and nuns. He highlights the susceptibility of monastic communities to diseases related to their particular lifestyle when he describes in an aphorism how fever swiftly destroys the vital spirit of those living frugal lives of penitence and study.[164] How are the special needs of monastic communities reflect-ed in Arnau's medical texts and those attributed to him? In view of the fear that a religious lifestyle is not always conducive to health, how did physicians cope with monastic regulations? And more specifically, if coition, in addition to being the divine means to ensure regeneration, is regarded as a necessary contribution to a healthy life, if it eases the strains of the body, mitigates fury, helps the melancholic, provokes lovers to nostalgic memory, eases longing, reduces lust, and makes one tame and timid even though one is frenzy-stricken before coitus,[165] how should one advise monks who suffer from melancholy? That this is not an artificial question clearly appears in *Breviarium practice*, which asserts that the retention of bodily fluids which should have been emitted is one of the causes of melancholy. 'And this we see often happening amongst these widows and religious men and women. For as Galen says, when the seed is retained longer than needed, it is converted into poison,' remarks the author of *Breviarium practice.*[166] A healthy regimen thus sometimes con-tradicted monastic practice.

Physicians prescribed diet or phlebotomy for monks to reduce the

---

[164] 'Qui multis temporibus penitentia vel labore studii in contemplatione vixerunt et maxime parcissimi celeriter eos febris vitali depauperat spiritu.' *Repetitio super can. Vita bre-vis*, fol. 278rb; *Afforismi*, fol. 122ra.

[165] 'Coitus solvit malam habitudinem corporis, furorem mitigat, melancholicis prodest et amantes ad memoriam provocat; et concupiscentiam solvit. Licet furoribundum est ante-quam coeat, postquam vero coierit, fit magis domesticm.' *De coitu*, fol. 273va. On the neces-sity of coition for health see also *Speculum medicine*, fol. 26$^{rb–va}$; D. Jacquart and C. Thomasset, *Sexuality and Medicine in the Middle Ages* (Cambridge, 1988), 117–18; Cadden, *Meanings of Sex Difference*, ch. 6 and esp. 271–7; P. Gil-Sotres, 'Les normes de vida per a mantenir-se continent', in *AVOMO*, x. 1, 305–7.

[166] 'Et hoc in istis viduis religiosis viris et mulieribus sepe accidere videmus. Nam ut ait Galenus, sperma cum plus debito retinetur convertitur in venenum.' *Breviarium practice*, fol. 161rb. Cf. fol. 162ra which adds after a discussion of musical therapy for melancholy: 'And specifically these well fit the needs of people who suffer from these passions because of excessive abstinence like these religious monks (*religiosi monachi*), widows and the like and also those who study too much and who because of such study (*studium*) and passions of the soul and abstinence become mad and melancholic.' The term *studium* may also denote (religious) devotion. For the Arab roots of the notion linking extreme religious piety and excess study to melancholy, see R. Klibansky, E. Panowsky, and F. Saxl, *Saturn and Melancholy: Studies in the History of Natural Philosophy, Religion and Art* (London, 1964), 82–6.

quantity of semen, not masturbation.[167] Cataleptic epilepsy (all epileptic fits originating from various members of the body except for the brain and the stomach) may arise among men from 'poisonous soot generated by retention of a large quantity of cold semen in the male's vessels'.[168] For unmarried men, masturbation would be a logical therapy; yet the author of *De epilepsia* recommended that the treatment be the same as that prescribed to those who feel pain in coitus. Citing religious (Augustine's *Confessions* and possibly Bernard of Clairvaux) and not medical authorities to support his position, he emphatically cautions not to masturbate under medical guise. Masturbation, being a counter-natural practice, is abhorrent, and is one of the reasons why God smote Sodom. A physician who encourages it sins mortally, since the patient's soul is destroyed by it.[169]

Similar attitudes arise when the *Breviarium practice* discusses women's masturbation.[170] The natural cure for hysteria or suffocation of the womb (*suffocatio matricis*, an illness believed to be frequently caused by corrupt feminine seed or menstrual blood) is coition (within the marital contract), which is indeed prescribed to lay patients.[171] For widows, nuns, and other women vowed to chastity, the author of the *Breviarium* offers a chemical treatment to induce them to emit the seed without coition. A concoction made of finely ground sage and natron mixed with vinegar or salt water is prepared. Silk worm is dipped into the concoction, which is then inserted into the womb. The resulting gripping leads to emission of the superfluous seed. He then mentions a despicable habit of widows and wives of merchants who are sometimes absent from home for years. They yearn for coition, but, fearing pregnancy, they masturbate. He points out the women of Tuscany, especially the Florentines, who excelled in that practice. His attitude towards these practices is as harsh as those expressed by the author of *De epilepsia* against male masturbation.

---

[167] *Breviarium practice*, fol. 161[rb]; *De regimine sanitatis*, fol. 75[vb]; Cadden, *Meanings of Sex Difference*, 267, 275, 277, and Jacquart and Thomasset, *Sexuality and Medicine*, 146–55.

[168] *De epilepsia*, fol. 315[ra].

[169] 'Nihil enim mortalius medico, vel pernecabilius egro, ergo nihil fedius Deo, quam cuius ob depulsionem languoris, semina detestabitur provocare. Iuxta illud Bernardi: Vindictam peccati Sodomam, qui fundebat semen in terra percussit Dominus: quia rem detestabilem faciebat. Cui alludit Augustinus tertio Confessionum: Flagrantur qui sunt contra naturam ubique atque semper detestanda sunt, qualia Sodomitarum fuerunt.' Ibid. fol. 315[ra]; cf. Augustine, *Confessionum libri xiii*, III. viii.15, in *CCSL* 27, 35: 3–5.

[170] On female masturbation and the *suffocatio matricis*, see Jacquart and Thomasset, *Sexuality and Medicine*, 152–5, 173–7, and H. Rodnite Lemay, 'William of Saliceto on Human Sexuality', *Viator*, 1 (1981), 165–81, at 177–8.

[171] *Breviarium practice*, 190[vb].

The reasoning is again religious and not medical: 'these are all sodomic practices that are forbidden by the Church. It is therefore a grave sin to act this way and they should rather copulate with men and thus commit a lesser sin.'[172] As with the previous example, his solution complied with the ecclesiastical prohibition on masturbation and subordinated medical practice to religious considerations. It thus seems that physicians usually chose to subject themselves to self-censorship, in this way reaching a working relationship with the clergy in spite of the potential tensions. However, medical research on pathological discharges was impeded by these religious sensibilities.

Can one talk of special medical treatments which were applied specifically to members of the monastic orders? Those engaged in theological contemplation were encouraged to consume good wine, which clarified the mind and rendered the intellectual spirits clearer, subtler, and more numerous.[173] According to the *Breviarium*, it was the physician's role also to solve the sexual anxieties of those bound by monastic vows of abstinence. The chapter discussing how to extinguish the libido is directed at monks who suffer from *satyriasis* (a permanent erection accompanied by strong desire, usually assuaged by the performing of the sexual act) caused by the instigation of the devil or desire-inducing diet. Because the whole book was written in a Carthusian house (*Scala Dei*), the author recites the experience of its various members. Among the recommended remedies were the cooling of the testicles, proper diet which desiccates the seed and relieves the body of wind, fasting, hard labour, rough beds, and vehement contemplation of the First Cause.[174] The prescribed therapies coincided with those of theologians, who believed that virginity was lost only if involuntary emission occured after thoughts about coitus or the pudenda. In this case diet or phlebotomy were of no use; one must undergo fasting and flagellation. The most common therapy to curb extreme sexual desire among monks was phlebotomy, which was compatible with the monastic rule as well as with mainstream medical theory.

Arnau himself tells of a monk (*religiosus*) who has been treated with

---

[172] 'sed predicta omnia Sodomitica sunt et ab ecclesia prohibita. Est enim maximum peccatum hoc facere, unde potius consulo quod cum viris coeant et minus peccatum committent.' Ibid. fol. 191[ra]. On the other hand, Albertus Magnus held that female masturbation was often a physical necessity which may even help to preserve chastity. Jacquart and Thomasset, *Sexuality and Medicine*, 152.

[173] *Commentum super regimen salernitanum*, fol. 133[va–b].

[174] *Breviarium practice*, fol. 176[vb]–177[ra].

phlebotomy against frequent and annoying nocturnal pollutions, yet with no results.[175] The monk's complexion and especially that of his testicles was hot and humid. He complained that not only was the treatment ineffective, it even seemed to increase the intensity of the pollutions. The bewildered physician of this unfortunate monk sought advice from Arnau, who asked what the patient had eaten after the treatment. The physician replied that easily digestible food which generated good blood was suitable for those who had undergone phlebotomy. However, the monk confessed that for three days after the treatment he did not eat the ordinary monastic food, but what was prescribed in the infirmary instead. This reply provided Arnau with the solution to the enigma. If the ordinary diet (based on beans, cabbage, and low-fat cheese) in the monastery generated a pathological abundance of seed, it was not surprising that the far richer diet in the infirmary (based on mutton, wine, juices of meat, and full-fat cheese) generated even more of it.

Recourse to the expertise of medical practitioners became general in the first half of the fourteenth century in all lawsuits and discussions of offences that could require their art (such as legal questions related to the consummation of marriage). Often physicians acted as a complement to or a check on the examinations carried out by midwives.[176] *Astesana*, for example, discusses states of health which constitute an impediment to marriage and might lead to break up of the marital contract. Two such cases were when a woman complained that coitus could not take place due to a defect in the man's reproductive organ, or when she suffered from excessive bodily heat and complained that her husband could not satisfy her. Henry of Susa (Hostiensis) determined that the man should be investigated by expert and honest men (*per viros expertos et honestos*), and may have meant physicians as forensic experts. Similarly, action should be taken in the case of a woman who was tight or narrow (*arta*). To the question what would happen if the woman could not admit the man's penis owing to its size, *Astesana* replied:

Some say that she should be heard. Avicenna said that where the woman is not tight but her man is incompatible with her both need a change. But Hostiensis says that he has heard from a woman expert that this can hardly or never happen.

---

[175] *De consideracionibus operis medicine*, *AVOMO*, iv. 256–7.
[176] On the acceptance of medical judgement as a legitimate part of the Church's investigation of sexual dysfunction, see McVaugh, *Medicine before the Plague*, 202–7.

Yet some say that such things should be left to the judgement of experts, but Hostiensis says that he would consult the Pope in such a case.[177]

Thus the involvement of physicians in this type of litigation was possible, but not essential. The opinion of the expert would have to compete with clerical opinion, and *Astesana* leaves the issue undecided. Even by 1317 (by which time *Astesana* was completed), Hostiensis's opinion from the 1250s had not become redundant.

Whereas medical theory could prescribe therapy which was incompatible with a monastic lifestyle, the texts we have examined suggest that physicians tended to accommodate their therapies to the particular lifestyle of their clients and to the tenets of Christian ethics. On the basis of these texts it is possible to conclude that, despite the image of physicians as dangerous to the soul, awareness of the special needs of religious communities and submission to religious precepts characterized practical medicine.

In this chapter I set out to examine whether Arnau's medical texts, and those attributed to him, justified in any way the fears of some clerics about medicine and the human physician. My conclusion is that it was normal for physicians and priests to cooperate. Potentially, there was ground for friction on theoretical and practical issues: medical practice was not religiously neutral. However, medical aetiology and the therapies which physicians offered were not usually a cause for an open conflict with the clerics. The one worry frequently expressed by priests was that medical practitioners would not always ensure that the seriously ill confessed before receiving treatment.

---

[177] 'Dicunt enim aliqui eam audiendam. dicit eciam Avic. quod mulier quanquam non est arta sed vir eius non convenit ei unde uterque indiget permutacione. Dicit autem host. se audivisse a femina experta quod hic vix aut nunquam accidere potest. quidam autem dicunt talia esse relinquenda iudicio expertorum. host. vero dicit quod ipse consulet papam in hoc casu.' *Astesana* viii. 26, *De frigiditate*. Jacquart and Thomasset, *Sexuality and Medicine*, 171–2.

6

Conclusions

This book has two foci. First, it examines the specific case of Arnau de Vilanova, a theologizing physician, and the impact of his medical background on his spiritual activity; and second, it investigates the cultural role of medicine in a period in which learned, rational medicine was beginning to win greater social acceptance. These topics are interrelated, and the first sheds light on the second.

I have found fusion rather than disjunction between Arnau's medical and spiritual writings. Arnau kept his medical science largely insulated from supernatural concerns; magical therapies hardly appeared there, and he was hostile to or at least ambivalent about alchemy.[1] His medical writings were generally devoid of religious allusions. Although there was nothing medical about his eschatology or his Franciscan-like reformist ideas, his movement to the theological field was also influenced by his medical background.

Arnau did see a medical purpose in contemplating spiritual matters, namely to ensure the spiritual health of his audience, and when he entered the spiritual realm he brought a medical frame of mind to bear on it. This frame of mind was founded on four essentials. First, his medical language was shared partly with the clergy, which thus enabled him to perceive his art as quasi-religious. This affinity between the two languages made him feel at home in the field of metaphysical speculation. Second, he was convinced that medicine and medical knowledge could deliver a spiritual message, giving its practitioners access to secret spheres of knowledge. Third, his emphasis on the virtue of Christian love (*caritas*) as an essential characteristic of the perfect physician allowed him to approach divine matter since, in his view, *caritas* was the key to metaphysical knowledge. And finally, his definition of medicine allowed him to treat the soul and its passions in as much as they affect the body. Eventually he went further and offered medical treatment to improve the patient's adaptability to the monastic lifestyle. Medicine, even in the eyes

---

[1] See M. Pereira, 'Arnaldo da Vilanova e l'alchimia. Un'indagine preliminare', *ATIEAV* ii. 95–174.

of an orthodox Galenic physician like Arnau, was not merely a therapeutic art for the preservation or restoration of bodily health.

Arnau's medical frame of mind is expressed in a high-level medical language characterized by dense medical imagery, rich with the tropes of anatomy and disease, intercalated spontaneously into the text without moralization and without citing specific medical authorities. This type of imagery is overwhelmingly dominant in his figurative language. He uses medical knowledge in a spiritual context in a neutral way without moral and theological assumptions, and the physical body as a starting-point for discussing the spiritual body. Arnau extended his professional preoccupation with purging the body of its malignant humours to the mystical body of the Church, which he diagnosed as diseased and to which he offered remedies that would guarantee its full recovery. He also offered cures for unbalanced mental composition or complexion and suggested means for maintaining healthy souls. The therapeutic certainty which characterized his spiritual cure may have derived from the medical certainty so important for him as a physician.

Arnau maintained that divine revelation was a possible (though not very common) source of medical knowledge, and regarded the physician as a specially chosen divine agent who was a vessel of medical truth. This assumption was probably subconsciously linked to his self-portrait as a watchman who had special access to divine knowledge and who could cure the disease of human ignorance. Common traits connected Arnau the physician, who believed in the divine origin and usefulness of medical knowledge, with Arnau the spiritual speculator, who attributed exactly the same characteristics to theological knowledge.

As a theologizing physician, Arnau saw himself following the footsteps of Christ and Luke, Cosmas and Damian, all of whom provided both spiritual and physical health. He was thus utterly convinced that by engaging in spiritual matters he was fulfilling the biblical idea of the perfect physician as expressed in Ecclesiasticus 38. He believed that his behaviour had historical precedence and was religiously licit and even desirable. Moreover, the juxtaposition of his medical and spiritual writings reveals an acrobatic ability to adapt medical theory to the desired theological argument. He uses medical metaphors based on Aristotelian theories, despite his Galenic affiliation, and, while there is little trace in his medical writings of any moral or religious significance to diseases, in his spiritual writings he explicitly allots God an active role in giving health.

I have not established a causal relationship between Arnau's medical background and his spirituality. A physician by virtue of his occupation did not necessarily slide into the spiritual or theological realms, and his medical practice was usually executed unhampered by ecclesiastical restrictions and constrictions. I have found no evidence to support the hypothesis that Arnau's success at harmonizing his ecstatic experiences with his critical science is one of the keys to the appeal of his religious ideas for his followers.[2] What I have shown, however, is that the two aspects of Arnau's intellectual life were never disconnected and that his medical background facilitated his movement to the clerical domain.

There is no evidence that Arnau's exposure to natural philosophy and in particular to Aristotelian ideas led him into theological heterodoxy.[3] The esoteric textual knowledge of the physician, his access to powerful and dangerous medicines, his claimed mastery of natural forces, and his possible ties with Jewish physicians may have encouraged associations between medicine and magic, and made physicians an easy target for zealous inquisitors. Traces of these factors appear in Arnau's writings, but none can be shown to have caused his collision with the Church.

Arnau was not *sui generis* in this pattern of intellectual behaviour. I have shown that the emergence of academic medicine as a separate and socially recognized science and profession did not create barriers between medicine and a preoccupation with spiritual questions. While their medical theory and practice remained strictly instrumental, natural, and scientific, some physicians sought to use their expertise in the spiritual field as well. Like Arnau, Galvano da Levanto revealed a medical frame of mind when he ventured into spiritual matters. His spiritual writings were saturated with sophisticated medical allusions and images spontaneously intercalated in the text. Medicine in the broadest sense was the main source of his figurative language, which serves as a direct pointer to the sources and motivations of his spirituality. The human body was, for him, a starting-point and even a trigger for spiritual speculation, and his description of his transumption (*transumptio*) from the physical to the mystical body epitomized an intellectual process in which a physician might drift from the medical into the clerical domain. By merging the discussion of physical disease with its spiritual counterpart he, like Arnau, extended his medical knowledge and curative activities from body

---

[2] C. R. Backman, 'The Reception of Arnau de Vilanova's Religious Ideas', in S. L. Waugh and P. D. Diehl (ed.), *Christendom and its Discontents: Exclusion, Persecution and Rebellion*, 1000–1500 (Cambridge, 1996), 122.

[3] For similar conclusion concerning Florentine physicians see K. Park, *Doctors and Medicine in Early Renaissance Florence* (Princeton, 1985) 52–3.

to soul. By presenting himself as a herald (*preco*) armed with superior knowledge which he was obliged to divulge, Galvano shared with Arnau the belief that he was a divine agent.

Arnau and Galvano were not completely alike. Unlike Arnau, Galvano moralized on the body, offered explicit spiritual interpretation for medical subject matter and cited explicit medical sources in his spiritual writings. Whereas Arnau employed medical themes as exemplary models for the explanation of abstract religious truths, Galvano held that the body as such had a moral and spiritual significance. Unlike Arnau, Galvano did not separate his medical texts from his spirituality, and his piety influenced the style of his medical writing far more than in Arnau's case. Galvano's medical background was responsible for the way in which he described and explained key moral issues along orthodox Christian lines. In his own way he also analysed religious questions from an undoubtedly medical angle and frequently cited medical sources to buttress the arguments and descriptions in his spiritual treatises. For him, medical knowledge and practice fulfilled a distinctive spiritual purpose which extended beyond their therapeutic function. Galvano explicitly fused medicine and Christianity.

Galvano and Arnau do not provide a sufficient sample upon which to base a comfortable generalization. However, they offer a starting-point for further research into the works of other physicians who also ventured into Christian speculation and contemplation in that period, such as John of Toledo, Peter of Spain, Pietro d'Abano, Cecco d'Ascoli, Giacomo da Padua, and Johannes Basoles.[4] To these names, taken from Danielle Jacquart's analysis, it is possible to add others. Thus the Catalan physician Jacme d'Agramont referred in his *Regiment de preservació de pestilència* (possibly the earliest medical work written in response to the Black Death in 1348) to 'pestilence naturally understood' and 'pestilence morally understood'. The moral pestilence, defined as 'a contra-natural change in the spirit and in the thoughts of people, resulting in enmities and rancours, wars and robberies, destructions of places and deaths far beyond the ordinary in certain regions', was not just a metaphor for Jacme. However, unlike Galvano, he avoided discussion of moral pestilence, claiming that his understanding in these matters was not sufficient, and inviting others with more subtle minds to do so.[5] Despite the clear

---

[4] All appear in D. Jacquart, *Le Milieu médical en France du XIIᵉ au XVᵉ siècle* (Geneva, 1981), 223 n. 1.

[5] J. Arrizabalaga, 'Facing the Black Death: Perceptions and Reactions of University Medical Practitioners', in L. García-Ballester, R. French, J. Arrizabalaga and A. Cunningham (ed.), *Practical Medicine from Salerno to the Black Death* (Cambridge, 1994), 237–88 at 244–5.

inclination to expand his discussion, Jacme resisted the temptation to draw a moral interpretation from the medical discussion. Nevertheless, it is plausible that there were other physicians who would respond to his challenge.

By extending the research forward into later periods it may be possible to achieve further insight into patterns of change and continuity in physicians' extra-medical intellectual activity.[6] Another line for future research might be a comparative study of Christian and non-Christian theologizing physicians. A significant number of Jewish physicians in south-western Europe, from Maimonides to Profiat Duran, took part in extra-medical intellectual activity. Did they behave according to the pattern shown by Arnau and Galvano, or are we dealing here with a specifically Christian phenomenon? Maimonides seems to have endorsed the view that there is an essential similarity between the healthy soul and the healthy body and between the sick soul and the sick body.[7] The case of the physician and philosopher Moses Ben Joshua of Narbonne (*c.*1300–1362) suggests that Jewish physicians were also aware of the spiritual implications of their profession. Following his discussion of the moral education of children, he excuses himself for dedicating space to such a topic in what is largely a book of medical regimen: 'Our objective in healing of the body is the healing of the soul. Our first desire is the healing of the soul as God knows,' he declares, and preaches the combination of both forms of cure.[8]

André Vauchez, who examined the forms of lay piety in the late Middle Ages, ignored the learned laity as a category.[9] I would like to suggest that university graduates who did not hold ecclesiastical positions or benefices and whose professional career and private life can be characterized as lay deserve a special study. It would be illuminating to find out

[6] For instance, Johannes Spenlin (d. *c.*1456–1459), Nicholas Salicetus (d. 1494), and Raymond de Sebonde (d. 1436).

[7] A. Broadie, 'Medical Categories in Maimonidean Ethics', in F. Rosner and S. S. Kottek (ed.), *Moses Maimonides: Physician, Scientist, and Philosopher* (Northvale, NJ and London, 1993), 121; D. J. Eisenman, 'Maimonides' Philosophic Medicine', ibid. 145–50.

[8] G. Bos, 'R. Moshe Narboni: Philosopher and Physician, a Critical Analysis of *Sefer Orah Hayyim*', *Medieval Encounters*, 1(1995), 219–51 at 244.

[9] A. Vauchez, *The Laity in the Middle Ages: Religious Beliefs and Devotional Practices* (Notre Dame, Ind., 1993) treats mainly female and various forms of popular piety and religiosity. On the 'philosophical culture' of the laity in the 13th and 14th centuries see R. Imbach, *Laien in der Philosophie des Mittelalters: Hinweise und Anregungen zu einem vernachlässigten Thema* (Amsterdam, 1989). See also P. Biller, 'Popular Religion in the Central and Later Middle Ages', in M. Bentley (ed.), *Companion to Historiography* (London and New York, 1997), 221–46.

whether spiritualizing tendencies existed among the learned laity in general, or whether this tendency was peculiar to medical men. Such an investigation would add more answers to the question of what was specifically medical about Arnau's and Galvano's behaviour.

My second control—preachers' manuals and especially Giovanni da San Gimignano's *Sde*—has enabled a refinement of my assessment of Arnau's 'medical language'. Giovanni used medical language of a higher level than Arnau. He employed sophisticated medical similes adorned with frequent and accurate citations from medical authorities, and seems to have made a sincere attempt to convey a picture which was in accord with current scientific knowledge. Giovanni's text, supported by other contemporary sermon literature, might imply that at the turn of the thirteenth century there was a growing tendency among clerics in general and preachers in particular to substantiate their extensive use of medical metaphors, analogies, and *exempla* by specific medical authorities usually drawn from encyclopaedic collections.

Giovanni's text warns the modern commentator against uncritically overemphasizing the importance of language. High-level medical language cannot by itself serve as an efficient litmus test for the identification of a medical background in the author's career. Three characteristics seem to distinguish Arnau's use of medical language from that of preachers. First, Arnau's spiritual language was 'medical' both in employing dense anatomical metaphors and in reflecting his medical approach to spiritual questions. It reveals the forces motivating him to theologize in a manner unparalleled among preachers. Second, he neither relied on encyclopaedias nor gave a moral interpretation to the medical examples that he used merely as exemplary metaphors. In using medical knowledge in a spiritual context, Arnau, unlike the preachers, avoided a mystical and moral approach to the body and its pathologies. Thirdly, unlike Giovanni, for whom medicine was only one of several sources of figurative language (albeit a very important one), Arnau was overwhelmingly loyal to medicine as the main source. *Sde*, like the texts by Servasanto and Bersuire discussed in this book, is encyclopaedic in character, and the high density of medical matter in those of its sections dedicated to the human body is not surprising. Giovanni's sermons are far less saturated with medical allusions than his encyclopaedia.

By highlighting the elaborate use of medical matter in sermons Giovanni and other preachers of that period shed a different light on physicians who were inclined to theologize. For when high-level medical language becomes a commonplace in religious discourse, the entrance of physicians to the clerical realm is understandable and even natural. Giovanni provides us with a powerful example of the fusion between religion and medicine, and reinforces from the clerical angle my conclusion that conjunction rather than disjunction characterized the relationship between them at the turn of the thirteenth and fourteenth centuries. Furthermore, my findings concerning Arnau, Galvano, and Giovanni suggest that intellectual developments which sixteenth-century historians link to the impact of the Reformation on medicine[10] represent a continuation of, rather than a break with, the medieval past. The body as displaying the design, plan, and workmanship of the Creator in the high point of His creation, the physician as a follower of the Apostles, a chosen divine agent who reveals the arcane,[11] advocating a 'religion' of medicine and giving primacy to the medical knowledge of the laity,[12] and the extensive use of medical imagery in religious discourse,[13] are all patterns identifiable at the turn of the thirteenth century.

This study demonstrates that the institutional demarcation of disciplines, one of the intellectual hallmarks of the turn of the thirteenth century, failed to curb reciprocal movements between medicine and theology. While the universities as ecclesiastical institutions were founded on the idea of separation, the actual boundaries between disciplines were not impenetrable, especially outside the university system. Arnau and Galvano demonstrate how a movement between medicine and theology could take place. Giovanni, Servasanto, and Bersuire show that clerics also breached the boundary from the opposite side, venturing into medicine not in order to take part in medical practice but in order to borrow efficient figurative terms and sometimes to substantiate arguments.

The borrowing of medical terminology and medicine's role as a cultural

---

[10] O. P. Grell and A. Cunningham (ed.), *Medicine and the Reformation* (London, 1993); M. van Lieburg, 'Religion and Medical Practice in the Netherlands in the Seventeenth Century: An Introduction', in *The Task of Healing: Medicine, Religion and Gender in England and the Netherlands*, ed. H. Marland and M. Pelling (Rotterdam, 1996), 135–43; A. Wear, 'Religious Beliefs and Medicine in Early Modern England', ibid. 145–69.

[11] Often associated with Paracelsus; see e.g. K. Golammer, *Der Göttliche Magier und die Magier in Natur* (Kosmosophie, v; Stuttgart, 1991), esp. 75–96; J. J. Bono, *The Word of God and the Languages of Man* (Madison, 1995), 123–66.

[12] C. Webster, 'Paracelsus: Medicine as Popular Protest', in Grell and Cunningham (ed.), *Medicine and the Reformation*, 57–77.

[13] Almost every medical metaphor which English Calvinists used had already been used by preachers around 1300. D. Harley, 'Medical Metaphors in English Moral Theology, 1560–1660', *Journal of the History of Medicine and Allied Sciences*, 48 (1993), 396–435, and 'Spiritual Physic, Providence and English Medicine, 1560–1640', in Grell and Cunningham (ed.), *Medicine and the Reformation*, 101–17.

agent need further elaboration. My observation was founded on a specific literary genre—that of moralized preachers' manuals and some sermon collections. Yet these texts portray attitudes (such as the apparent medicinalization of the explanation of abstinence) communicated by the learned clerics to their fellow clerics and to the unlettered or the laity. A more systematic study of actual sermons, Latin and vernacular, academic[14] and directed at the laity, is essential so that these findings might be substantiated. However, beyond this, what role did medicine play when learned people discussed moral and theological questions among themselves? Here it is necessary to look more closely at other literary genres, and particularly at scholastic texts, barely touched upon in the present study. A fuller consideration of these sources will bring further clarification of the extent to which medical knowledge penetrated the non-medical milieu.

It has been convincingly shown how medical theory penetrated the vocabulary and contents of religious and ideological polemics concerning prophecy, enthusiasm, and claims to divine inspiration in the seventeenth century.[15] The medical concept of 'religious melancholy', which goes back to Greek medical and philosophical discourse, and which was known to medieval physicians like Bernard de Gordon, became a key argument in the critique of Nonconformist religious groups in the early modern period. The general question of the 'medicalization' of religious language needs further refinement, for it seems that certain domains of religious language absorbed medical theory and knowledge from the latter part of the thirteenth century whilst others had to wait for later periods. Thus, while sermon literature and preaching manuals of around 1300 were saturated with medicine, other domains of religious language (such as the explanation of religious behaviour deemed devious or heretical) were 'medicalized' much later.

Arnau's case provides little evidence in support of the contention that inherent tensions characterized the relationship between physicians and clerics. Encyclopaedias, sermons, biblical commentaries, and other clerical sources occasionally hint at suspicion about the religious reliability of physicians. Yet medical questions hardly became an issue in Arnau's protracted conflict with the Church. On the practical level, his medical texts

---

[14] For medical analogies (including a comparison of theological contemplation to the radical humour) in an academic sermon, see S. Wenzel, 'Academic Sermons at Oxford in the Early Fifteenth Century', *Speculum*, 70 (1995), 325, 327.

[15] M. Heyd, *'Be Sober and Reasonable': The Critique of Enthusiasm in the Seventeenth and Early Eighteenth Centuries* (Leiden, 1995), *passim.* and esp. 44–108, 191–210.

and those attributed to him suggest that physicians regularly adapted and accommodated their therapeutic advice to their patients' lifestyle. These texts do not justify the fear, usually articulated in monastic contexts, that physicians undermined their patient's religiosity. On the theoretical level, Arnau was reluctant to involve divine power as an active factor in any phase of the disease, differing from clerics, who regularly stressed the moral significance of disease and God's role in curing it. However, except for the one practical consequence of the need for priest and physician to cooperate when assisting the acutely ill, this difference did not create a visible tension between the two professions. But Arnau provides evidence that they did not always cooperate; he does not mention the priest in his didactic medical treatises, and in his spiritual texts he expresses strong reservations about the notion that a last-moment confession expiates all sins.

In many respects this book does not have a firm conclusion. Producing a manifesto from historical research is a sign that the investigation has ended. As far as the particular topic of this book is concerned, however, exactly the opposite applies. What I offer the reader is an incomplete and imperfect, provisional synthesis; I ask many questions and leave them unanswered; I leave ample space for myself and others to fill the gaps and correct the errors. The study of more cases of theologizing physicians will make it possible to determine whether the pattern of intellectual behaviour detected in Arnau and Galvano was regionally confined to southern Europe. Nevertheless, one conclusion is paramount: physicians and clerics around 1300 did not confine the role of medical knowledge to its therapeutic function. An understanding of the cultural role of medicine, the deciphering of its patterns of interaction with religious and social needs, and an analysis of its non-medical functions are all necessary for a balanced and refined presentation of the medieval medical milieu.

Appendix I[a]

Medical Analogies in Giovanni da San Gimignano,
Summa de exemplis et rerum similitudinibus locuplentissima (Antwerp, 1583)

A. The Medical Model

Signifier	Signified	Reference	Source
Medical effects of seasonal changes	**4 *status anime* on the way to perfection**	*Sde* i. 74, 92⁴–94².	
winter—1. increase in phlegmatic humours. 2. choleric people (young) can sustain winter better than phlegmatic (old) who easily succumb to phlegmatic diseases (quotidian fever). 3. recommended diet—warm and dry food	*status tribulationis* characterized by: 1. abundance of the humour of tears. 2. those who lament sin but are not inflamed with celestial love are vulnerable to sin like the phlegmatic who easily succumb to disease in winter. 3. love for eternal things will dry the humours of carnal desire and cure the pathological condition	"	
spring—1. increase in density of blood. 2. dangerous exposure (particularly of the young) to continuous fever (*synochus*). 3. recommended diet—cold and dry food. 4. meteorological instability (March in particular) as a cause for disease	*status conversionis* characterized by: 1. elated soul. 2. tumour of pride; old people can better withstand the temptations which accompany conversion. 3. fasting and hard labour. 4. inconstancy of the newly converted	"	*physici.*
summer—1. abundance of heat. 2. phlegmatics are better off. 3. recommended diet of cold and moist food	*status sub fervore dilectionis* characterized by: 1. anger towards sin and increasing love. 2. tears of contrition	"	
autumn—1. increase in melancholy. 2. youth of sanguine complexion are better off than the elderly melancholics. 3. recommended diet of warm and moist things	*status sub maturitate discretionis* characterized by: 1. sadness over sins committed. 2. young enjoy the happiness of love, the old are left with sadness. 3. one must dry the humour of desire and cool down the heat of vices	"	

Signifier	Signified	Reference	Source
Treatments which heal the body	**Treatments which heal the soul**	*Sde* ix. 53, 477[1-2]	**Bible**
plaster	word of God	"	Isa. 38: 21 (corrupt) 'Iussum est ut super ulcus Ezechie cataplasmaretur massa ficuum que dulcedinem verbi Dei significat'
sweat which expels harmful humours	fear of God (*timor Dei*)	"	Ecclus. 1: 27, 'Timor Dei expellit peccatum'; Prov. 3: 7-8, 'Time Dominum et recede a malo, sanitas quippe in umbilico tuo erit'
baths	compunction through *effusio lacrimarum*	"	2 Kgs. 5: 10, 'Vade lavare septies in Iordane et recipiet sanitatem caro tua'
vomit	confession	"	Ecclus. 31: 25, 'Si coactus fueris in edendo multum, surge de medio et evome'
diet	abstinence from sin	"	1 Thess. 4: 3 'abstinetis vos a fornicatione'; Ecclus. 37: 34, 'qui abstinens est addiciet vitam'
removal of putrid organs (*putridorum resecatio*)	Job-like tribulations	"	Job, 5: 17, 'Increpetionem Domini ne reprobes, quia ipse vulnerat et medetur'
medicinal unction	devotion and piety which alleviate the soul	"	Mark. 6: 13, 'Ungebant oleo multos egrotos et sanabantur'
Hippocrates's nine signs for medical prognosis	**Prognosis of the sinner's chance to overcome his state**	*Sde* x. 74, 485[3]–487[4]	**Hippocrates, *De prognosticis* [Galen, *In Hipp. prog.*]**
weakness/strength (*fortitudo/debilitas*)	sin accompanied by temptation and despair (weakness of the soul) will lead to death; if accompanied by continuous good deeds and faith is curable	"	"
manœuverability/ exhaustion (*levitas infirmi/gravitas infirmi*)	convertibility / intransigence	"	"

Signifier	Signified	Reference	Source
Hippocrates's nine signs for medical prognosis (*cont.*)	Prognosis of the sinner's chance to overcome his state	*Sde* x. 74, 485³–487⁴	Hippocrates, *De prognosticis* [Galen, *In Hipp. prog.*]
healthy or diseased form of the organs (*effigies membrorum*)	actions follow the temperaments of religious soul or perverse inclination	"	"
good appetite and healthy mind (*sana mens / facilis appetitus*) versus *perturbatio mens* or *difficilis appetitus*	appetite for the word of life and following just counsels	"	"
quality and timing (night) of sleep	tranquillity of soul and degree of indulgence in God or in temporalities	"	"
easy / short breath (*suavitas / angustia spiritus*)	inhaled air is the consoling word; the different tones of reproaching sinners	"	" Ezek. 34: 4, 'vos autem cum austeritate imperabitis eis et cum potentia'
irregularity of pulse beat (*inequalitas pulsus*) which measures the flow of blood in the arteries.	irregularity of soul (*inequalitas mentis*)	"	"
proper functioning of digestive system in primary (stomach, liver) and secondary digestive organs	food of soul is digested in the stomach of memory through remembrance, in the heat of the liver through love, in the remaining organs through action	"	"
quality of sweat which purges the body; when it is only local=an evil omen	sweat of confession must be total; otherwise it signifies grave sin	"	"

ᵃ The 'signifier' rubric includes a highly condensed version of the specifically medical topics in each article. The 'source' rubric mentions only the specific source for the medical analogy as it is cited in the text. This may be a medical, philosophical, or biblical authority. Whenever I refer the reader to a more specific reference (preceded by cf.) I attempt to locate the source from which the writer acquired the medical material. This relates to two sources: Bartholomaeus Anglicus, *Venerandi patris Bartholomei Anglici . . . opus de rerum proprietatibus* (Nuremberg, 1519) (*Barth.* in the table) and Avicenna, *Liber canonis* (Venice, 1507). Square brackets signify the titles of works which do not appear in the original text but were either added by the Renaissance editor or by me. The few biblical references mentioned are a selection of verses (as they appear in the text) directly linked to the medical content of the analogy. Many more biblical, patristic, and exegetical references are mentioned.

B. The Vocabulary of Disease

Signifier	Signified	Reference	Source
Disease	**Sin**		
characteristics of nightmare (*incubus*); announces impending epileptic, apoplectic, or maniacal fits; signifies a complexional imbalance of the brain which is weakened and excessively hot	characteristics of temptation to sin; the inability of the sinner to remain morally upright	*Sde* vi. 72, 358$^{1-3}$	Avicenna (6x); Aristotle, [*De somn. et vig.*]
seven characteristics of dropsy as a liver disease which destroys its digestive powers; resulting from the corrupt complexion which is diagnosed by discoloured skin; corruption of digestion, avid thirst, accumulation of water and swelling body	damaged liver ruins discretion and disturbs the complexion of the soul; exterior signs betray the interior corruption of the sinner; hypocrisy, pride (*tumefactio anime*) and intemperate illicit love	*Sde* vi. 62, 330^4–332^1	Avicenna (5x); Johannitius; Bede; Ps. 106: 5, 'Esurientes et sitientes anima eorum in ipsis deficit'; Matt. 23: 27, 'Ve vobis hypocryte qui similes estis sepulchris dealbatis'
fever: exterior heat kindled in the heart and transferred by the spirits and blood through arteries and veins to the whole body which is inflamed and whose natural operations are damaged	sin as exterior non-natural heat which disrupts reason	*Sde* vi. 52, 332^1–333^2	Avicenna (2x); cf. *Barth.* vii. 32–40 (Hippocrates, Galen, Constantinus, Isaac); Matt. 15: 19 'De corde exeunt cogitationes male'
febris etica, originating from the radical organs and of which there are three kinds: 1. consumes the nutritive moisture (*ros*). 2. consumes transformable matter (*cambium*). 3. consumes moisture assimilated into the organs and responsible for their cohesion (*glus*).	sins of prelates and clergy who are the principal organs of the Church of which there are three kinds respectively: 1. disordered love for family and friends which desiccates piety. 2. carnal love which destroys spiritual devotion. 3. simony destroying spiritual grace which is the glue of the soul	" 332$^{2-4}$	
febris putrida originating from putrefied humours and of which there are three types: continuous, tertian, quartan	sin of the laity which is infected with corrupt desires. Its three types, avarice, anger, sloth, correspond respectively to types of putrid fever	" 332^4–333^2	Damascenus

Signifier	Signified	Reference	Source
Disease	**Sin**		
febris ephimera from over-heated spirits	sins of members of the monastic orders	*Sde* vi. 52, 333[2]	
paralysis: partial or full immobility; weak pulse	sin in general, which varies in intensity	*Sde* vi. 52, 333[2]–334[1]	Avicenna (2x); John 5: 1-10; Matt. 8: 5-13, 9: 1-9
epilepsy: partial privation of sense and motion accompanied by spasm, falling, tremor and mental disturbances and originating from an obstruction in the interior ventricle of the brain	sin which deprives the person of spiritual prudence and not necessarily of secular wisdom (*prudentia sive astutia secularis*); mental instability	*Sde* vi. 52, 334[1–2]	Avicenna (2x)
lethargy: putrefied, phlegmatic, cranial abscess (*apostema*) accompanied by a feverish fit and excessive sleep; has a debilitating effect and corrupts the memory	sin brought by intemperate, unreasonable love and a cold soul leads to persist in immoral behaviour and to forget God	*Sde* vi. 52, 334[2–4]	Avicenna (3x)
apoplexy: 1. causes laziness of organs and 2. breathing difficulties. 3. is incurable when fit is violent. 4. patient resembles a corpse. 5. sometimes resolved only to become paralysis	sin which corresponds to the five types of physical apoplexy: 1. sloth and laziness. 2. gluttony and lust. 3. avarice. 4. envy. 5. pride and anger. The sins are interconnected; one leads to the other	*Sde* vi. 53, 337[3–4]	Avicenna; Hippocrates; Prov. 14: 30 'Putredo ossium invidia'
umbilical cord: nourishing the foetus; the location of female genitals; clinical description of cutting off, washing, drying and binding the umbilical cord after delivery	opportunities for sinning; the foetus of interior sin conceived by ill-will and nourished by exterior actions; woman as source for man's sin; one should treat opportunities of sinning like umbilical cord; model for treating the newly reformed sinner	*Sde* vi. 47, 325[4]–326[2]	Constantinus (2x); cf. *Barth.* v. 47 (verbatim, includes Jerome's commentary on Ezek. 16: 4 ('non est praecisus umbilicus tuus') as well as St Gregory's gloss on Job 40: 11, 'Virtus in lumbis eius et fortitudo illius in umbilico ventris eius'

Signifier	Signified	Reference	Source
Disease	**Sin**		
viscera: 1. *Intestinum subtilium* also called *duodenum*. 2. *Intestinum ieiunium* always empty. 3. *Intestinum simillimum*. 4. *Intestinum orbum* has one opening only. 5. *Intestinum ilium* the origin of iliac passion. 6. colon (the lowest part of viscera)	plurality of sinners: 1. proud (12 degrees of *superbia*). 2. prodigal. 3. gluttonous. 4. avaricious. 5. invidious. 6. lustful (the basest)	*Sde* vi. 53, 336⁴–337²	*quidam sapiens*
dental medicine and the radical treatment necessary for toothache	desired treatment of sinners	*Sde* vi. 33, 321²	Avicenna; Gal. 5: 12, 'Abscindantur qui vos conturbant'; 1 Cor. 5: 7, 'Expurgate vetus fermentum'
melancholy	sloth (*acedia*)	*Sde* vi. 1, 292⁴–293²	Avicenna (2x); cf. *Liber canonis* III fen I, tract. IV, c.18–20
back pain caused by cold complexion, crude phlegm, excessive coitus or surfeit of the vein above the back	inability or unwillingness of the slothful to bear heavy loads	*Sde* vi. 36, 321⁴–322¹	Avicenna; cf. *Liber canonis* III, fen XXII tract. II, c.1, p. 380ᵛᵇ
dropsy causes violent accumulation of fluids and swelling of the organs; 3 types: *hydropisis hyposarcha* generated from phlegmatic material which penetrates the organs and inflates the whole body; *hydropisis alchites* generated from the accumulation of watery matter in the belly; *hydropisis timpanites* generated from flatulent matter	*superbia* caused by uncontrolled self-love; the three types correspond to avarice, lust, and pride	*Sde* vi. 5, 296¹–297¹	Avicenna (2x); cf. *Liber canonis* III, fen XIV, tract. IV, c.4, p. 300ʳᵇ; (different from *Barth*. vii. 59 (*Viaticum*), which divides the disease into four species. Isa. 16: 11 'venter meus ad Moab quasi cythara sonabit'

Signifier	Signified	Reference	Source
Disease	**Sin**		
loss of appetite caused by: 1. viscous phlegm. 2. catarrh descending from the head. 3. malfunction of evacuation (constipation). 4. weakening of the liver 5. intestinal worms. 6. pregnancy and retention of menstrual blood. 7. excessive physical exercise or inordinate labour	loss of appetite for spiritual food due to: 1. carnal love. 2. pomposity, pride, and ambition. 3. avarice. 4. tepid love toward God. 5. harmful care (*sollicitudo*) for temporalities. 6. rancour. 7. inordinate penitence, abstinence and excessive spiritual exercise	*Sde* vi. 8, 2984–300[1]	Avicenna (6x); cf. *Liber canonis* III, fen XIII, tract. II c.7, p. 275[ra–vb]. Prov. 12: 10 'Viscera impiorum crudelia'
headache caused by excessive heat or tumour and ruins the appetite; therapy: 1. if caused by heat: smear head with oil of roses, shave hair (disposing of superfluities), poultice of cold oil, avoid heat and light. 2. when caused by tumour smear head with oil of violets	appetite for mundane delight caused by cupidity or pride; therapy: 1. suffering of the Saints. 2. oil of humility and love	*Sde* vi. 8, 300[1–2]	2 Kgs. 4: 19 'Caput meum doleo, caput meum doleo; Ps. 7: 17, 'Convertetur dolor eius in caput eius'
cold flatulence rising from the toes to the brain as precursor to an epileptic fit	ruin caused by *superbia*	*Sde* vi. 71, 357[3–4]	Avicenna; Prov. 16: 18, 'Ante ruinam exaltatur spiritus'
stomach ache above the right leg accompanied by a swollen bladder will lead to death within 27 days	pride invading the pious and penitents, torturing the soul and ruining spiritual love	*Sde* vi. 71, 357[4]	Avicenna; Prov. 17: 16 'Qui altam facit domum suam querit ruinam'
leprosy: *lepra elephantia* (melancolic), *leonina* (choleric), *tyria* (or *serpentina*), *allopicia* (or *vulpina*)	avarice and its putrefying effects	*Sde* vi. 10, 301[1–3]	*medici*
throat: the two-way system of swallowing and breathing, which cannot be performed simultaneously and are regulated by the *epiglotum*; fatness which impedes health, intellectual performance, and female fertility	gluttony which impedes spirituality	*Sde* vi. 32, 320[2–4]; *Conciones*, 101	Constantinus; Galen, *In Hip. aphorismi*; cf. *Barth.* v. 63 (verbatim). 1 Cor. 2: 14, 'Animalis homo non percipit que sunt spiritus Dei'; Ps. 5: 10, 'Sepulchrum patens est guttur eorum'; Phil. 3: 12 'Quorum Deus venter est'

Signifier	Signified	Reference	Source
Disease	**Sin**		
toothache: originating in the teeth, in their roots (nerves), and in ulcerated gums	3 reasons for the sadness of the envious	*Sde* vi. 37, 322[1-2]	Avicenna; Prov. 14: 30, 'Putredo ossium invidia'

C. The Anatomy of Christian Practice

Signifier	Signified	Reference	Source
Organs	**Virtues**		
upper/lower jaw	contemplative/active life	*Sde* vi. 2, 293[2-4].	Constantinus; cf. *Barth.* v. 16, 'De Mandibulis'
chin and its essential role in opening the mouth	*dilectio caritatis*	*Sde* vi. 23, 314[4]-15[2]	Constantinus; cf. *Barth.* v. 18, 'De mento'
legs: 44 bones in each leg (2 heel bones, 2 *manicule*, 10 leg bones, 30 bones in the toes); Galen's test for the gender of the foetus— right leg of the pregnant woman stretched first predicts a male child	*amor caritatis* as the moving agent of the soul; like the leg, *caritas* is the foundation of moral stability and behaviour; 2 legs = 2 kinds of love (God and one's neighbour); the heel signifies death which 2 sacraments (baptism and penitence) can overcome; 10 commandments; the toes are *doctores* whose minimal age is 30; the right leg in Galen's test is *amor spiritualium*	*Sde* vi. 4, 295[1-4]	Constantinus; Galen. Cf. *Barth.* v. 54
back bears all bodily weight and is the foundation of all bones	love (*caritas*)	*Sde* vi. 13, 304[3]-305[1]	Isidore; Ps. 65: 10, 'Posuit tribulationes in dorso nostro'
sense of touch centred around the heart and not in the flesh	love (*caritas*)	*Sde* vi. 13, 305[1]-306[2]	Aristotle [*De animalibus*]; [*De sen. et sen.*]; Deut. 6: 5, 'Diliges dominum deum tuum ex toto corde tuo'
the utility of hot and moist flesh as fuel for natural heat, and as preserver of bones, nerves and muscles and as a tempering element against cold	spiritual love has a nutritive effect on soul and body	*Sde* vi. 18, 312[3]	Constantinus; Aristotle [*De animalibus* xii]. Cf. *Barth.* v. 62, Ecclus. 38: 29 (corrupt), 'Fervor ignis id est fervor divini amoris, urit carnes eius'

Signifier	Signified	Reference	Source
Organs	**Virtues**		
clay (*argilla*) which restrains haemorrhage and especially nasal bleeding	vinegar of compunction mixed with the clay of love restrains the flow of sin	*Sde* i. 13, 263^{-4}	Constantinus
podagra, sciatica and other arthritic diseases are caused by excessive rest, exercise, coition (esp. on a full stomach), and drunkenness (esp. after fasting)	spiritual excess which harms the joints of the soul; temperance as the desirable disposition in spiritual regimen	*Sde* vi. 50, 3283^{-4}	Avicenna
Organs	**Christian Practice**		
bone marrow: generated in the hollowness of the bones, which are refreshed by it, is warm and humid, nourished by the purest of all matters, its quantity varies with the lunar cycle	grace generated out of humility, ignites love and moistens the arid soul into a state of piety	*Sde* vi. 30, 319^4–320^1	Constantinus (2x); Varro. Cf. *Barth.* v. 58
bile, choler: bitterness; the gall-bladder (*cistula fidelis*) and its double function—to carry choler to the intestine (expulsion of super-fluities) and to the stomach (aid to digestion); the strengthening effect of hawks' (and other prey-birds') bile on the eyesight; attracts sweetness around it and purifies the blood	the bitterness of penitents; the fortifying power of penitence; the double-sided penitence which relates to past deeds and includes commitments toward future behaviour	*Sde* vi. 3, 294^1–295^1	Constantinus; Tob. 6: 9, 'Fel eius valet ad inungendos oculos'; Deut. 32: 32, 'uva eorum uva fellis et botrus amarissima'; Ps. 68: 22, 'Dederunt in escam meam fel'
lungs produce a foamy humour (*spumosa*); mitigate the heat of the heart; create voice	compunction accompanied by tears of penitence as spiritual humour; voice of confession mitigates concupiscence	*Sde* vi. 54, 338$^{1-2}$	Constantinus; Aristotle. Cf. *Barth.* v. 35, 'De pulmone'
eyelids defend the eyes from air and move concurrently	True penitents must perform both interior and exterior penitence	*Sde* vi. 54, 338$^{2-4}$	Constantinus; Aristotle [*De animalibus*]

Signifier	Signified	Reference	Source
Organs	**Christian Practice**		
eyelashes defend the eye and are dry of all fleshly superfluities	examples of saints who often experienced conversion	*Sde* vi. 54, 338[4]	Constantinus; cf. *Barth.* v. 8
conception and gradual foetal formation (*gradus formationis*) involve: 1. *materia conveniens* (menstrual humour/female seminal humour). 2. *locus expediens* (the womb). 3. efficient cause (male semen). 4. instrumental cause (the heat of nature). 4 stages of foetal formation (*lacti vicinus*, mixing of semen and blood, formation of three principal organs, completion of the body which is ready to accept the soul); duration of formation and pregnancy	penitence 1. *recordatio peccati*. 2. mind. 3. fear of God (*timor Dei*). 4. stages toward perfection of penitent (*recognitio peccati, detestatio peccati, peccati confessio*, satisfaction); three principal organs signify the three theological virtues	*Sde* vi. 54, 338[4]–340[4]	Galen; Aristotle; Constantinus. Cf. *Barth.* vi. 4 (*De creatione infantis.*) Isa. 26: 18 (corrupt), 'A timore tuo Domine concepimus et peperimus spiritum salutis'
black choler, melancholy (positive) which originates in spleen (source of laughter): (negative) it dominates the left side of the body, is cold and dry, causes anger, timidity, wakefulness, and occasional sleepiness	sadness accompanying penitence; hope in future favour is always mixed with this sadness	*Sde* vi. 74, 359[1–2]	*physici*
four kinds of stomach ache: 1. pain which appears after the meal. 2. that which appears during the meal. 3. that which can be removed by vomiting. 4. or that which will disappear only after a total scouring of the stomach	four kinds of penitence 1. after comiting sin. 2. during sin and as a result of spiritual food (sermons). 3. the penance violently extracted in purgatory. 4. sadness and anger followed by the evacuation of memories of sin	*Sde* vi. 74, 359[2–4]	Avicenna [*Liber canonis* III, fen. XIII, Tract. II, c.1, p. 373[vb]–374[ra]]

Signifier	Signified	Reference	Source
Organs	**Christian Practice**		
stomach as the locus of primary digestion; its digestive capability varies according to its complexion; when warm and humid it seeks and easily digests fat food, and generally digests more than its appetite demands; if cold, it cannot bear fat food which corrupts its humours; if dry, creates severe thirst	spiritual digestion of divine word; those who are hotter in spiritual love better understand subtle and elevated teaching	*Sde* vi. 14, 306^2–307^3	Constantinus; Aristotle. Cf. *Barth.* v. 38, 'De stomacho'
mouth	preachers of God's word	*Sde* vi. 59, 343$^{1-3}$	
food: 1. *cibus substantialis*. 2. *cibus subtilis* (easily digested and dispersed throughout the organs). 3. *cibus grossus* (slowly digested, nourishing and blood-producing). 4. *cibus temperatus*—(in quantity and quality the preferred food)	knowledge: 1. *doctrina sana et catholica*. 2. refined teaching of the ignorant which sinks to oblivion. 3. 'nourishing' doctrine. 4. balanced doctrine which is neither subtle nor crude and hence equally suits *simplices* and *sapientes*	*Sde* vi. 25, 315^4–316^2	Galen; Hippocrates; Avicenna [*Liber canonis* I, fen. II, doct.2, c.15, p. 33$^{va–b}$]. Cf. *Barth.* vi. 21
three kinds of drink: 1. without nutritional value (water). 2. nutritional (wine). 3. medicinal (syrup)	three kinds of spiritual drink: 1. secular (product of vain curiosity). 2. scriptural. 3. compunction and penitence	*Sde* vi. 58, 342^4–343^1	Constantinus (2x). Cf. *Barth.* vi. 22 'De potu'
voice	the way in which the divine word should be preached for effective impact	*Sde* vi. 25, 316^4–317^3	Constantinus (2x) [*Viaticum* II, 'De amore']. Cf. *Barth.* v. 20 'De voce'
sense of hearing, ear: the movement of sound via the two nerves which connect the brain with the ears; the air's mediating role	interior sense of hearing; sound of spiritual doctrine transferred through the mediation of an exterior teacher or preacher	*Sde* vi. 11, 301^4–303^2	Constantinus (4x); Aristotle [*De sens. & sens., De animalibus*]. Cf. *Barth.* iii. 18; v. 12 'De auribus'
breathing	necessity of prayer and graceful actions	*Sde* vi. 49, 327^4–328^2	

Signifier	Signified	Reference	Source
Organs	**Christian Practice**		
female breast: defends the heart and the chest; maternal milk made of cooked, digested purest sanguine matter; larger right breast is a sign for male foetus; mollified breast is a sign for impending miscarriage	pastoral care; the priest offers blood (tasteful and life-giving doctrine) which must be sweetened, purified, and thickened for willing reception; right breast is *rigor* discipline; left is *dulcor* misericordie; both are necessary for efficient correction but the first should prevail	*Sde* vi. 19, 313[1-4]	Constantinus (2x); Aristotle (3x) [*De animalibus*]; Galen, *Super Aphor.* Cf. *Barth.* v. 34
regulated wakefulness (*vigilia*); excessive wakefulness increases the heat	care for spiritual things; excessive care for temporalities increases avarice	*Sde* vi. 58, 356[2-3]	Constantinus. Cf. *Barth.* vi. 27 'De vigilia'

D. The Anatomy of the Christian Body

Signifier	Signified	Reference	Source
symmetry of the body's side (*latus*); 14 ribs (*coste*) defending interior organs; lying in times of acute disease on the right side is a good omen signifying that the region of the heart is not obstructed	double perfection (in this world and in *status glorie*) of apostles and their followers who share 7 virtues (3 theological, 4 cardinal) and 7 gifts (3 of soul and 4 of the body); they are vulnerable to the sin of pride; the absolute preference of contemplative over active life	*Sde* vi. 9, 300[3]–301[1]	Hippocrates, [Galen, *In Hipp. prog.*]; Constantinus. Cf. *Barth.* v. 31
spleen: located at the body's left side, defends the heat of the stomach (by emitting invigorating humours into it) and mitigates the heat of the liver (by drawing black choler and melancholy from it), purifies the blood, its composition is hard and enables it to sustain the liver's corrosive humour; source of laughter	patience of saints	*Sde* vi. 51, 329[1-2]	Aristotle; Isidore. Cf. *Barth.* vi. 41

Signifier	Signified	Reference	Source
Organs	**Christian Practice**		
liver: the lobes (*fibre*) through which it supplies heat to the stomach; locus of secondary digestion which turns the digested food into sanguine mass which is then separated into the four natural humours; emits as urine the impure superfluities with the aid of the kidneys through the bladder; failure of the liver which involves loss of heat may result in dropsy	the just and perfect who make a vital contribution to the common good; compunction as a secondary stage in purifying the soul after penance; the just and spiritual should beware of *indiscretus fervor presumptionis*	*Sde* vi. 38, 322²⁻⁴	Aristotle [*De animalibus*]
heart: the fountain of bodily heat and humour (blood); concave, fleshy, full of spirits first to be formed; 2 ventricles; quality of breathing and pulse as signs of testing the heart's powers; diseases of the heart	perfection of saintly people who are the fountain of the heat of love (*calor caritatis*) and whose concave mind is filled with humility and devotion and solidified by patience	*Sde* vi. 64, 352²⁻353³	Constantinus; Galen; Haly; Augustine; Aristotle (4x); cf. *Barth.* v. 37, 'De corde' (verbatim)
eyes, pupils, the two nerves which transmit the visual spirit from the brain to the crystalline humour of the eye, are situated in a form of a cross; the necessity of light for the sight; three humours (*albugineus, cristallinus, vitreus*) and seven tunics (*retina, secundina, sclirotica* and four in front of the crystalline humour *aranea, uvea, cornea, coniunctiva*)	preachers totally attached to Christ; necessity of Scripture as light or mirror; seven gifts of Holy Spirit which are arranged in pairs (e.g. wisdom and understanding are like the retina which is connected to the *aranea*) except for the last (*timor*) which is on its own like the *coniunctiva tunica*	*Sde* vi. 59, 344³⁻345²	Haly; *auctor perspective*; cf. *Barth.* v. 5, 7, 'De oculis', 'De pupila'; Isa. 11: 2-3, 'Requiescet super eum spiritus Domini, spiritus sapientie et intellectus, spiritus consilii et fortitudinis, spiritus scientie et pietatis, et replebit eum spiritus timoris Domini'
kidneys attract the four humours from the concave liver, purify the blood and transmit urine to the bladder, generate seminal matter and temper the coolness of the back	saintly teachers of the Church and the effect of their teaching (based on the 4 senses of Scripture) which should purify the sinners and bring about their conversion	*Sde* vi. 26, 317³⁻⁴.	Constantinus; Isa. 11: 5; Aristotle [*De animalibus*]. Cf. *Barth.* v. 43, 'De renibus'
thighs are the founda-	virgins (nuns) who	*Sde* vi. 76, 361²	Constantinus. Cf.

Signifier	Signified	Reference	Source
Organs	**Christian Practice**		
tion of the body; composed of the largest bones in the body, rich in muscles and nerves, their upper part is concave	need special powers to sustain chastity; characterized by extreme humility		*Barth.* v. 51 'De femoribus'
treatment of newly born babies: 1. rub them with roses and salt to strengthen their fluid organs and to purge viscous matter. 2. rub their gums and palate with a finger smeared with honey to cleanse the interior of the mouth and to provoke the appetite. 3. frequent baths followed by ointment of myrtle and roses. 4. avoid excessive light and prefer dark surroundings. 5. avoid at any cost corrupt milk; no medicine should be given directly to the baby who should be cured through a medicinal regimen prescribed to the wet-nurse. 6. bandage the limbs to avoid deformity. 7. frequent sleep to revive the interior heat and further the digestion; songs and gentle movement of the cradle	treatment of new converts by: 1. *exempla* of saints. 2. moderate penitential duties. 3. tears of compunction accompanied by teaching temperance and patience. 4. they should rather be kept ignorant (*simplicitas, obscurantia*) of certain aspects of doctrine and avoid its subtleties. 5. they must be defended at all cost from heretical doctrine. 6. laws and rules must be given to them. 7. they must be provided with occasional periods of vacation for quiet meditation and contemplation and they must avoid idleness	*Sde* vi. 76, 311$^{1-4}$	Constantinus (2x). 1 Pet. 2: 2, 'Quasi modo geniti infantes lac concupiscite'
head as the seat of the four sense-faculties (*communis, imaginativa* (preserves the form perceived by the senses), *estimativa, memorativa*), neck (divided into throat—*guttur*, which is one of several organs of the voice and responsible for its beauty and strength, and nape—*cervix*); the structure and composition of the brain (3 ventricles enclosed by 2 protective membranes—*pia* and	prelate who needs 4 perfections: 1. *peritia divinarum scripturarum* from which all secular sciences emerge. 2. *cura et custodia animarum*. 3. *prudentia et discretio*. 4. remembrance of one's flaws and blemishes; the hair is the family and friends of the prelate, who like the brain must be white (morally pure), bloodless (free of consanguine love), and full of spirits; the *dura mater* represents his austere	*Sde* vi. 60, 345^2–348^2	Averoes; Algazel; Avicenna; Constantinus (2x); Aristotle. Cf. *Barth.* v. 2, 'De capite' (where the description is attributed to Haly's commentary on Galen's *Tegni*; *Barth.* v. 25 (neck)

Signifier	Signified	Reference	Source
Organs	**Christian Practice**		
dura mater); diseases of the head	side, the *pia mater*, his kind and liberal side; like the neck, he is an intermediary between God and the people and characterized by doctrinal authority and solidity of life		
nerves which originate in the brain and introduce motion to the body via the spine	prelates and political leaders (*rectores*) who derive their power from God through human intermediary	*Sde* vi. 61, 350$^{2-4}$	
cartilage: soft, flexible yet powerful defence of the joints	prelates and *rectores* should be temperate and mix correction with compassion	*Sde* vi. 62, 350^{2}–351^{1}	Aristotle [*De animalibus*]
32 teeth: *quadrupli, incisores, canini, molares*	members of the Orders	*Sde* vi. 63, 351$^{1-4}$	Cf. *Barth.* v. 20
shoulders which defend the spiritual organs, composed of various bones of which the major ones are the *spatule* and the *furcule*	princes who must defend the *religiosi*	*Sde* vi. 56, 341^{3}–342^{1}	Isa. 9: 6 'Factus est principatus super humerum eius'
forehead neither hard nor soft, little flesh or fat, which hampers the intelligence	government (*regimen*) of princes and prelates should be neither rough nor soft; they should refrain from focusing on carnal things	*Sde* vi. 62, 350$^{1-2}$	Constantinus; Aristotle (3x). Cf. *Barth.* v. 10, 'De fronte'
hands, fingers (*pollex, index, impudicus, annularis, auricularis*, each composed of three bones); pulse as a diagnostic tool	human actions and virtues; *justicia* (*commutativa, distributiva, vindicativa*), the most powerful of moral virtues; *prudentia, temperantia* (abstinence, sobriety, chastity), *fortitudo, obedientia*; human actions as indicator of their internal thoughts	*Sde* vi. 48, 326^{2}–327^{2}	Constantinus; Aristotle; Avicenna [*Liber canonis* I, fen I, doct.5, c.23, p. 12vb–13ra]. Cf. *Barth.* v. 29 'De digitis'
arms: linked to the heart and hence teach about the heart's condition and alert us to consult the physician; defensive function; position of arms in times of acute disease as a sign for approaching death	political power (*potestas humana*) which should be oriented to promote public good and which should in emergency consult wise experts in order to defend properly the public good	*Sde* vi. 57, 342$^{1-4}$	Galen, *In pronosticis*; cf. *Barth.* v. 27

E. The Anatomy of the Mind

Signifier	Signified	Reference	Source
hair defends the brain; produced from cranal thick vapour which originates in burnt humours; boldness; white hair which is the result of cooling down of nutrimental humour or domination of cold phlegmatic humour	thoughts as the dress of the mind, the defence of the soul and a reflection of its internal constitution; penitence cools down the nutrimental humour of the soul and produces whiteness of the mind (*canities mentis*) which signify honesty and maturity	*Sde* vi. 15, 308^1–309^1	Constantinus; Isidore; Aristotle (2x). Cf. *Barth.* v. 66
sleep strengthens the natural virtue, restores the spirits which have been released, unifies the faculties of the body, an integral part of any therapy	contemplation which strengthens the powers of the interior soul	*Sde* vi. 16, 309$^{1-3}$	Aristotle (2x) [*De somn. et vigil.*]; Avicenna [*Liber canonis* I, fen II, doct.2, c.13, p. 33^{ra-b}]. Cf. *Barth.* vi. 25
physical vision, optics, perspective	contemplation	*Sde* vi. 16, 309^4–310^4	Aristotle
Aristotle's versus Galen's doctrine concerning the source of blood (heart or liver) and the harmonizing solution; hot and humid	the pleasant effect of contemplation (*dulcedo contemplationis*), when motivated by the heat of love and will and by the humidity of fear, renders the contemplator healthy	*Sde* vi. 16, 310^4–311^1	Aristotle, cf. *Barth.* iii. 7; Galen
chest: two concavities; the seat of two breasts; vulnerability to a variety of diseases	mind and its afflictions; two major faculties— will and intellect; two breasts of wisdom and eloquence	*Sde* vi. 43, 324$^{2-3}$	*physici*; Aristotle (2x) [*De animalibus*]. Cf. *Barth.* v. 33, 'De pectore'
taste and its organs: affected by the animal virtue through the animal spirits which reach the tongue (the visible taste-organ) via two specific nerves; the heart as the primary organ of taste which is transferred to it (like the sense of touch) through the medium of flesh (the tongue); the essential role of saliva (humid environment) for sensing taste and for evacuating cerebral and pulmonary superfluities	wisdom (*sapientia*) affected by faith through the articles of faith and fear of God; it expels inordinate thoughts; the 2 nerves signify 2 roles of the wise person: to defend truth and repel falsehood; saliva is Christian doctrine which directly flows from Christ's head and is essential as a medium for acquiring wisdom	*Sde* vi. 65, 353^3–354^4	Aristotle (2x) [*De animalibus, De sen. et sen.*]; Constantinus (2x). Cf. *Barth.* iii. 20, 'De gustu'. Prov. 14: 33, 'In corde requiescit sapientia prudentis'

Signifier	Signified	Reference	Source
tongue is warm and humid, wets the mouth, linked to 2 salivary veins, can be venomous amongst serpents and rabid dogs; saliva (always digested matter and a medium connecting between taste and its object); spitting (expels rheumatic superfluities and hence is useful to *phthisis* patients); an indicator for possible interior corruption in stomach, heart, or lungs	words of good people, of confessors, or venom of evil people	*Sde* vi. 75, 359^4–361^1	Avicenna; Aristotle [*De animalibus*], Damascenus, Constantinus, Galen (2x). Cf. *Barth.* v. 21-2
nose: two concavities separated by cartilage; air, spirits, and smell reach the brain through one; cerebral superfluities are expelled through the other; its aesthetic importance; exposed to cerebral and neural imbalance	speculative and practical human knowledge (*scientia humana*) is the way by which we grasp truth, reject falsehood, and supply the mind with infrastructure for sense-perception. It is vulnerable to error, vices, and sin	*Sde* vi. 66, 355$^{1-4}$	Constantinus (2x); Galen. Cf. *Barth.* v. 13

Appendix II

Medical Analogies in Pierre Bersuire, *Reductorium morale super totam bibliam* (Venice, 1583)

Signifier	Signified	Reference	Source
The physical senses (e.g sense of touch)	dispositions of the soul (touch signifies compassion)	*Reduct.* i. 7–11, 12[2]	Avicenna; cf. *Barth.* iii. 21
The three spirits of the body (natural, vital, and animal) which are formed in the liver from cooked blood	three species of grace and the Holy Spirit	*Reduct.* i. 12, 13[1]	*medici*; Avicenna; Constantinus
pulse which reveals the heart's complexion and which the physician must discreetly check	revealing the deeds and the interior feelings mainly through confession, whose contents must be kept private	*Reduct.* i. 13, 13[2]–14[1]	
four elements; four qualities	*ardor caritatis, nitor puritatis, timor divine maiestatis, fundamentum humilitatis*; 4 cardinal virtues	*Reduct.* i. 14, 14[1–2]	
heat	*ardor caritatis, caritas*	*Reduct.* i. 15, 14[2]–16[1]	
cold	*frigus divini timoris, frigus tribulationis*	*Reduct.* i. 16, 16[1]–17[1]	
dryness	death, penitence, abstinence, poverty	*Reduct.* i. 17, 17[1]–18[1]	
humidity	devotion, compassion, grace, doctrine	*Reduct.* i. 18, 18[1]–19[2]	
humours: their life-securing function which counters the effects of the natural heat on bodily humours; their production in the liver through heat: phlegm → blood → melancholy → choler (and not vice versa)	grace; four gospels, cardinal virtues (blood=temperance and modesty; choler=firmness, *iusticia*; melancholy= bravery; phlegm=prudence); by insufficient *calor / fervor contritionis* or *zelus iusticie* one can produce at the most *indevotio, morum indigestio, levitas iuvenilis* and not *sanguis devotionis* and *dulcedo compassionis*; excessive spiritual heat may irreversibly lead to *cholera*	*Reduct.* i. 19, 19[2]–20[2]	Constantinus, *In theorice*, c.25; cf. *Barth.* iv. 6 (attributes to Avicenna rather than to Constantinus the order of producing the humours); *Liber Pantegni*, Theorica i. 25, in Isaac Israeli, *Omnia opera ysaac* (Lyons, 1515), iv[va]–v[va]

Signifier	Signified	Reference	Source
	iracundie and *melancholica desperationis et tristitie*; malfunction of the humours (superfluity)=4 vices: *cruditas indevotionis, carnalitas luxurie infectionis, lenitas superbie et elevationis, gravitas avaritie et terrestris affectionis*		
blood: the result of perfect digestion; the disagreement between Aristotle and the *opinio medicorum* on the principality of the heart; curative effect; the corrupting effect of the retention of menstrual blood which indicates impending miscarriage	members of the Orders and clerics are like arteries which originate in the heart and through which most subtle blood flows; the veins are the lay people; the corrupting effect of lust	*Reduct*. i. 20, 20²–23¹	Constantinus; Aristotle, *De animalibus*; Solinus; cf. *Barth*. iv. 7
phlegm: imperfect humour, converts to blood when properly digested; four kinds of defects which are the outcome of an improper mixture with other humours (*phlegma acetosum, salsum calidum, dulce, vitreum*); signs of the phlegmatic according to Constantinus	newly converted who are imperfect, exposed to four kinds of spiritual indigestion such as excessive sadness, anger, exuberance; sinners whose thoughts and behaviour are not properly digested or composed	*Reduct*. i. 21, 23²–24¹	Constantinus; cf. *Barth*. iv. 9
choler: its double digestive function in the stomach and intestine; four species: *citrina, vitellina, prasina, eruginosa*; when corrupted in the body the side-effects include bitterness in the mouth, burning in the stomach, nausea, headache, dry tongue, insomnia, madness	4 kinds of choler equivalent to *ardor iracundie, luxurie, avaritie, invidie* which cloud and corrode the mind	*Reduct*. i. 22, 24¹⁻²	Constantinus, in *Pantechni*, lib. 10 Theorice c.2; cf. *Liber Pantegni*, x. 2, fol. 52ʳᵃ, 'De significatione plenitudinis et dominatione humorum'; *Barth*. iii. 10
melancholy: fear; peculiar, demented behaviour of the melancholic who lose reason and believe that they are dead	*spiritualis tristitia* and *timor Dei*; those who hold false, vain opinions	*Reduct*. i. 23, 24²–25²	Constantinus; Galen, *Liber passionum*; magister arnaldus de villa nova; cf. *Barth*. iv. 11; Arnau de Vilanova, *De parte operativa*, fol. 128ᵛᵇ

Signifier	Signified	Reference	Source
organs in general: distinction between organs composed of *similia* (blood, flesh etc.) and those composed of *dissimilia* (e.g. hand); further division into *membra animata* (brain, nerves, and sense organs), *spiritualia* (lung, heart, and arteries) and *naturalia* (stomach, liver, kidney); harmony; mutual aid	distinction between the clerics or contemplative people (who have one, simple *intentio*—God) and the laity or *activi*; the second distinction corresponds to the distinction between prelates, religious and clerics, and the laity	*Reduct.* ii. 1, 26[1]	Avicenna; Johannitius; cf. *Barth.* v. 1, 'De membrorum proprietatibus in generali'; Constantinus
head: bones' strength; fullness of marrow; lack of flesh; hair	prelate or any *capitaneus* who should be characterized by constancy, clemency, reject carnality	*Reduct.* ii. 2, 28[1]	Constantinus; Aristotle; Isidore
brain: while being humid, full of spirits and marrow, it has scarcely any blood; 3 ventricles responsible for imagination, reason, and memory; two defensive membranes—exterior *dura mater* and interior *pia mater*; cold and humid organ, the second to be formed; exposed to excessive heat which rises from the heart through the arteries	prelates or just people; 3 ventricles signify faith in the Trinity, and 3 theological virtues; the brain's (prelate's mind) membranes signify *iusticia* and clemency; as second organ to be formed it signifies the virgin who mitigates the severity of God's judgement; the prelate is exposed to *calor cupiditatis* through evil company	*Reduct.* ii. 3, 29[1]–30[1]	Constantinus, *Pantechni*, li. 3 c.12; Haly; Aristotle; cf. *Liber Pantegni* iii. 12, fols. x[va]–xi[rb], 'De compositis membris interioribus ut cerebro'; *Barth.* v. 3
eye, pupils: 3 humours, 7 tunics which serve the pupils where the source of vision is	3 theological virtues, 7 moral virtues; *complexio spiritualis, speculatores ecclesie, viri spirituales*; pupils are conscience	*Reduct.* ii. 4–5, 30[2]–32[2]	Haly; Isidore
eyelids	*virtus discretionis*	*Reduct.* ii. 6, 33[1]	
eyebrows	discloses information about the soul; *fortitudo animi*	*Reduct.* ii. 7, 33[2]	
forehead	apostles and martyrs; *virtus constantie et fortitudinis*	*Reduct.* ii. 8, 33[2]	Constantinus; Isidore; Aristotle
temples	*virtus fidei*	*Reduct.* ii. 9, 34[1]	
ears whose structure is like a wine- or oil-press (*torcular*); they prevent	hearing the divine word; preacher and confessor who must be	*Reduct.* ii. 10, 34[2]–35[1]	Constantinus, *Pantechni* li. 4 theorice c.12; cf. *Liber Pantegni* iv. 12,

Signifier	Signified	Reference	Source
damage to the nerves from sudden flow of air; cartilaginous, hard, equally receives noises from all directions	kind in attending, hard in their faith, and attentive in listening to everyone		fol. xvii[rb], 'De auditu'; *Barth.* v. 12
nose: purges superfluities from the mouth, transfers air to the brain and to the smell organs in it via *caruncule*; slenderness of nose ominous sign in times of acute disease	*virtus prudentie et discretionis*; temporal judges; prelates; reveals information concerning the dispositions of the soul—ignorance (slender nose), arrogance (excessively open nostrils)	*Reduct.* ii. 11, 35²–36¹	Constantinus, *in Pantechni*; Galen; cf. *Liber Pantegni* iii. 15, fol. xi [va–b], 'De naribus'; *Barth.* v. 13
cheeks: fleshy; changing colours	indicator of passions of the soul; exterior behaviour (*conversatio*) which reveals extent of interior beauty (*carnositas seu mollities pietatis, rubedo seu ignities caritatis, albedo seu florities puritatis*)	*Reduct.* ii. 12, 36¹	Constantinus; Isidore
beard: decoration; gender differentiation; absence amongst women and *castrati*	virtuous wisdom and bravery (*prudentia vel fortitudo virtuosa*)	*Reduct.* ii. 13, 32	Constantinus
jaws	teachers (*doctores*); sinners	*Reduct.* ii. 14, 37¹	Constantinus
lips	preachers and words of preachers as the lips of the Church; they act as intermediaries of the tongue of God; their softness mitigates the *duritia iusticie*; flatterers	*Reduct.* ii. 15, 37¹⁻²	Constantinus; Aristotle, *De part. anim.* 2
chin	perseverance and persistence	*Reduct.* ii. 16, 37²	
mouth: its role in the provision of nutrition, in formation of words, purgation of superfluous cerebral, pulmonary, or ventral humours, in respiration and in cooling down the heart	preachers or teachers who examine, masticate, and transfer the food of doctrine to every organ in the Church's body	*Reduct.* ii. 17, 37²	Constantinus (2x)
teeth: 32, names, function, order of growing, number of roots, ailments; men have more teeth than women	the mouth is *domus principium et prelatorum* where *simplices* (food) are checked; the incisors (one root and	*Reduct.* ii. 18, 38¹–39²	Constantinus, *Pantechni*, li.II, theorice iii. Constantinus (2x). Vincentius, li.30, c.44; cf. *Liber Pantegni* ii. 3,

Appendix II

Signifier	Signified	Reference	Source
	hence easily removed) are the extortionist bailiffs; canine teeth (two roots hence harder to remove) are the insatiably avaricious lesser judges; molar teeth (three roots hence most firm) are the intimate advisors and masters; teeth also represent words of wisdom which are more abundant among *prudentes* (virile beings) than the *simplices* (women); they need fundamental virtue (devotion) to flourish; healthy teeth are the teeth of Christ or of the *viri iusti*		fol. vi^{ra}, 'De ossibus capitis'; Vincent de Beauvais, *Speculum naturale* xxviii. 67
tongue, saliva: saliva as tasteless humour mediating between the taste organ and its object; sanguine, fetid saliva as a sign of injured lungs; retention of saliva may cause death by suffocation as is the case with phthisis patient	preacher or teacher; healthy saliva is divine grace which originates from good actions and refraining from evil	*Reduct.* ii. 19, 39^2–40^2	Constantinus (2x)
voice: throat as vocal instrument; gender differences in voice	*locutio viri iusti*; preachers=throat; air=Holy Spirit	*Reduct.* ii. 20, 40^2–42^1	Constantinus (2x); cf. *Liber pantegni* iii. 19, fols. xi^{vb}–xii^{rb}, 'De gutture'
throat: its parts: *lingua gutturis* which blocks corrupt air, fluid or dust; the danger of suffocation when food deviates from the gullet (*isophagus*) into the trachea (*trachea arteria*); *squinantia* (quinsy) and the suffocation brought by its ulcers; it can be cured if the ulcers are exterior; otherwise it is lethal	will be defended by the fear of God and the virtues of prudence or temperance (*lingua gutturis*); mind which cannot be open concomitantly to spiritual and carnal things; the humours causing quinsy are the humours of vice which prevent confession and hamper the activity of the jaws of devotion	*Reduct.* ii. 21, 42^1–43^1	Constantinus (5x). Cf. *Barth.* vii. 27; *Liber pantegni* ix. 20, fol. xliv^{vb}; *Viaticum* iii. 1, fol. cli^{rb} (for quinsy)
neck: mediates between head and body	hope which mediates between God and the mind	*Reduct.* ii. 22, 43$^{1-2}$	Constantinus; Isidore

Signifier	Signified	Reference	Source
shoulders: dislocation of the shoulder and malignant humours between the joints that cause gout (*gutta*) are usually treated with a soothing ointment	*humeres ecclesie*=knights who occupy a superior place in the church after the prelates (head) and the priests (neck); *humeres anime*=obedience, courage, and constancy; the sinner suffers from *delocatio inconstantie* and the malignant effects of bad company, excessive wealth, and pleasures	*Reduct.* ii. 23, 43²–44¹	Constantinus
arms: phlebotomy executed from the hand opposite to the ailment (unless it's poison); special relationship with the heart	the virtue of good action, and resolution of the soul; just people, prelates and preachers in particular	*Reduct.* ii. 24, 44¹–45¹	Constantinus; Isidore; Galen, *sicut in prognosticis*
hands: men are more liable than women to be ambidextrous (because of their complexion), passions of *contractio, arefactio, postulatio, scissio, vermium corrosio, pruritum, titilatio, tremor et vacillatio, iuncturarum dislocatio, chiragrica*	good actions, prelates preforming a plurality of actions which fit the diversity of people (hit, caress etc.); religious people are God's palm (*vola Dei*) represented by the left hand (which is usually weaker since they live outside this world); the secular clerics are the right hand; right side represents contemplative virtue, the left is active (and hence inferior); left-handedness represents sinners, right-handedness represents *simplices* and *religiosi* who are spiritually strong, and ambidexterity represents the prelates, the perfect and the just; each of the passions corresponds to another sin	*Reduct.* ii. 25, 45¹–46²	Isidore; Constantinus; Solinus; Aristotle, *De part. anim.* 4; Galen; *In aphorismis*; cf. Galen, *In Hipp. aph.* vii, no. 43, in *Opera omnia*, ed. Kühn, xviiia, 147–9
fingers: thinness of skin, scarcity of flesh, richness of nerves; high sensibility; tendency to shrink after eating	faithful people, *boni viri* who are free of carnality; the effect of Eucharist and the word of God	*Reduct.* ii. 26, 46²–47¹	Isidore; Constantinus; *ut dicitur super Aphorismos*
fingernails: produced from fumes of the heart and hence reveal its physical disposition	actions which reveal the fumes and affections of the heart	*Reduct.* ii. 27, 47¹⁻²	Constantinus

Signifier	Signified	Reference	Source
ribs: may be inflicted with pleurisy (*pleuresis*) which is revealed through sanguine spitting; lying on the right side in times of acute fever is a good sign that the lung is not inflamed; other ailments of the ribs include *ventositas, opilatio, contractio, duritia inflatura et distensio, spasmus*	two spiritual parts of the virtuous soul— seven gifts and seven virtues; pleurisy and its symptoms represent the abscess of sin lurking in the heart	*Reduct.* ii. 28, 47^2–48^1	Isidore; Constantinus; *sicut dicitur in prognosticis*
back	*fortitudo mentis*	*Reduct.* ii. 29, 48^{1-2}	
chest	*mens humana*	*Reduct.* ii. 30, 48^2–49^1	
breasts: if softened in pregnancy they are sign of approaching miscarriage; blood which is not converted into milk foretells approaching mania; tight, firm, and round breasts are sign of healthy foetus and its gender (right is male); the production of milk may be impeded by windiness and the corrupting effect of retention of menstrual blood	preachers and teachers; breast is doctrine and the foetus represents the soul, or human actions; abundant carnality (blood in breast) rather than spirituality characterizes many of the clergy	*Reduct.* ii. 31, 49^1–50^1	Isidore; Constantinus; Hippocrates (2x, one mentioning *Apho.* 30) with Galen's commentary on it; cf. Hippocrates, *Aphorismi*, v. 39, in Kühn, xviiib, 828–9; *Barth.* v. 24
lungs: soft, fleshy, full of air; ulcerated by cerebral humours, the air exits through the perforation, the heart is not properly cooled and phthisis is caused	will or mental condition (*mentis affectio*) which should be benign, serene, and pure, yet is exposed to corruption	*Reduct.* ii. 32, 50^1	Constantinus
heart: tilted to the left; two ventricles—the right is fuller with blood than spirits and left vice versa; vital spirit is generated in the left ventricle whence it is transferred to the rest of the organs via the arteries; *sedes cordis* is the bony, cartilaginous part of the heart to which *cordis auricule* and *cordis capsula* are attached; the	prelates who rule the church; two kinds of love: in prosperity (more carnal and profit oriented) and in adverse situation (more spiritual); confession operates like the openings of the heart which shut after emission; *mens anime* which should be characterized by constancy (bony), promptness of obedience (*auricule*), and *caritas*; faith which	*Reduct.* ii. 33, 50^2–52^2	Isidore; Constantinus, *Pant.* li.4; Aristotle; Galen; Haly (2x one of which *Super techni*); cf. *Liber Pantegni*, iii. 22, fol. xii^{va}, 'De corde et cerebro'; *Barth.* v. 36

Signifier	Signified	Reference	Source
origin of life and the first organ to be formed; it may suffer excessive heat or cold, abscess in the *capsula cordis*; the pulse reveals its health	is the principal virtue; the uncompassionate, harsh, cold prelate is like the heart which may suffer from excessive cold and dryness		
breath	divine grace	*Reduct.* ii. 34, 52²–53¹	
stomach: aids the liver in digestion and uses its heat; the liver attracts the stomach's juices which flow into it through the mesenteric veins; by digesting the juices it turns them into blood; a warm stomach demands a lot of food and drink, efficiently digests fat food and utterly consumes subtle food; the opposite applies to a cold stomach; all passions of the stomach are related to evacuation and repletion; they include indigestion, diarrhoea, hiccups (*singultus*), flatulence, belching (*eructatio*), voracious appetite (*bulimus*), and aversion	prelates or preachers; good subject who receives and accepts the doctrinal food; gluttonous, avaricious; stomach signifies the temporal philosophers who relate philosophy, whilst the liver signifies theologians who, aided by the former, produce clarity and theological doctrine; like the liver, prelates need fervent people near them; the liver can denote a heretic who corrupts and totally alters everything he has received from the stomach of scripture; fat-rich food is will motivated by avarice and temporal goods; subtle food signifies spiritual goods	*Reduct.* ii. 35, 53¹⁻²	Constantinus, li.1 Theorice c.15; cf. *Liber Pantegni* I.15, fol. iii^rb, 'De complexione stomachi'; *Barth.* v. 38
liver: five ways through which it aids the stomach; converts and alters humours received from the stomach. The heart tempers it from above	mind which must be fervent and warm by devotion, red and sanguine by the memory of Christ's passion, and concave by humility; the 5 powers of the senses through which the mind is directed; the preacher who generates the blood of doctrine	*Reduct.* ii. 36, 53²–54²	Haly
gall: cleanses impure blood, sends choler to the stomach to aid digestion, and to the intestine to strengthen its expulsive powers	bitter contrition	*Reduct.* ii. 37, 54²–55¹	Constantinus
spleen: enlarged spleen makes leaner and vice	love of God	*Reduct.* ii. 38, 55¹⁻²	Hippocrates

Signifier	Signified	Reference	Source
versa. Moderately sized spleen is thus a sign of good health			
viscera: intestines are divided into 3 parts: *Intestinum ieiunium, duodenum, orbum seu saccus*. Among the ailments of the viscera are *passio collica vel Iliana*, flatulence, constipation, dryness, dysentery, abscesses, choleric corrosion	priests and confessors who have their place in the *ecclesia intestinorum*; they receive therefore faeces (sins) from the whole body of the church; one can also speak of *intestina mentis*; the open ended intestines signify pious people who relinquish to poorer people all temporal goods they have received from God; conversely, they may signify perverse listeners who do not retain any of the good words; the 3 intestines signify 3 cardinal virtues	*Reduct.* ii. 39, 55^2–56^2	Constantinus; Isidore
kidney	spiritual people, priests, confessors and good preachers; *boni affectus*	*Reduct.* ii. 40, 56^2–57^1	Isidore; Haly; Aristotle
bladder (*vesica*)	*virtus confessionum in anime*	*Reduct.* ii. 41, 57^{1-2}	Constantinus
urine: a major source of knowledge concerning the internal body	sins omitted through confession	*Reduct.* ii. 42, 57^2	Constantinus; Isidore; Isaac; Theophilus
belly: stronger appetite in winter due to warmer belly and vice versa	prelates who supply spiritual food for the whole body; mind	*Reduct.* ii. 43, 57^2–58^1	Constantinus; Hippocrates
umbilical cord	*voluptas carnis*	*Reduct.* ii. 44, 58^{1-2}	Same as *Sde* vi. 47, 325^4–326^2
genitalia: castration	*virtus bona opera generandi et foetum virtutum et meritorum producendi*; spiritual castration like physical deprives of constancy (virile powers) and effeminates	*Reduct.* ii. 45, 58^2–59^1	Aristotle
womb: among the mentioned diseases suffocation of the matrix and *mola*, which is a tumour hardened by corrupt	will which receives the semen of word or grace; once a foetus has been conceived it is nourished by Christ's blood;	*Reduct.* ii. 46, 59^{1-2}	

Signifier	Signified	Reference	Source
humours; it creates the false impression of pregnancy. The story of a woman who was thus three years 'pregnant' and when she delivered, the extruded flesh could hardly be cut by a knife	as long as it is preserved in the mind, conception of good actions lasts. Those conceived on the right side are the contemplative people (males), those on the left are the imperfect and active (female)		
buttocks	patience and courage which are fundamental to the moral body; carnal riches and delights; farmers who support the body of the church in temporal matters	*Reduct.* ii. 47, 59[2]	Constantinus
thighs	princes and prelates; carnal desires	*Reduct.* ii. 48, 59[2]–60[1]	
knees	humility, fear	*Reduct.* ii. 49, 60[1–2]	
shin	preachers and doctors of the church who build the *columna fidei*	*Reduct.* ii. 50, 60[2]	
legs: 44 bones; the pregnant woman who is suddenly called—the gender of the foetus is revealed by her first leg to be stretched out	*affectus*; farmers or merchants who are at the extreme end of the body of the church	*Reduct.* ii. 51, 60[2]–62[1]	Constantinus; Galen, *Super aphor.*; Aristotle, *De anim.* and *De part. anim.*; cf. *Sde* vi. 4, 295[4]
bones	just and perfect men—preachers, prelates, and religious in particular; virtues	*Reduct.* ii. 52, 62[1–2]	Constantinus
marrow	divine grace	*Reduct.* ii. 53, 62[2]–63[1]	Constantinus; Varro; Dioscorides. Cf. *Sde* vi. 30, 319[4]–320[1]
cartilage	*flexibilitas ad bonum*; obedient men versus *cartilegia diaboli*	*Reduct.* ii. 54, 63[1–2]	Constantinus
nerves: originate from the brain and the spinal cord (*nucha*); irreversible damage when a nerve is cut	just men—religious, preachers, prelates in particular; virtues which originate from Christ (brain) and Mary (*nucha*), schismatics can hardly rejoin the Church	*Reduct.* ii. 55, 63[2]	Constantinus; Isidore; Aristotle
veins	pious men, preachers who carry the blood of doctrine from the liver	*Reduct.* ii. 56, 64[1]	

Signifier	Signified	Reference	Source
flesh	*conditio nature carnis*	*Reduct.* ii. 57, 64$^{1-2}$	Constantinus; Remigius
fat (*pinguedo*): fat people are cured more slowly, are more liable to suffocate and lack the ability to move easily; fat women can hardly conceive	lust, pleasure; grace, *caritas*, devotion which nourishes the fire of good desires	*Reduct.* ii. 58, 64^2–65^1	Constantinus; Isidore; Aristotle, *De part. anim*
skin	*exterior conservatio*	*Reduct.* ii. 59, 65$^{1-2}$	
hair: grows out of interior fumes	interior affections, moral condition; riches and temporal substance	*Reduct.* ii. 60, 65^2–66^2	
head-hair: in *Alopicia* hair falls off due to blocking the channels or to corrupt humours. Baldness suffered by men only, as a result of old age and excessive sexual activity (introduces dryness and cold)	*casus virtutum* by sinners; spiritual baldness caused by *humanis abundantia et frigiditas*; conversely, it signifies *nuditas confessionis, flebilitas contritionis, largitas possesionis* among perfect people	*Reduct.* ii. 66, 66$^{1-2}$ *Repertorium*, i. fol. cxlvi^{rb}–cxlviii^r	Galen; Constantinus; Avicenna
conception: need of *locus competens, materia obediens, semen viri infusus, calor operans*; *pellicula secundina*—the membrane wrapping the embryo and which must be expelled at birth lest it harms the woman; gradual formation of the embryo, longer period of formation for female; duration of pregnancy: seven months—every embryo has *motus* and may survive early birth; eight-months-old embryos cannot survive, for they need a month rest; the treatment of the newly born involves frequent baths, wrapping in clean cloths, bandaging, wiping the mouth with honey to entice the appetite; they are most vulnerable to corrupt milk	penitence; need of faith (uterus), good obedient will (female semen), divine word and preacher's teaching, grace of the Holy Spirit; the embryo represents sin, the membrane is evil carnal satisfaction which should be utterly expelled by confession; male foetus represents good spiritual actions, female foetus signifies *opera inutilia et terrena*; 7 months = 7 virtues and perfection; 8, which is the first number to transgress 7, represents the condition of sin; 9 signifies the 9 orders of angels, and 10 the perfection of the decalogue; the young, penitent, new converts and newly appointed prelates are to be treated like newly born children	*Reduct.* iii. 2, 67^2–69^1	Constantinus; Galen, *Super aphor.*; Hippocrates; Constantinus, *li. Pantechni* 5, c. 34 (*sic*) and 3, c. 34; cf. *Liber Pantegni* iii. 34, fols. xiii^{vb}–xiv^{va}, 'De genitalibus'; *Barth.* vi. 4
seven natural things necessary for life	spiritual life also needs: *aer puritatis*=innocence, *cibus*	*Reduct.* iii. 14, 77^1	Johannitius

Signifier	Signified	Reference	Source
	devotionis=Eucharist, *potus scripture*=grace and wisdom, *exercitatio laboris et diligentie, quies tranquilitatis mentis conscientie, vigilia medicationis et providentie, somnum contemplationis supernaturalis glorie et eminentie*		
food: converted into the substance of the body; physician must be aware of the *conditiones* of a specific food (its essentiality, quality, quantity, and time restrictions) lest pestiferous food is used; he also should adapt the food to the condition of the eater; distinction between subtle food which is not nutritive (but generates blood that dissolves and evaporates quickly) and nutritive food (rich in fats) which contributes substantially to the body; rejection of fresh, crude vegetables and new fruits; recommending a uniform diet and avoiding mixing a large variety of food	spiritual food converted into the substance of the moral person; the cure of the soul must entail refraining from damaging spiritual food; distinction between subtle and sophisticated doctrine which does not survive the test of time, and fat, simple doctrine which settles firmly into the heart; students should avoid mixing too many kinds of doctrines, books, and disciplines;. erratic movement between the disciplines may corrupt the existing knowledge	*Reduct.* iii. 15, 77[1]–78[2]	Constantinus; Galen; Avicenna; Hippocrates
drink: three kinds: simple drink, which has no nutritional value (water), drink and food (wine), and neither drink nor food (syrup); the various qualities of water (rain is purest, lake and river water is the worst and must be boiled before drinking); the medicinal effects of wine	different kinds of sciences: *phisica* (medicine)—reveals the truth yet does not induce to perform good deeds; theology nourishes the virtues; law—renders the learner neither trained in speculation nor morally good; the secular sciences should be boiled before being taken in; Christ's blood has medicinal effects like wine	*Reduct.* iii. 16, 79[1]–81[1]	Constantinus (2x); Avicenna; *Magister de proprietatibus rerum;* cf. *Barth.* vi. 22
diseases (general): divided into causes (e.g.	vices (general); divided into *causa vitiorum,*	*Reduct.* iv. 1	

Signifier	Signified	Reference	Source
non-natural disposition like *mala complexio*, over-filling or defect in evacuation), affliction itself (e.g. fever, abscess) and the accidents of the disease (e.g. thirst, swelling)	vices themselves (*calor avaritie, apostema superbie*), and the accompanying side-effects like *parcitas, pompositas*		
diseases of the head: (1) *cephala*—by an overflow of one of the humours in the head: blood at the front, choler at the right, melancholy at the left, and phlegm at the back	prelates; the mind which is divided into four *status*, youth, old age, prosperity, and adversity, each dominated respectively by carnality and lust, laziness, avarice, and pride, fear, despair, and sadness	*Reduct.* iv. 2, 86²–88¹	Galen, *in libro institutionum (sic)*; cf. *Barth.* vii. 1
(2) *hemicrania* (migraine) is the outcome of a cold choleric fume which causes pricking and ringing in the head; the patient cannot stand, sleep	*iracundia*	"	Constantinus
(3) *tinea, squama* (ringworm, scale) is a phlegmatic disease that affects children in particular; causes itching and leaves scars if skin does not heal; the cure for breast-fed children is phlebotomy from the back of the head and besmearing the head with the warm blood, together with austere diet	simple, ignorant person who is inflicted with lust	"	Constantinus; cf. *Barth.* vii. 2
(4) *eruginosa squamositas* which involves lice, spots, and the loss of hair (*fluxus capillorum*) as a result of corrupt fumes	*squamositas male conversationis, squama malorum exemplorum*; the loss of hair is *defectus virtutis*; hair signifies clerics who lapse as the result of the evil examples (fumes) of prelates (head)	"	
catarrh which is an immoderate flow of humours into the head. As long as the fit of catarrh is violent, no poultice should be used lest it obstruct rather	mind which suffers from the flow of evil thoughts and desires. Sometimes one should not castigate the sinner on the spot (it may prove counterproduc-	"	Magister; Constantinus; cf. *Barth.* vii. 3

Signifier	Signified	Reference	Source
than aid the destruction of the disease	tive) but allow him to persevere in his evil behaviour until he is ready to be corrected; this should especially be applied to the lustful and angry		
phrenesis: a hot abscess in the membranes of the brain; its symptoms include insanity, pathological wakefulness, mad look in the eyes; remedies should be applied quickly: the shaved head should be washed with tepid vinegar, poulticed with beef-lung, phlebotomy must be performed through the frontal vein; he should be locked, tied, and not heeded to; he should be encouraged to sleep, not be shown any pictures and be maintained on a diet of bread and water; if the symptoms do not disappear after three days one should give up any hope of a cure	sinner and the proud in particular whose brain is infested with tumours of pride, and hence loses his reason, the ability to sleep; the therapy of bloodletting represents confession, vinegar the memory of Christ; the sinner should be segregated from society and temporalities and withdraw to a secluded environment so that the fury of his cupidity may be extinguished	*Reduct.* iv. 3, 88[1–2]	Constantinus
madness (*amentia*): mania which is the result of infection in the anterior ventricles of the brain; it deprives the patient of the imaginative power; the remedy involves music, purgative medicines and surgery as a last resort—all to remove the alien thoughts, fears, and worries	those infected with such a love for the pleasures of this world that they lose any *spiritualis imaginatio et meditatio*	*Reduct.* iv. 4, 88[2]–89[2]	Constantinus; Platearius
numbness (*stupor*): when a specific organ falls asleep; sensual blindness; loss of sense of judgement with respect to sensible things; may be caused by superfluous humours blocking the channels of the spirits (drunkards) or by	the *sapientes* of this world who are spiritually blinded and ignore the things useful to their souls; the lethargic is the evil rich man whose mind is occupied with evil desires and feelings; he can also be the hypocrite who is secretly evil and who is	"	Constantinus

Signifier	Signified	Reference	Source
excessive cold which suppresses the nerves; may be a sign for a graver approaching disease such as lethargy which is caused by phlegmatic humours flooding the brain and creating abscess at its posterior part; false sleep is its hallmark and it is treated by moving the patient to a well-lit place, talking to him constantly, fumigating the room, cold water, clyster, purgation and evacuation, shaving the head, provoking sneezing; *phrenesis* which develops into lethargy is an evil omen and vice versa	much worse than he who commits sins overtly (represented by the *phrenesis* stricken person)		
vertigo: corruption of visual spirit caused by windy humour which is mixed with the spirit of vision	*falsi iudicatores et opinatores*, infected by flatulence of pride	"	Constantinus
falling disease (*morbus caducus*): *sacra passio*, epilepsy, apoplexy, analepsy, catalepsy; some can foresee the approaching fit, others collapse suddenly	pride	*Reduct.* iv. 5, 89^2–90^2	Galen (2x)
sneezing: when happens naturally, it is a good sign of proper expulsion of superfluous cerebral humours	contrition which purges the soul; when pathological, signifies diabolical temptation	*Reduct.* iv. 6, 90^2	Constantinus
shaking (*tremor*): paralysis accompanied by tremor is better than without it	the upwards movement (*ab natura*)=*motus rationis, virtutis, gratie*; downward movement (*ab morbo*)=*motus sensualitatis, culpe, carnalis*; *tremor* may mean fear (*timor*) which shows that the organ (the sinner) is not devoid of any natural power (God)	*Reduct.* iv. 7, 90^2–91^1	Constantinus
spasm: violent contraction of the nerves	laziness caused by repletion of riches, lack	*Reduct.* iv. 8, 91^{1-2}	

Signifier	Signified	Reference	Source
destroying any voluntary movement and sense and caused by repletion, emptiness, and excessive cold; one should not suddenly warm cold fingers lest the nerves be damaged	of virtues, and the cold of irreverence. The desirable and more effective procedure of correction should be gradual		
paralysis: caused by superfluous food and drink which create humour that causes the nerves to wrinkle and the spirits to solidify and thus hampers the motion; can strike the nerves in general or a specific organ	the nerves are the prelates; when they abuse their function through avarice, ambition, envy, or despair, the other organs of the Christian body lose their motion as well	*Reduct.* iv. 9, 91²–92¹	Galen, *primo de locis affectis*; cf. Galen, *De locis affectis* I.6 in *Opera omnia*, ed. Kühn, viii, 56–7; *Barth.* vii. 13
eye diseases: *apostema=albugo* caused by humours flowing to the pupils; cured by salve made up of female milk and rosewater which restrains the tears; it should not be used violently lest it get into the optic nerve and cause total blindness; *lippitudo*: viscous superfluity which hits the eyelids; red eye is cured by egg-white mixed with rose-oil; tela caused by solidified viscous humour; it can be restrained by the blood from wings of pigeons and hoopoes; involuntary flow of tears; *caligatio*	diseases of the mind (the will and understanding in particular); *apostema superbie et congregatio humoris carnalitatis et luxurie* is cured by the sweet milk of doctrine and by the rosewater of devotion which restrain the tears of despair; as noble organs, eyes represent the princes and nobles of this world (*sapientes mundi*) who, even though they have a healthy *pupilla intellectus*, yet suffer from *lippitudo carnalitatis*. The flow of tears represents the various forms of compunction	*Reduct.* iv. 10, 92¹–93¹	Constantinus
blindness: the worst possible affliction	ignorance, obstinacy, and malice	*Reduct.* iv. 11, 93¹–94²	Constantinus
deafness	abstinence and lack of patience	*Reduct.* iv. 12, 94²–95¹	
fetor (stench) strikes the nose and the mouth; in the nose caused by *polypus* which is a corrosive disease that disfigures the whole face	*polypus* represents lust; mouth-stench represents the deformity of speech of those who spread base, false, and disreputable words	*Reduct.* iv. 13, 95¹	
speaking difficulties, hoarseness	impediments on the speaking of prelates and preachers	*Reduct.* iv. 14–15, 95¹–²	

Signifier	Signified	Reference	Source
heart disease (*cardiaca*): *syncopis* is a motive flaw in the heart caused by lack of inhaled spirits; *margarite* (pearls) are a possible therapy which expels the damaging material	sadness and despair which are caused by the lack of Holy Spirit and the numerous vices; recourse to Mary is one of the cures	*Reduct.* iv. 16, 95²–96¹	
fevers: 3 kinds: *ephemera* (caused by dissolution and heating up of spirits), *putrida* (caused by humoral corruption which debilitates the body, tends to recur), *ethica* (caused by consumption of organs; the patient hardly feels ill); 4 species of fever: quotidian (caused by phlegmatic humours, lasts for a day), continuous (caused by corrupt blood), tertian (caused by corrupt choler), and quartan (caused by corrupt melancholy); constipation in acute fevers is an ominous sign, *fluxus ventris aut naris* is a positive sign; simple fever demands simple medicine, composite demands composite	*concupiscentia mentis* and *intemperantia desideriorum* which include pride (corresponds to ephemeral because caused by vain spirits), lust (corresponds to putrid because its substance are corrupt humours, it debilitates the soul, recurs even after penitence), and avarice (which corresponds to hectic since its object is solid matter); 4 species of fever correspond respectively to sloth, lust, avarice, and despair or sadness; *venter conscientie* should wash away corrupt humours through confession	*Reduct.* iv. 17, 96¹–97²	Constantinus; Galen
stomach conditions: *fastidium* (aversion) in which the nutritive power is damaged by a failure of spirits, obstruction of nerves which transmit the sense or humoral repletion; *bulismus* caused by cold which suppresses the food at the stomach's bottom, thus creating a sensation of emptiness, or by immoderate heat which passes to the stomach from the liver through the mesenteric veins; hiccough (*singulatus*), spasmodic activity of the stomach which	abhorrence towards the divine word and spiritual goods, caused by lack of grace and devotion, prudence and discretion, or by the affluence of pleasures, riches, and earthly possessions; bulimia represents avarice caused by *frigiditas indevotionis* and by *caliditas aliene voracis affectionis*; *singulatus* is the vice of indignation, grumbling, quarrelsome dissatisfaction, caused by the *frigus indevotionis, calor concupiscentie et ambitionis, inanitio paupertatis et repletio mundane tem*	*Reduct.* iv. 28, 97²–98¹	

Signifier	Signified	Reference	Source
causes compressed air to create violent sound; can be cured by inducing sneezing, sudden shocks, recoil from some shameful thing	*poralitatis* which damage the *stomachus voluntatis*; fear of damnation, creating feelings of shame and *sternuatio contritionis et confessionis* may cure it		
vomit: can be sign of pregnancy	expelling vices through confession from the stomach of conscience; can be provoked by the pain of contrition (*mordicatio nervorum*), by medical intervention of the word of God, by fervour of love (*calor stomachi*), or by the conception of grace and devotion (*gravitas matrix*); it can also represent kind distribution of alms or, conversely, evil language	*Reduct.* iv. 19, 98[1–2]	Galen
stomach ache: windiness (*ventositas*) which is more harmful to the stomach than corrupt humours, and more painful in the subtle parts of the intestines (the six kinds of ache related to this cause: *dolor infixus, extensivus, aggravativus, congelativus, deambulativus*); *tortura viscerum; tortiones intestinorum; passio colica*—intestines blocked by viscous matter may lead to death; *fecis desiccatio in colone*; worms; *fluxus ventris* which is divided into diarrhoea, lyenteria, dysenteria	pain to the soul (the stomach) may be caused by the cold of irreverence and sloth, by the tumour of pride, and by the faeces of lust; pride (*ventositas*) is worse than lust (the humours of carnal infection) and is more detrimental and painful to the wise; the grip of envy tortures the soul like *tortura intestinorum*; the evil solidified viscous habit to indulge in vices cannot be simply expelled by penitence; constipation in the intestines of conscience impedes confession; sins corrode the conscience like worms; 3 kinds of *fluxus ventris* represent moral inconstancy and weakness in speaking, listening, and doing	*Reduct.* iv. 20, 98[2]–100[2]	Constantinus (2x); *commentator super Ioannitium; ut dicunt medici*
dropsy: defective digestive power	pride caused by defective reason and discretion; avarice caused by defective evacuation	*Reduct.* iv. 21, 100[2]–101[1]	

Signifier	Signified	Reference	Source
jaundice (*ictericia*) caused by mixture of superfluous choler and infected blood from the liver; it is divided into three kinds (according to colour of choler involved), *crocea*, *viridis*, *negra*; infection of the skin is one of its symptoms; haemorrhoids	the interior affections which are corrupted by the mind (liver) and infested with triple concupiscence (choler); the infected skin represents corrupt behaviour and speaking; 5 veins which may develop haemorrhoids are the simple, secular, lay people who are lowest in the hierarchy of the Church; governed by sensual appetite, and ignoring the poor, they refrain from expelling the superfluities of the riches given to them by God	*Reduct.* iv. 22, 101^{1-2}	
kidney and bladder conditions: stones, *passio ex defectu contentive virtutis*, hernia (rupture of a membrane named *siphach*, which is located between the nutritive and the generative organs)	The bladder is supposed to collect superfluous vices but may be hampered by obstinacy and interior hardening; conversely, involuntary emission of urine represents prodigality; hernia represents the vice of *discordia* caused by the rupture of *caritas*	*Reduct.* iv. 23, $101^{2}-102^{1}$	
gout: disease of the joints divided into *chiragra* (strikes the fingers), *schiatica* (hips and shins), *podagra* (all the limbs); women, children, and castrati do not develop podagra	triple concupiscence (*carnis, oculorum, superbie vite*); simple and innocent people (children), chaste (castrati), and pious and merciful (women) are immune to it	*Reduct.* iv. 24, 102^{1-2}	Hippocrates
abscess (*apostema*): corrosive abscesses cancer, *lupus, erispelas/sacer ignis; fistula*, corrupting and putrefying abscess; anthrax (*carbunclus*) can be cured by theriac, warm medicinal wine, and phlebotomy in acute cases; *ulcera vesicule*, superficial skin disease; *postula/variole=vesicule puerorum* is the result of corruption of menstrual blood; impetigo as choleric disease	sin in general; corrosive abscess represents the inflated arrogant; *fistulae* signify the lustful. Carbuncles signify the angry ones; one should treat the *carbones peccatorum* or the *postula venialium peccatorum* in a gradual manner; pustule is venial sins; *scabies malorum exemplorum* is caused by the heat of concupiscence and humours of evil desires; impetigo represents *pruritum et appetitum luxurie*	*Reduct.* iv. 32, $102^{1}-104^{2}$	Constantinus

Signifier	Signified	Reference	Source
leprosy: four kinds: *alopecia, serpentina, leonina, marphea*	sin and corruption in general; malice, lust, pride	*Reduct.* iv. 26, 104²–106¹	
poisons: 3 sources: teeth and humours of reptiles, juices of plants, minerals; poisons extracted from females are stronger than those of males; the devastating effect of rabid dog's poison; the symptoms of poisoning (inner burning, spasms, tumours on the finger-nails, heat in the tongue, sweat, cloudiness in the eyes) and the antidotes (vomit and evacuation, medicinal oils, phlebotomy, diet and theriac, e.g. *theriaca rusticorum* composed of balsam, women's milk, and juice of a cooked fat chicken)	words of demons and malignant people, heretics, flatterers and deceivers, the liqueur of carnal delights and riches—all have poisonous effect over the soul; confession, memory of Christ's death and passion, *unctuositas misericordie, elemosyne et compassionis*, self-mortification and abstinence are the cures parallel respectively to the cures of physical poison	*Reduct.* iv. 27, 106¹–108²	Avicenna (2x); Constantinus (2x one of which mentions *in Viatico*)

Appendix III

A Sermon for Students of Medicine[1]

Ad studentes in medicina LXVI

Notandum quod propter peccatum primorum parentum condicio humana deteriorata est in tribus; videlicet in rationis offuscatione et hoc quo ad animam; et contra hoc inventa sunt artes liberales que illuminant rationem. Item in morbositate propter corruptibilitatem et hoc quo ad corpus; et contra hoc inventa est ars medicine. Item in rerum proprietate; communes enim erant omnes res; et contra hoc inventa est scientia iuris per quam redduntur et conservantur unicuique sua.

Porro inter istas tres scientias medicina quo ad multa est melior; cognitio enim eius quod docent liberales scientie parum confert. Scientia autem iuris etsi confert, tamen plus valet illud quod confert medicina quanto plus valet corpus quam res. Sunt enim tria valde utilia ad que valet ista scientia medicine.

Primum est cognitio sue nature corporee. Ipsa enim est que docet quam misera, quam fragilis sit natura corporis humani.

Secundum est opus misericordie. Per ipsam enim possunt fieri multa opera misericordie circa infirmos qui subiacent magne miserie.

Tertium est medicina spiritualis animarum. Per artem enim scientie medicinalis multa habetur instructio circa medicinam spiritualem.

Sed notandum iterum quod sunt multi medici qui in operatione artis sue multotiens offendunt multum. Sunt enim aliqui qui quia nesciunt sufficienter quod est artis, omittunt in operatione et ideo rei sunt mortis multorum. Et hoc est peccatum homicidii. Alii sunt qui faciunt emere res caras a suis familiaribus cum per viliora possent infirmis interdum eque subvenire. Et hoc est infidelitas.

Alii sunt qui ea que ordinavit ecclesia facienda circa infirmos pro salute animarum ut confessio et communicatio et similia negligunt; et hoc est inobedientia ad ecclesie mandata.

Ve talibus medicis qui quos deberent sanare occidunt; et confidentibus in se sunt valde infideles; et salutaria ecclesie negligunt mandata.

Proinde notandum est quod ad hoc quod studium istud vertatur in bonum, debent huiusmodi studentes intentionem suam ad utilitates supradictas dirigere. Debent etiam cavere ne egrediantur ad practicam ante bonam sufficientiam artis adquisitam. In prosequendo vero practicam debent cauere ne in dubiis unquam procedant sine concilio vel delibratione multa. Sic etiam fideliter agant cum patientibus quod cum paucioribus expensis quantum poterunt eis subveniant; salarium sic temperatum recipiant quod suam conscientiam lesam non relinquent. Super omnia vero debent cavere ne occasione

---

[1] Humbert de Romans, *Sermones ad diuersos status* (Hagenau, 1508), tr. i. 66, 'Ad studentes in medicina'.

medicine aliquid faciant contra deum in se vel in aliis ne dum corporibus sanandis intendunt animas suas vel aliorum interficiant. Denique vero non debent tantum in arte confidere quantum in orationibus et magis in deo confidant. Unde Ecc. xxxviii dicitur de medicis quod ipsi orent pro infirmis.

Materia de predictis: Thema Honora medicum propter necessitatem etenim illum creauit altissimus; omnis medela a deo est.

Nota quod ars medicine in hoc verbo commendatur a tribus, videlicet ab actore, scilicet deo, ab utilitate cum dicitur propter necessitatem. Item a fructu cum dicitur: honora.

Notandum autem quod propter peccatum ut supra.

BIBLIOGRAPHY

PRIMARY SOURCES

Manuscripts

MS Basel, Universitätsbibliothek, B VIII 30 (*Sde*).
MS Berlin, Staatsbibliothek PK, lat. quart. 773 (Galvano).
MS Berlin, Staatsbibliothek PK, Theol. lat. fol. 219 (*Sde*).
MS London, BL, Addit. 24998 (Giovanni).
MS London, BL, Arundel 198 (Servasanto).
MS Oxford, Bodl. Lib., Laud. Misc. 41 (Aldobrandinus Tusculanus, *De scala fidei*).
MS Oxford, Bodl. Lib., Bodley 315 (Pierre de Limoges, *De oculo morali*).
MS Oxford, Bodl. Lib., Douce 177 (Bersuire).
MS Oxford, Bodl. Lib., Laud Misc. 278 (Johannes von Freiburg).
MS Paris, BN, lat. 486ᵃ (Gorranus).
MS Paris, BN, lat. 2338 (Servasanto).
MS Paris, BN, lat. 3181 (Galvano).
MS Paris, BN, lat. 3436 (Servasanto).
MS Paris, BN, lat. 3642 (Servasanto).
MS Paris, BN, lat. 15956 (Guillaume de Mailly)
MS Paris, BN, nouv. acq. lat. 259 (Servasanto).
MS Paris, BN, nouv. acq. lat. 669 (Galvano).
MS Rome, Archivio Generale dei Carmelitani, III Varia 1 (Arnau).
MS Vat. lat. 2463 (Galvano).
MS Vat. lat. 3824 (Arnau).

Printed Primary Sources

ALBERTUS MAGNUS, *Commentarium in II Sententiarum*, in *Opera Omnia*, 27, ed. A. Borgnet. Paris, 1894.
—— *Super Matthaeum*, in *Opera Omnia*, 21/1, ed. B. Schmidt. Münster, 1987.
Annales Ordinis Cartusiensis, i. Correira, 1687.
ANTONIO DA PADOVA, *Sermones dominicales et festivi ad fidem codicum recogniti*, eds. B. Costa, L. Frasson, and I. Luisetto. 3 vols., Padua, 1979.
ARNAU DE VILANOVA, *Alia informatio beguinorum* = Perarnau, *L'"Alia informatio beguinorum"*.
—— *Allocutio christini* = Perarnau, 'La *Allocutio christini*', 75–117.
—— *Allocutio super tetragrammaton* = Carreras i Artau, 'L'*Allocutio*'.
—— *Ars catholicae philosophiae* = Perarnau, 'L'*Ars catholicae philosophiae*', 57–162.
—— *Confessió de Barcelona* = Arnau de Vilanova, *Obres Catalanes*, i. 101–39.

—— *De esu carnium* = Bazell, 'Christian Diet'.

—— *De helemosina et sacrificio* = Perarnau, 'Dos tratados', 609–30.

—— *De prudentia catholicorum scholarium* = Graziano di Santa Teresa, 'Il *Tractatus de prudentia*'.

—— *De zona pellicea* = Perarnau, 'Troballa de tractats espirituals', 508–12, and Cartaregia and Perarnau, 'El text sencer'.

—— *Dyalogus de elementis catholice fidei* (*Alphabetum catholicorum*) = Burger, 'Beiträge', 173–94.

—— *Epistola ad priorissam de caritate* = Manselli, 'La religiosità', 60–76.

—— *Eulogium de notitia verorum et pseudo-apostolorum* = Carreras i Artau, 'La polémica gerundense'.

—— *Informació espiritual* = Arnau de Vilanova, *Obres Catalanes*, i. 223–43.

—— *Interpretatio de visionibus in somniis* = Menéndez y Pelayo, *Historia de los heterodoxos españoles*, iii. pp. liii–lxxiii.

—— *Introductio in librum Ioachim De semine scripturarum* = Manselli, 'La religiosità', 43–59.

—— *Per ciò che molti* = Ibid. 92–100.

—— *Raonament d'Avinyó* = Arnau de Vilanova, *Obres Catalanes*, i. 167–221.

—— *Tertia denunciatio gerundensis* = Carreras i Artau, 'La polémica gerundense'.

—— *Tractatus de mysterio cymbalorum* = Perarnau, 'El text primitiu', 53–107.

—— *Tractatus de tempore adventus Antichristi et fine mundi* = Ibid. 134–69.

—— *Obres Catalanes*, ed. M. Batllori. 2 vols., Barcelona, 1947.

—— *Opera*. Lyons, 1520.

—— *Opera Medica Omnia*, eds. L. García-Ballester, J. A. Paniagua, and M. R. McVaugh. Barcelona, 1975– .

—— Raymund de Moleris and Jordan de Turre (attr.), *Tractatus de sterilitate*, ed. E. Montero Cartelle. Valladolid, 1993.

ASTESANO DI ASTI, *Summa de casibus*. Strasbourg, 1474.

AVICENNA, *Liber canonis*. Venice, 1507.

BARTHOLOMAEUS ANGLICUS, *Venerandi patris Bartholomei Anglici . . . opus de rerum proprietatibus*. Nuremberg, 1519.

BERNARD OF CLAIRVAUX, *S. Bernardi opera*, ed. J. Leclercq, C. H. Talbot, and H. M. Rochais. Rome, 1957–77.

—— *The Steps of Humility*, tr. G. B. Birch. Cambridge, Mass., 1942.

BERTRAND DE LA TOUR, *Sermones quadragesimales epistolares*. Strasbourg, 1501/2.

Biblia sacra, cum glossa ordinaria . . . et postilla Nicolai Lyrani, 6 vols. Lyons, 1589.

BONAVENTURA, *Opera Omnia*. 10 vols. Quaracchi, 1882–1902.

—— *Sermons De Diversis*, ed. J. G. Bougerol. 2 vols., Paris, 1993.

Capitula Regni Sicilie que ad hodiernum diem lata est, i. ed. F. Testa. Palermo, 1741.

Cartulaire de l'Université de Montpellier, i. ed. A. Germain. Montpellier, 1890.

Chartularium Universitatis Parisiensis, ii. ed. H. Denifle and E. Chatelain. Paris, 1891.

Fasciculus morum: A Fourteenth Century Preacher's Handbook, ed. and tr. S. Wenzel. University Park, Pennsylvania, 1989.

GALEN, *Opera omnia*, ed. C. G. Kühn. 20 vols. Leipzig, 1821–33.

GERSON, JEAN, *Oeuvres complètes*. 10 vols., ed. P. Glorieux. Paris, 1960–73.

GIORDANO DA PISA, *Quaresimale Fiorentino 1305–1306*, ed. C. Delcorno. Florence, 1974.

GIOVANNI DA SAN GIMIGNANO, *Summa de exemplis et rerum similitudinibus locuplentissima*. Antwerp, 1583.

—— *Conciones funebres*. Paris, 1611.

—— *Convivium quadragesimale hoc est conciones et sermones tam sacri quam suaves singuli totius quadragesimae feriis et dominicis . . .* Paris, 1611.

GUILLAUME DE SAINT-THIERRY, *De natura corporis et animae*, ed. M. Lemoine. Paris, 1988.

HENRI DE MONDEVILLE, *Die Chirurgie des Heinrich von Mondeville*, ed. J. L. Pagel. Berlin, 1892.

HUGUES DE FOUILLOY (FOLIETO), *De medicina anime*. *PL* 176: 1183–1202.

HUGUES DE SAINT-CHER, *Pars prima (-sexta) huius operis continens textum Biblie, cum postilla Hugonis*, iii. Paris, 1533.

HUMBERT DE ROMANS, *Sermones ad diuersos status*. Hagenau, 1508.

ISAAC ISRAELI, *Omnia opera ysaac*. Lyons, 1515.

JACOPO DA VORAGINE, *Sermones aurei ac pulcherrimi variis scripturarum doctrinis referti de sanctis per anni totius circulum concurrentibus*. Cologne, 1478.

—— *Ordinis predicatorum fratris Iacobi de Voragine sermones dominicales per anni circulum predicabiles alphabetico ordine magistraliter registrati*. Ulm, 1484.

JOHN BROMYARD (JOANNES DE BROMYARD), *Summa predicantium*. Nuremberg, 1518.

JOHANNES VON FREIBURG, *Summa confessorum*. Augsburg, 1476.

JOHN OF SALISBURY, *Ioannis Saresberiensis Policraticus I–IV*, ed. K. S. B. Keats-Rohan. *CCCM* 118. Turnhout, 1993.

—— *Ioannis Saresberiensis Metalogicon*, ed. J. B. Hall. *CCCM* 98. Turnhout, 1991.

LLULL, RAMON, *Ars abbreviata praedicandi*, in *Opera Latina*, 208, ed. A. Soria Flores, F. D. Reboiras, and M. Senellart, *CCCM* 80. Turnhout, 1991, 50–158.

—— *Declaratio Raimundi*, in *Opera Latina*, 80, ed. M. Pereira and Th. Pindl-Büchel, *CCCM* 79. Turnhout, 1989, 219–402.

—— *Liber de praedicatione*, in *Raimundi Lulli Opera Latina*, 118, ed. F. Stegmüller. Palma de Mallorca, 1961–3.

—— *Liber de virtutibus . . . Ars maior praedicationis*, in *Opera Latina*, 205, ed. F. D. Reboiras and A. Soria Flores, *CCCM* 76. Turnhout, 1986, 103–432.

—— *Quattuor libri principiorum*, with an introduction by R. D. F. Pring-Mill. Paris, 1969. [reprint from the *Opera Omnia*, i. Mainz, 1721].

—— *Selected Works of Ramon Llull (1232–1316)*, ed. and tr. A. Bonner. 2 vols., Princeton, 1985.

LLULL, RAMON, *Principes de médecine*, tr. A. Llinares. Paris, 1992. [Collection 'Sapience', 5, ed. B. Ribémont.]

MARTIN VON TROPPAU, *Sermones Martini ordinis predicatorum penitentiarii domini pape de tempore et de sanctis super epistulas et euangelia*. Strasbourg, 1483/4.

NICOLAUS EYMERICUS, *Directorium Inquisitorum*, ii. Rome, 1578.

PETRARCA, F., *Contra medicum objurgantem invectivarum libri IV*, ed. P. G. Ricci and B. Martinelli. Storia e letteratura, 32. Rome, 1978.

PIERRE BERSUIRE (PETRUS BERCHORIUS), *Reductorium morale super totam bibliam*. Venice, 1583.

RAMON DE PENYAFORT, Summa S^ti raymundi de Peniafort Barcinoneusis . . . De poenitentia, et matrimonio cum glossis Ioannis de Friburgo. Rome, 1603.

RAMON MARTÍ, *Pugio fidei adversos Mauros et Judaeos*. Leipzig, 1687.

RABANUS MAURUS, *De universo VI*, in *PL* 111: 137–80.

—— *Commentarium in Ecclesiasticum*, in *PL* 109: 1030–3.

ROBERT HOLCOT, *In librum sapientie regis Salomonis prelectiones ccxiii*. Basel, 1586.

SERAPION, *De simplicibus medicinis*. Strasbourg, 1531.

SERVASANTO DA FAENZA, *Liber aureus qui antidotarius animarum dictus est*. Leuven, *c.*1485.

THOMAS LE MYÉSIER, *Questiones dubitabiles super quattuor libris sententiarum cum questionibus solutiuis magistri Thome Attrabatensis*. Lyons, 1491.

VICENT FERRER, *Sermons*. 6 vols., ed. J. Sanchis Sivera (i–ii) and G. Schib (iii–vi). Barcelona, 1932–88.

—— *Sermons de Quaresma*. 2 vols., ed. M. Sanchis Guarner. Valencia, 1973.

VINCENT DE BEAUVAIS, *Speculum maius*. Venice, 1591.

SELECT SECONDARY SOURCES

Actes de la I Trobada Internacional d'Estudis sobre Arnau de Vilanova, ed. J. Perarnau. 2 vols., Barcelona, 1995.

AGRIMI, J. and CRISCIANI, C., *Medicina del corpo e medicina dell'anima: Note sul sapere del medico fino all'inizio del secolo XIII*. Milan, 1978.

—— *Malato, medico e medicina nel medioevo*. Turin, 1980.

——'Savoir médical et anthropologie religieuse: Les représentations et les fonctions de la *vetula* (xiiie–xve)', *Annales Économies Sociétés Civilisations*, 48 (1993), 1281–1308.

—— 'Charité et assistance dans la civilisation chrétienne médiévale', in Grmek (ed.), *Histoire de la pensée médicale*, i. 151–74.

ALSZEGLY, Z., 'L'effetto corporale dell'Estrema Unzione', *Gregorianum*, 38 (1957), 385–405.

AMUNDSEN, D. W., 'Medieval Canon Law on Medical and Surgical Practice by the Clergy', *Bulletin of the History of Medicine*, 52 (1978), 22–44 [also in id., *Medicine, Society and Faith*, 222–47].

—— 'Casuistry and Professional Obligations: The Regulation of Physicians by the Court of Conscience in the Late Middle Ages', *Transactions and Studies of the College of Physicians of Philadelphia*, n.s., 3 (1981), 22–39, 93–112 [also in id., *Medicine, Society and Faith*, 248–88].

AMUNDSEN, D. W., 'The Medieval Catholic Tradition', in R. L. Numbers and D. W. Amundsen (ed.) *Caring and Curing*, 65–107 [also in id., *Medicine, Society and Faith*, 175–221].

—— *Medicine, Society, and Faith in the Ancient and Medieval Worlds*. Baltimore and London, 1996.

—— and FERNGREN, G. B., 'Medicine and Religion: Early Christianity through the Middle Ages', in M. E. Marty and K. L. Vaux (ed.), *Health/Medicine and the Faith Traditions*, 93–131.

—— 'The Early Christian Tradition', in R. L. Numbers and D. W. Amundsen (ed.), *Caring and Curing*, 40–64.

ARRIZABALAGA, J., 'Facing the Black Death: Perceptions and Reactions of University Medical Practitioners', in L. García-Ballester *et al.* (ed.), *Practical Medicine*, 237–88.

BACKMAN, C. R., 'Arnau de Vilanova and the Franciscan Spirituals in Sicily', *Franciscan Studies*, 50 (1990), 3–29.

—— *The Decline and Fall of Medieval Sicily: Politics, Religion, and Economy in the Reign of Frederick III, 1296–1337*. Cambridge, 1995.

—— 'The Reception of Arnau de Vilanova's Religious Ideas', in S. L. Waugh and P. D. Diehl (ed.), *Christendom and its Discontents: Exclusion, Persecution and Rebellion, 1000–1500*. Cambridge, 1996, 112–31.

BALDWIN, J. W., *The Language of Sex: Five Voices from Northern France around 1200*. London and Chicago, 1994.

BATAILLON, L.-J., '*Similitudines* et *exempla* dans les sermons du XIIIe siècle', in *The Bible in the Medieval World: Essays in Memory of Beryl Smalley*, ed. K. Walsh and D. Wood, Studies in Church History—Subsidia, 4. Oxford, 1985, 191–205.

—— 'Les images dans les sermons du xiiie siècle', *Freiburger Zeitschrift für Philosophie und Theologie*, 37/3 (1990), 327–95.

BATLLORI, M., 'Els textos espirituals d'Arnau de Vilanova en lengua grega', *Quaderni Ibero-americani*, 14 (1953), 358–61.

—— 'Dos nous escrits espirituals d'Arnau de Vilanova', *AST* 28 (1955), 45–70.

BAZELL, D. M., 'Christian Diet: A Case Study Using Arnald of Vilanova's *De esu carnium*'. Ph.D. thesis, Harvard, 1991.

—— '*De esu carnium*: Arnald of Vilanova's Defence of Carthusian Abstinence', in *ATIEAV* ii. 227–48; also in *ATCA* 14 (1995).

BERGDOLT, K., *Arzt, Krankheit und Therapie bei Petrarca*. Darmstadt, 1992.

BÉRIOU, N., (ed.) 'La Prédication au béguinage de Paris pendant l'année liturgique 1272–1273', *Recherches Augustiniennes*, 13 (1978), 105–229.

—— 'La confession dans les écrits théologiques et pastoraux du XIIIe siècle: Médication de l'âme ou démarche judiciaire', in *L'Aveu: Antiquité et Moyen Âge*. Collection de l'école française de Rome, 88, Rome, 1986, 261–82.

—— (ed.), *La Prédication de Ranulphe de la Houblonnière*. 2 vols., Paris, 1987.

—— 'La Prédication synodale au xiiie siècle d'après l'exemple Cambrésien', in *Le Clerc séculier au Moyen Âge*. Paris, 1993, 229–47 [xxiie congrès de la S.H.M.E.S., Amiens, Juin, 1991].

—— and F.-O. TOUATI., *Voluntate dei leprosus: les lépreux entre conversion et exclusion au XIIème et XIIIème siècles*. Spoleto, 1991.

—— and D. L. D'AVRAY, *Modern Questions about Medieval Sermons: Essays on Marriage, Death, History, and Sanctity*. Spoleto, 1994.

BILLER, P., '*Curate infirmos*: The Medieval Waldensian Practice of Medicine', in W. J. Sheils (ed.), *The Church and Healing*, 55–77.

—— 'Words and the Medieval Notion of "Religion" ', *Journal of Ecclesiastical History*, 36 (1985), 353–69.

—— 'Views of Jews from Paris around 1300: Christian or Scientific', in *Christianity and Judaism*, ed. D. Wood. Studies in Church History, 29; Oxford, 1992, 187–207.

—— 'Popular Religion in the Central and Later Middle Ages', in M. Bentley (ed.), *Companion to Historiography*. London and New York, 1997, 221–46.

—— 'Introduction: John of Naples, Quodlibets and Medieval Theological Concern with the Body', in P. Biller and A. J. Minnis (ed.), *Medieval Theology and the Natural Body*. York, 1997, 3–12.

BLOOMFIELD, M. W., *The Seven Deadly Sins*. East Lansing, Mich., 1952.

BØRRESEN, K. E., *Anthropologie médiévale et théologie Mariale*. Oslo, 1971.

BOYLE, L. E., 'The Date of the *Summa praedicantium* of John Bromyard', *Speculum*, 48 (1973), 533–7.

—— *Pastoral Care, Clerical Education and Canon Law, 1200–1400*. London, 1981.

BRÉMOND, C., LE GOFF, J., and SCHMITT, J.-C., *L' "Exemplum"*. 'Typologie des sources de Moyen Âge occidental', 40; Turnhout, 1982.

BROWN, P. R. L., *The Body and Society: Men, Women and Sexual Renunciation in Early Christianity*. London and Boston, 1987.

BRUNDAGE, J. A., *Law, Sex and Christian Society in Medieval Europe*. Chicago and London, 1987.

BURGER, C., *Aedificatio, Fructus, Utilitas: Johannes Gerson als Professor der Theologie und Kanzler der Universität Paris*. Tübingen, 1986.

BURGER, W., 'Beiträge zur Geschichte der Katechese im Mittelalter', *Römische Quartalschrift* (Geschichte), 21/4 (1907), 163–94.

BYLEBYL, J. J., 'The Medical Meaning of *Physica*', *Osiris*, 2nd ser., 6 (1990), 16–41.

BYNUM, C. WALKER, *Holy Feast and Holy Fast: The Religious Significance of Food to Medieval Women*. Berkeley, 1987.

—— 'The Female Body and Religious Practice in the Later Middle-Ages', in *Fragmentation and Redemption*, 222–35 [also in M. Feher *et al.* (ed.), *Fragments for a History of the Human Body*, i. 161–219].

—— *Fragmentation and Redemption: Esssays on Gender and the Human Body in Medieval Religion*. New York, 1991.

CADDEN, J., *Meanings of Sex Difference in the Middle Ages: Medicine, Science, and Culture*. Cambridge, 1993.

CAMBELL, J., *Vies Occitanes de Saint Auzias et de Sainte Dauphine*. Bibliotheca Pontificii Athenaei Antoniani, 12; Rome, 1963.

CAMPBELL, S. D., HALL, B. B., and KLAUSNER, D. N. (ed.), *Health, Disease and Healing in Medieval Culture*. Toronto, 1992.

CARRERAS I ARTAU, J., 'Una versió grega de nou escrits d'Arnau de Vilanova', *AST* 7 (1932), 127–34.

—— 'Arnaldo de Vilanova, apologista antijudaica', *Sefarad*, 7 (1947), 49–61.

—— 'Del epistolario espiritual de Arnaldo de Vilanova', *Estudios Franciscanos*, 49 (1948), 79–94, 391–406.

—— 'La *Allocutio super Tetragrammaton* de Arnaldo de Vilanova', *Sefarad*, 9 (1949), 75–105.

—— 'La polémica gerundense sobre el Anticristo entre Arnau de Vilanova y los dominicos', *Anales del Instituto de Estudios Gerundenses*, 5/6 (1950/1), 5–58.

—— *L'epistolari d'Arnau de Vilanova*. Barcelona, 1950.

CARTAREGIA, O. and PERARNAU, J., 'El text sencer de l'*Epistola ad gerentes zonam pelliceam* d'Arnau de Vilanova', *ATCA* 12 (1993), 7–42.

CATTO, J. I. and EVANS, R. (ed.), *The History of the University of Oxford*, ii. *Late Medieval Oxford*. Oxford, 1992.

CHABÀS, R. 'Inventario de los libros, ropas y demás efectos de Arnaldo de Villanueva', *Revista de Archivos, Bibliotecas y Museos*, 9 (1903), 189–203.

CLARK, D. L., 'Optics for Preachers: The *De oculo morali* by Peter of Limoges', *Michigan Academician*, 9/3 (1977), 329–44.

CONRAD, L. I., NEVE, M., NUTTON, V., PORTER, R., and WEAR, A., *The Western Medical Tradition 800 BC to AD 1800*. Cambridge, 1995.

COURTENAY, W. J., '*Antiqui* and *moderni* in Late Medieval Thought', *Journal of the History of Ideas*, 48 (1987), 3–10.

—— 'Inquiry and Inquisition: Academic Freedom in Medieval Universities', *Church History*, 58 (1989), 168–81.

CRISCIANI, C., '*Exemplum Christi* e sapere. Sull'epistemologia di Arnaldo da Villanova', *Archives Internationales d'Histoire des Sciences*, 28 (1978), 245–92.

—— 'History, Novelty, and Progress in Scholastic Medicine', *Osiris*, 2nd ser., 6 (1990), 118–39.

D'AVRAY, D. L., *The Preaching of the Friars: Sermons Diffused from Paris before 1300*. Oxford, 1985.

—— 'The Comparative Study of Memorial Preaching', *Transactions of the Royal Historical Society*, 40 (1990), 25–42.

—— 'Sermons on the Dead before 1350', *Studi Medievali*, 31 (1990), 207–23 [also in Bériou and D'Avray, *Modern Questions*, 175–93].

—— 'Some Franciscan Ideas about the Body', *AFH* 75 (1991), 343–63 [also in Bériou and D'Avray, *Modern Questions*, 155–74].

—— *Death and the Prince: Memorial Preaching before 1350*. Oxford, 1994.

—— 'Philosophy in Preaching: The Case of a Franciscan Based in Thirteenth-Century Florence (Servasanto da Faenza)', in *Literature and Religion in the Latter Middle Ages: Philological Studies in Honor of Siegfried Wenzel*, ed. R. G. Newhauser and J. A. Alford. Binghamton, NY, 1995, 263–73.

DELCORNO, C., 'La predicazione volgare in Italia (sec. XIII–XIV). Teoria, produzione, ricezione', *Revue Mabillon*, 65 (1993), 83–107.

DEMAITRE, L. E., *Doctor Bernard de Gordon: Professor and Practitioner*. Toronto, 1980.

—— 'The Description and Diagnosis of Leprosy by Fourteenth-Century Physicians', *Bulletin of the History of Medicine*, 59 (1985), 327–44.

—— 'The Relevance of Futility: Jordanus de Turre (fl. 1313–1335) on the Treatment of Leprosy', *Bulletin of the History of Medicine*, 70 (1996), 26–81.

DE RIDDER-SYMOENS, H. (ed.), *A History of the University in Europe*, i. *Universities in the Middle Ages*. Cambridge, 1992.

DIEPGEN, P., *Arnald von Villanova als Politiker und Laientheologe*. Berlin and Leipzig, 1909.

—— *Studien zur Geschichte der Beziehungen zwischen Theologie und Medizin im Mittelalter: Die Theologie und der ärztliche Stand*. Berlin, 1922.

—— *Medizin und Kultur: Gesammelte Aufsätze*, ed. W. Artelt, E. Heischkel, and J. Schuster. Stuttgart, 1938.

DONDAINE, A., 'La vie et les oeuvres de Jean de San Gimignano', *AFP* 9 (1939), 128–83.

DOWTRY, A. F., 'The *Modus Medendi* and the Benedictine Order in Anglo-Norman England', in W. J. Sheils (ed.), *The Church and Healing*, 25–38.

DULIEU, L., *La Médecine à Montpellier*, i. Montpellier, 1975.

DU PLESSIS D'ARGENTRÉ, C., *Collectio judiciorum de novis erroribus qui ab initio duodecimi saeculi ad anum 1735 in Ecclesia proscripti sunt et notati*, pt. 1/1. Paris, 1728.

DURLING, R. J., 'A Chronological Census of Renaissance Editions and Translations of Galen', *Journal of the Warburg and Courtauld Institutes*, 24 (1961), 230–305.

—— 'Corrigenda and Addenda to Diel's Galenica', *Traditio*, 23 (1967), 461–6.

EDELSTEIN, L., 'The Relation of Ancient Philosophy to Medicine', *Bulletin of the History of Medicine*, 26 (1952), 299–316. Also in *Ancient Medicine: Selected Papers of Ludwig Edelstein*, ed. O. Temkin and C. Lilian Temkin. Baltimore, 1967.

EHRLE, F., *Historia bibliothecae Romanorum pontificum*, i. Rome, 1890.

—— 'Arnaldo de Vilanova e i *Thomatiste*: Contributo alla storia della scuola Tomistica', *Gregorianum*, 1 (1920), 475–501.

ELL, S. R., 'Concepts of Disease and the Physician in the Early Middle Ages', *Janus*, 65 (1978), 153–65.

ENGELS, J., 'Berchoriana', *Vivarium*, 2 (1964), 62–124.

ENGELS, J., 'La lettre dédicace de Bersuire à Pierre des Prés', *Vivarium*, 7 (1969), 62–72.

FEHER, M., NADDAFF, R., and TAZI, N. (ed.), *Fragments for a History of the Human Body*. 3 vols., New York, 1990.

FERNGREN, G. B., 'Early Christianity as a Religion of Healing', *Bulletin of the History of Medicine*, 66 (1992), 1–15.

FICHTNER, G., 'Christus als Arzt. Ursprünge und Wirkungen eines Motivs', *Frühmittelalterliche Studien*, 16 (1982), 1–18.

FINKE, H., *Aus den Tagen Bonifaz VIII*. Münster, 1902.

—— *Acta Aragonensia*. 2 vols., Leipzig, 1908.

—— *Papsttum und Untergang des Templerordens*, vol. ii. Münster, 1907.

FINUCANE, R., *Miracles and Pilgrims: Popular Beliefs in Medieval England*. London, 1995.

—— *The Rescue of the Innocents: Endangered Children in Medieval Miracles*. New York and London, 1997.

FLINT, V. I. J., *The Rise of Magic in Early Medieval Europe*. Oxford, 1991.

—— 'The Early Medieval 'Medicus', the Saint—and the Enchanter', *Social History of Medicine*, 2 (1989), 127–45.

FORTUNY, F. J., 'Arnau de Vilanova: Els límits de la raó teològica. Arnau en oposició a Averrois, Maimònides i Tomàs d'Aquino', in *El debat intercultural als segles XIII i XIV*, ed. M. Salleras. Barcelona, 1989, 31–59.

FRENCH, R. and CUNNINGHAM, A., *Before Science: The Invention of the Friars' Natural Philosophy*. Aldershot, 1996.

FUNKENSTEIN, A., *Theology and Scientific Imagination from the Middle Ages to the Seventeenth Century*. Princeton, 1986.

GARCÍA-BALLESTER, L., *Historia social de la medicina en la España de los siglos xiii al xvi*. Madrid, 1976.

—— 'Arnau de Vilanova (*c*.1240–1311) y la reforma de los estudios médicos en Montpellier (1309): el Hipócrates latino y la introducción del nuevo Galeno', *Dynamis*, 2 (1982), 97–158.

—— 'Soul and Body, Disease of the Soul and Disease of the Body in Galen's Medical Thought', in *Le opere psicologiche de Galeno (Atti del terzo colloquio Galenico internazionale: Pavia, 10–12 Settembre, 1986)*, ed. P. Manuli and M. Vegetti. Naples, 1988, 117–52.

—— 'Dietetic and Pharmacological Therapy: A Dilemma among Fourteenth Century Jewish Practitioners in the Montpellier Area', *Clio Medica*, 22 (1991), 23–37.

—— 'Changes in the *Regimina sanitatis*. The Role of the Jewish Physicians', in S. Campbell, B. Hall, and D. Klausner (ed.), *Health, Disease and Healing in Medieval Culture*, 119–40.

—— 'On the Origin of the "six non-natural things" in Galen', in *Galen und das Hellenistische Erbe*, ed. K. Kollesch and D. Nickel. Stuttgart, 1993, 105–15.

—— 'Medical Ethics in Transition in the Latin Medicine of the Thirteenth and

Fourteenth Centuries: New Perspectives on the Physician–Patient Relationship and the Doctor's Fee', in *Doctors and Ethics: The Earlier Historical Setting of Professional Ethics*, ed. A. Wear, J. Geyer-Kordesch, and R. French. Amsterdam, 1994, 38–71.

—— 'The Construction of a New Form of Learning and Practicing Medicine in Medieval Latin Europe', *Science in Context*, 8 (1995), 75–102.

——, SÁNCHEZ-SALOR, E., MCVAUGH, M. R., and TRIAS, A., 'Las ediciones renacentistas de Arnau de Vilanova: su valor para la edición crítica de sus obras médicas', *Asclepio*, 37 (1985), 39–66.

——, MCVAUGH, M. R., and RUBIO-VELA, A., 'Medical Licensing and Learning in Fourteenth-Century Valencia', *Transactions of the American Philosophical Society*, 79/6 (1989).

——, FERRE, L., and FELIU, E., 'Jewish Appreciation of Fourteenth-Century Scholastic Medicine', *Osiris*, 2nd ser., 6 (1990), 85–117.

——, FRENCH, R., ARRIZABALAGA, J., and CUNNINGHAM, A. (ed.), *Practical Medicine from Salerno to the Black Death*. Cambridge, 1994.

GARCÍA Y GARCÍA, A., (ed.), *Constitutiones concilii quarti Lateranensis una cum commentariis glossatorum*. Monumenta iuris canonici, ser. A: Corpus Glossatorum. Vatican City, 1981.

GARCÍAS PALOU, S., *La Formación científica de Ramón Llull*. Mallorca, 1989.

GERWING, M., *Vom Ende der Zeit. Der Traktat des Arnald von Villnova über die Ankunft des Antichrist in der akademischen Auseinandersetzung zu Beginn des 14 Jahrhunderts*. Münster, 1996.

GETZ, F., 'The Faculty of Medicine before 1500', in Catto and Evans (ed.), *The History of the University of Oxford*, ii. 373–406.

GIL-SOTRES, P., 'Modelo teórico y observación clínica: Las pasiones del alma en la psicología medica medieval', in *Comprendre et maîtriser la nature au Moyen Age: Mélanges d'histoire des sciences offerts à Guy Beaujouan*. Geneva, 1994, 181–204.

GLORIEUX, P., *Répertoire des Maîtres en Théologie de Paris au XIIIe siècle*. Paris, 1933.

—— 'Gerson et les Chartreux', *RTAM* 28 (1961), 115–53.

GOUREVITCH, D. (ed.), *Maladie et maladies: histoire et conceptualisation. Mélanges en l'honneur de Mirko Grmek*. Geneva, 1992.

GOURON, A., 'Deux universités pour une ville', in *Histoire de Montpellier*, ed. G. Cholvy. Montpellier, 1985, 103–25.

GRABMANN, M., 'Der *Liber de exemplis naturalibus* des Franziskanertheologen Servasanctus', *Franziskanische Studien*, 7 (1920), 85–117.

GRAZIANO DI SANTA TERESA, 'Il *Tractatus de prudentia catholicorum scolarium* di Arnaldo da Villanova', in *Miscellanea André Combes*, ii. Rome and Paris, 1967, 425–48.

GREEN, M. H., 'Constantinus Africanus and the Conflict between Religion and Science', in G. R. Dunstan (ed.) *The Human Embryo: Aristotle and Arabic and European Traditions*. Exeter, 1990, 47–69.

GRELL, O. P. and CUNNINGHAM, A., (ed.) *Medicine and the Reformation*. London and New York, 1993.

GRMEK, M. D. (ed.), *Histoire de la pensée médicale en Occident, i: Antiquité et Moyen Âge*. Paris, 1995.

HARNACK, A., 'Medizinisches aus der ältesten Kirchengeschichte', in *Texte und Untersuchungen zur Geschichte der Altchristlichen Literatur*, 7/4, ed. O. v. Gebhardt and A. Harnack. Leipzig, 1892, 37–147.

HARVEY, B., *Living and Dying in England 1100–1540: The Monastic Experience*. Oxford, 1993.

HARVEY, E. R., *The Inward Wit: Psychological Theory in the Middle Ages and the Renaissance*. London, 1975.

HEIN, W.-H., *Christus als Apotheker*. Frankfurt am Main, 1974.

HENRY, J., 'Doctors and Healers: Popular Culture and the Medical Profession', in *Science, Culture and Popular Belief in Renaissance Europe*, ed. S. Pumfrey, P. L. Rossi, and M. Slawinski. Manchester, 1991, 191–221.

HEWSON, M. A., *Giles of Rome and the Medieval Theory of Conception: A Study of the De formatione corporis humani in utero*. London, 1975.

HILLGARTH, J. N., *Ramon Lull and Lullism in Fourteenth-Century France*. Oxford, 1971.

―― *The Spanish Kingdoms 1250–1516*, i. Oxford, 1976.

HINNEBUSCH, W. A., *The History of the Dominican Order*, ii. New York, 1973.

HUIZINGA, J., *The Waning of the Middle Ages*. London, 1955.

HUMPHREYS, K. W., 'The Medical Books of the Mediaeval Friars', *Libri*, 3 (1954), 95–103.

IANNELLA, C., 'Malattia e salute nella predicazione di Giordano da Pisa', *Rivista di Storia e Letteratura Religiosa*, 31 (1995), 177–216.

JACQUART, D., *Supplément* to Ernest Wickersheimer, *Dictionnaire biographique des médecins en France au Moyen Âge*. Geneva, 1979.

―― *Le Milieu médical en France du XIIᵉ au XVᵉ siècle*. Geneva, 1981.

―― 'The Influence of Arabic Medicine in the Medieval West', in *Encyclopedia of the History of Arabic Science*, iii, ed. R. Rashed. London and New York, 1996, 963–84.

―― and THOMASSET, C., *Sexuality and Medicine in the Middle Ages*. Cambridge, 1988.

―― and MICHEAU, F., *La Médecine arabe et l'Occident médiéval*. Paris, 1990.

JEHL, R., *Melancholie und Acedia: ein Beitrag zu Anthropologie und Ethik Bonaventuras*. Paderborn, 1984.

JOHNSTON, M. D., *The Evangelical Rhetoric of Ramon Llull: Lay Learning and Piety in the Christian West around 1300*. New York and Oxford, 1996.

JORDAN, M. D., 'Medicine and Natural Philosophy in Aquinas', in *Thomas von Aquin―Werk und Wirkung im Licht neuerer Forschungen*, ed. A. Zimmermann. Miscellanea Mediaevalia, 19; Berlin, 1988, 233–46.

―― 'The Disappearance of Galen in Thirteenth-Century Philosophy and

Theology', in *Mensch und Natur im Mittelalter*, ed. A. Zimmermann and A. Speer. Miscellanea Mediaevalia, 21/2; Berlin and New York, 1992, 703–13.

KAEPPELI, T., *Scriptores Ordinis Praedicatorum Medii Aevi*. 4 vols., Rome, 1970–93.

KEIL, G., 'Galen's Religious Belief', in *Galen: Problems and Prospects*, ed. V. Nutton. London, 1981, 117–30.

KIPLE, K. F. (ed.) *The Cambridge World History of Human Disease*. Cambridge, 1993.

KLIBANSKY, R., PANOWSKY, E., and SAXL, F., *Saturn and Melancholy: Studies in the History of Natural Philosophy, Religion and Art*. London, 1964.

KOHLER, CH., 'Traité de recouvrement de la Terre Sainte adressé vers l'an 1295 à Philippe le Bel par Galvano de Levanto, médicin génois', *Revue de l'Orient Latin*, 6/3 (1898), 343–69.

KÖPKE, E., *Iacobus de Cessolis*. Brandenburg a.d. Havel, 1879.

KROLL J., and BACHRACH, B., 'Sin and Etiology of Diseases in Pre-Crusade Europe', *Journal of the History of Medicine and Allied Sciences*, 41 (1986), 395–414.

KRUITWAGEN, B., 'Das *Antidotarium animae* von Fr. Servasenctus, O.F.M. (Lovanii, Joh. de Westfalia, c. 1458)', in *Wiegendrucke und Handschriften: Festgabe Konrad Haebler*. Leipzig, 1919, 80–106.

KUDLIEN, F., 'Der Arzt des Körpers und der Arzt der Seele', *Clio Medica*, 3 (1968), 1–21.

LAKOFF, G., and JOHNSON, M., *Metaphors We Live By*. Chicago and London, 1980.

LECLERCQ, J., 'Textes contemporains de Dante, sur des sujets qu'il a traités', *Studi Medievali*, ser. 3, 6/2 (1965), 531–5.

—— 'Galvano da Levanto e l'Oriente', in *Venezia e l'Oriente fra tardo medioevo e rinascimento*, ed. A. Petrusi. Civiltà Europea e Civiltà Veneziana, Aspetti e Problemi, 4. Venice, 1966, 403–16.

LEE, H., '*Scrutamini Scripturas*: Joachimist Themes and *Figurae* in the Early Religious Writing of Arnold of Vilanova', *Journal of the Warburg and Courtauld Institutes*, 37 (1974), 33–56.

——, REEVES, M., and SILANO, G., *Western Mediterranean Prophecy: The School of Joachim of Fiore and the Fourteenth-Century Breviloquium*. Toronto, 1989.

LE GOFF, J., 'Body and Ideology in the Medieval West', in id., *The Medieval Imagination*. Chicago and London, 1985, 83–5.

—— 'Head or Heart: The Political Use of Bodily Metaphors in the Middle-Ages', in M. Feher *et al.* (ed.), *Fragments for a History of the Human Body*, iii. 12–27.

LERNER, R. E., 'The Pope and the Doctor', *The Yale Review*, 78 (1988–9), 62–79.

—— 'Ecstatic Dissent', *Speculum*, 67 (1992), 33–57.

—— 'Writing and Resistance among Beguins of Languedoc and Catalonia', in *Heresy and Literacy 1000–1530*, ed. P. Biller and A. Hudson. Cambridge, 1994, 186–204.

Lexikon des Mittelalters. Zurich and Munich, 1977–.

LINDBERG, D. C., *Theories of Vision from Al-Kindi to Kepler*. Chicago, 1976.

LONGÈRE, J., *La Prédication médiévale*. Paris, 1983.

LUPTON, D., *Medicine as Culture: Illness, Disease and the Body in Western Societies*. London, 1994.

McGINN B. (ed.), *Three Treatises on Man: A Cistercian Anthropology*. Kalamazoo, 1977.

McVAUGH, M. R., 'Theriac at Montpellier 1285–1325', *Sudhoffs Archiv*, 56 (1972), 113–24.

—— 'The *Humidum Radicale* in Thirteenth-Century Medicine', *Traditio*, 30 (1974), 259–83.

—— 'The Nature and Limits of Medical Certitude at Early Fourteenth-Century Montpellier', *Osiris*, 2nd ser., 6 (1990), 62–84.

—— *Medicine before the Plague: Practitioners and their Patients in the Crown of Aragon 1285–1345*. Cambridge, 1993.

—— 'Medical Knowledge at the Time of Frederik II', *Micrologus*, 2 (1994), 3–17.

—— 'Two Texts, One Problem: the Authorship of the *Antidotarium* and *De venenis* Attributed to Arnau de Vilanova', in *ATIEAV* ii. 75–94; also in *ATCA* 14 (1995).

—— 'Bedside Manners in the Middle Ages', *Bulletin of the History of Medicine*, 71 (1997), 201–23.

MANSELLI, R., 'La religiosità d'Arnaldo da Villanova', *Bullettino dell'Istituto Storico Italiano per il Medio Evo e Archivio Muratoriano*, 63 (1951), 1–100.

—— *Spirituali e Beghini in Provenza*. Rome, 1959.

MANSI, J. D., *Sacrorum conciliorum nova et amplissima collectio*. Florence and Venice, 1759–98.

MARLAND, H. and PELLING, M. (ed.), *The Task of Healing: Medicine, Religion and Gender in England and the Netherlands, 1450–1800*. Rotterdam, 1996.

MARTIN, H., *Le Métier de prédicateur à la fin du Moyen Âge 1350–1520*. Paris, 1988.

MARTINELLI, B., 'Il Petrarca e la medicina', in F. Petrarca, *Contra medicum*, 201–49.

MARTY, M. E. and VAUX, K. L. (ed.), *Health / Medicine and the Faith Traditions: An Inquiry into Religion and Medicine*. Philadelphia, 1982.

MAURER, A., *St Thomas Aquinas: The Division and Methods of the Sciences*. 4th rev. edition, Toronto, 1986.

MENÉNDEZ Y PELAYO, M., *Historia de los heterodoxos españoles*, iii. Buenos Aires, 1951.

MENSA I VALLS, J., *Arnau de Vilanova, espiritual: Guia bibliogràfica*. Barcelona, 1994.

—— 'Sobre la suposada paternitat arnaldiana de l'*Expositio super Apocalypsi*', in *ATIEAV* i. 105–205; also in *ATCA* 13 (1994).

MICHELONI, P., *La medicina nel primi tremita codici del fondo vaticano latino.* Rome, 1950.

MONTOLIU DE, M., *Ramon Llull i Arnau de Vilanova.* Barcelona, 1958.

MOORE, R. I., 'Heresy as Disease', in *The Concept of Heresy in the Middle Ages (11th–13th c.)*, ed. W. Lourdaux and D. Verhelst. Leuven and The Hague, 1976, 1–11.

—— *The Formation of a Persecuting Society.* Oxford, 1987.

MÜLLER, R. A., *Der Arzt im Schachspiel bei Jakob von Cessolis.* Munich, 1981.

MURDOCH, J. E., 'Philosophy and the Enterprise of Science in the Later Middle Ages', in *The Interaction between Science and Philosophy*, ed. Y. Elkana. Atlantic Highlands, NJ, 1974, 51–74.

—— 'From Social into Intellectual Factors: An Aspect of the Unitary Character of Late Medieval Learning', in *The Cultural Context of Medieval Learning*, ed. J. E. Murdoch and E. D. Sylla. Boston Studies in Philosophy of Science, 26; Dordrecht and Boston, 1975, 271–339.

MURRAY, A., *Reason and Society in the Middle Ages.* Oxford, 1978.

—— 'Religion among the Poor in Thirteenth-Century France: The Testimony of Humbert de Romans', *Traditio*, 30 (1974), 285–324.

—— 'The Epicureans', in *Intellectuals and Writers in Fourteenth-Century Europe*, ed. P. Boitani and A. Torti. Tübingen and Cambridge, 1986, 138–63.

NEBBIANI-DALLA GUARDA, D., 'Les livres de l'infirmerie dans les monastères médiévaux', *Revue Mabillon*, 66 (1994), 57–81.

NEWMAN, JOHN HENRY CARDINAL, 'Christianity and Medical Science. An Address to the Students of Medicine', in *The Idea of a University* (New York, 1968), 380–91.

NICAISE, E. (tr.), *Chirurgie de Maître Henri de Mondeville.* Paris, 1893.

NOORDA, S., 'Illness and Sin, Forgiving and Healing: the Connection of Medical Treatment and Religious Beliefs in Ben Sira 38. 1–15', in *Studies in Hellenistic Religions*, ed. M. J. Vermaseren. Leiden, 1979, 215–24.

NOYE, I., 'Maladie', in *DS* x (1980), 137–52.

NUMBERS, R. L., and AMUNDSEN, D. W. (ed.), *Caring and Curing: Health and Medicine in the Western Religious Traditions.* New York and London, 1986.

NUTTON, V., 'Murders and Miracles: Lay Attitudes towards Medicine in Classical Antiquity', in *Patients and Practitioners*, ed. R. Porter (Cambridge, 1985), 23–53. [Also in Nutton, *From Democedes to Harvey*, essay VIII].

—— 'From Galen to Alexander: Aspects of Medicine and Medical Practice in Late Antiquity', *Dumbarton Oaks Paper*, 38 (1984), 1–14. [Also in Nutton, *From Democedes to Harvey*, essay X].

—— *From Democedes to Harvey: Studies in the History of Medicine.* London, 1988.

—— 'From Medical Certainty to Medical Amulets: Three Aspects of Ancient Therapeutics', *Clio Medica*, 22 (1991), 13–22.

NUTTON, V., 'Medicine in Medieval Western Europe, 1000–1500', in Conrad *et al.*, *The Western Medical Tradition*, 139–205.

O'BOYLE, C., 'Medicine, God and Aristotle in the Early Universities: Prefatory Prayers in Late Medieval Medical Commentaries', *Bulletin of the History of Medicine*, 66 (1992), 185–209.

OLDONI, M., *Giovanni da San Gimignano. Un enciclopedico dell'anima*. San Gimignano, 1993.

—— 'Giovanni da San Gimignano', in *L'enciclopedismo medievale*, ed. M. Picone. Ravenna, 1994, 213–28.

OLIGER, L., 'Servasanto da Faenza OFM e il suo *Liber de virtutibus et vitiis*', in *Miscellanea Francisco Ehrle: Scritti di storia e paleografia*, i. Studi e testi, 37; Rome, 1924, 148–89.

OLIVIERI, A., 'I'sermones e la cultura dal '200 al '400: indagini sulla metaphora dell'occhio', *Il Santo*, 26/2 (1986), 425–36.

PANIAGUA, J. A., *Estudios y notas sobre Arnau de Vilanova*. Madrid, 1963.

—— *El Maestro Arnau de Vilanova médico*. Valencia, 1969; 2nd edition in Paniagua, *Studia Arnaldiana*, 49–143.

—— 'Cronología de los hechos conocidos de la vida de Arnau de Vilanova', in Paniagua, *Studia Arnaldiana*, 465–81.

—— 'Abstinencia de carnes y medicina', *Scripta Theologia*, 16 (1984), 323–46.

—— *Studia Arnaldiana: Trabajos en torno a la obra médica de Arnau de Vilanova, c. 1240–1311*. Barcelona, 1994.

—— 'En torno a la problemática del corpus científico arnaldiano', in *ATIEAV* ii. 9–22; also in *ATCA* 14 (1995).

PARAVICINI-BAGLIANI, A., *Medicina e scienze della natura alla corte dei papi nel Duecento*. Spoleto, 1991.

—— *Il corpo del Papa*. Turin, 1994.

PARK, K., *Doctors and Medicine in Early Renaissance Florence*. Princeton, 1985.

—— 'Medicine and Society in Medieval Europe, 500–1500', in *Medicine in Society: Historical Essays*, ed. A. Wear. Cambridge, 1992, 59–90.

—— 'The Criminal and the Saintly Body: Autopsy and Dissection in Renaissance Italy', *Renaissance Quarterly*, 47 (1994), 1–33.

—— 'The Life of the Corpse: Division and Dissection in Late Medieval Europe', *The Journal of the History of Medicine and Allied Sciences*, 50 (1995), 111–32.

PAXTON, F. S., 'Curing Bodies—Curing Souls: Hrabanus Maurus, Medical Education and the Clergy in Ninth-Century Francia', *Journal of the History of Medicine and Allied Sciences*, 50 (1995), 230–52.

—— 'Liturgy and Healing in an Early Medieval Saint's Cult: The Mass *in honore sancti Sigismundi* for the Cure of Fevers', *Traditio*, 49 (1994), 23–43.

—— 'Anointing the Sick and the Dying in Christian Antiquity and the Early Medieval West', in S. D. Campbell *et al.* (ed.), *Health, Disease and Healing*, 93–102.

PEASE, A. S., 'Medical Allusions in the Works of St Jerome', *Harvard Studies in Classical Philology*, 25 (1914), 73–86.

PELSTER, H., 'Die Quaestio Heinrichs von Harclay über die zweite Ankunft Christi und die Erwartung des baldigen Weltendes zu Anfang des XIV Jahrhunderts', *Archivio Italiano per la storia della Pietà*, 1 (1951), 25–82.

PERARNAU, J., 'Dos tratados "espirituales" de Arnau de Vilanova en traducción castellana medieval: *Dyalogus de elementis catholice fidei* y *De helemosina et sacrificio*', *Anthologica Annua*, 22–3 (1975–6), 476–630.

—— 'Troballa de tractats espirituals perduts d'Arnau de Vilanova', *Revista Catalana de Teologia*, 1 (1976), 489–512.

—— L' *"Alia informatio beguinorum" d'Arnau de Vilanova*. Barcelona, 1978.

—— 'El text primitiu del *De mysterio cymbalorum ecclesiae* d'Arnau de Vilanova', *ATCA* 7/8 (1988/9), 7–182.

—— 'L'*Ars catholicae philosophiae*: primera redacció de la *Philosophia catholica et divina*', *ATCA* 10 (1991), 7–223.

—— 'L'*Allocutio Christini* . . . d'Arnau de Vilanova', *ATCA* 11 (1992), 7–117.

—— 'Problemes i criteris d'autenticitat d'obres espirituals atribuïdes a Arnau de Vilanova', in *ATIEAV* i. 25–103; also in *ATCA* 13 (1994).

—— and Santi, F., 'Villeneuve (Vilanova, Arnaud de)', *DS* 16 (1994), 785–97.

PEREIRA, M., 'Le opere mediche di Lullo in rapporto con la sua filosofia naturale e con la medicina del xiii secolo', *Estudios Lulianos*, 23 (1979), 5–35.

—— *The Alchemical Corpus Attributed to Raymond Lull*. Warburg Institute Surveys and Texts, xviii. London, 1989.

—— 'Arnaldo da Vilanova e l'alchimia. Un indagine preliminare', *ATIEAV* ii. 95–174; also in *ATCA* 14 (1995).

PETTI BALBI, G., 'Arte di governo e crociata: Il *Liber sancti passagii* di Galvano da Levanto', *Studi e Ricerche. Istituto di Civiltà Classica Cristiana Medievale (Genoa)*, 7 (1986), 131–68.

—— 'Società e cultura a Genoa tra due e trecento', *Atti dela Società Ligure de Storia Patria*, n.s. 24/2, *Genoa, Pisa e il Mediterraneo tra due e trecento*, (1984), 123–49.

POLO DE BEAULIEU, M.-A. (ed.), *La 'Scala Dei' de Jean Gobi*. Paris, 1991.

PONS I GURI, J. M., 'Constitucions Conciliars Tarraconenses (1229–1330)', in *Recull d'estudis d'història jurídica catalana*, ii. ed. J. M. Pons i Guri, Barcelona, 1989.

PORTER, R., 'Religion and Medicine', in *Companion Encyclopedia of the History of Medicine*, ed. W. F. Bynum and R. Porter, London and New York, 1993, ii. 1449–68.

POSCHMANN, B., *Penance and the Anointing of the Sick*, tr. F. Courtney. Freiburg and London, 1964.

POUCHELLE, M.-C., 'La prise en charge de la mort: médecine, médicins et chirurgiens devant les problèmes liés à la mort à la fin du Moyen Âge (XIIIe–XVe siècles)', *Archives européenes de sociologie*, 17/2 (1976), 249–78.

POUCHELLE, M.-C., *The Body and Surgery in the Middle Ages*. Cambridge, 1990.

RANGER, T. O. and SLACK, P. (ed.), *Epidemics and Ideas: Essays on the Historical Perception of Pestilence*. Cambridge, 1992.

RATH, G., 'Gilles de Corbeil as Critic of his Age', *Bulletin of the History of Medicine*, 38 (1964), 133–8.

RAWCLIFFE, C., *Medicine and Society in Later Medieval England*. Stroud, 1995.

REEVES, M., *The Influence of Prophecy in the Later Middle Ages*. Oxford, 1969.

RENGSTORF, K. H., *Die Anfänge der Auseinandersetzung zwischen Christusglaube und Asklepiosfrömmigkeit*. Schriften der Gesellschaft zur Förderung der Westfälischen Landesuniversität zu Münster, 30; Münster, 1953.

RODNITE LEMAY, H., 'William of Saliceto on Human Sexuality', *Viator*, 1 (1981), 165–81.

ROSEN, G., 'The Historical Significance of some Medical References in the *Defensor Pacis* of Marsilius of Padua', *Sudhoffs Archiv*, 37 (1953), 350–6.

ROSNER F. and KOTTEK, S. S. (ed.), *Moses Maimonides: Physician, Scientist and Philosopher*. Northvale, NJ and London, 1993.

ROUSE, R. H. and ROUSE, M. A., *Preachers Florilegia and Sermons: Studies on the Manipulus florum of Thomas of Ireland*. Toronto, 1979.

SALVADOR DE LES BORGES, *Arnau de Vilanova moralista*. Barcelona, 1957.

SAMARAN, C., 'Pierre Bersuire, prieur de Saint Éloi de Paris', *Histoire littéraire de la France*, 39 (1962), 259–450.

SANTI, F., 'Gli *Scripta spiritualia* di Arnau de Vilanova', *Studi Medievali*, 26 (1985), 977–1014.

—— *Arnau de Vilanova: L'obra espiritual*. Valencia, 1987.

—— 'La vision de la fin des temps chez Arnaud de Villeneuve. Contenu théologique et expérience mystique', in *Fin du monde et signes des temps*. Cahiers de Fanjeaux, 27; Paris, 1992, 107–27.

—— 'Arnaldo da Villanova. Dal potere medico al non potere profetico', in *Poteri carismatici e informali: chiesa e società medioevali*. Palermo, 1991, 262–86.

SCHIPPERGES, H., 'Krankheit IV, V', in *TRE* 19/5, 686–94.

SCHMITT, J.-CL., 'Religion et guérison dans l'Occident médiéval', in *Historiens et sociologues aujourd'hui: Journée d'études annuelles de la Société Française de Sociologie. Université de Lille 1—14–15 Juin 1984*. Paris, 1986.

SELGE, K.-V., 'Un codice quattrocentesco dell'Archivio Generale dei Carmelitani contente opere di Arnaldo da Villanova, Gioacchino da Fiore e Guglielmo da Parigi', *Carmelus*, 36 (1989), 166–76.

—— 'Ancora a proposito del codice III Varia I dell'Archivio Generale dei Carmelitani', *Carmelus*, 37 (1990), 170–2.

SEYMOUR, M. C., *Bartholomaeus Anglicus and his Encyclopedia*. London, 1992.

SHARPE, W. D., 'Isidore of Seville: The Medical Writings', *Transactions of the American Philosophical Society*, 54/2 (1964), 1–75.

SHATZMILLER, J., *Jews, Medicine and Medieval Society*. Berkeley, Los Angeles, London, 1994.

SHEILS, W. J. (ed.), *The Church and Healing.* Studies in Church History, 19; Oxford, 1982.

SIGERIST, H. E., 'Bedside Manners in the Middle Ages: The Treatise *De cautelis medicorum* Attributed to Arnold of Villanova', in *Henry E. Sigerist on the History of Medicine*, ed. F. Martí-Ibáñez. New York, 1960, 131–40.

SIRAISI, N. G., *Arts and the Sciences at Padua: The Studium of Padua before 1350.* Toronto, 1973.

—— 'The Medical Learning of Albertus Magnus', in *Albertus Magnus and the Sciences*, ed. J. A. Weisheipl. Toronto, 1980, 379–404.

—— *Medieval and Early Renaissance Medicine.* Chicago and London, 1990.

—— 'The Faculty of Medicine ', in H. de Ridder-Symoens (ed.), *A History of the University in Europe*, 360–87.

SMALLEY, B., 'Glossa Ordinaria', in *TRE* 13, 452–7.

SONTAG, S., *Illness as Metaphor.* London, 1978.

—— *AIDS and its Metaphors.* London, 1989.

SOSKICE, J. M., *Metaphor and Religious Language.* Oxford, 1985.

—— 'Metaphor and Realism: An Argument for Science and Religion'. Science and Theology Seminar Papers i, The Farmington Institute for Christian Studies; Oxford, 1987.

SOUTHERN, R. W., 'The Changing Rôle of Universities in Medieval Europe', *Historical Research*, 60 (1987), 134–46.

—— *Scholastic Humanism and the Unification of Europe*, i. Oxford, 1995.

STOLL, U., *Das 'Lorscher Arzneibuch'.* Sudhoffs Archiv, Beiheft 28; Stuttgart, 1992.

TANNER, N. P. (ed.), *Decrees of the Ecumenical Councils.* 2 vols., London, 1990.

TEMKIN, O., *The Falling Sickness: A History of Epilepsy from the Greeks to the Beginning of Modern Neurology.* Baltimore, 1945.

—— *Hippocrates in a World of Pagans and Christians.* Baltimore and London, 1991.

THIJSSEN, J. M. M. H., 'Academic Heresy and Intellectual Freedom at the University of Paris, 1200–1378', in *Centres of Learning: Learning and Location in Pre-Modern Europe and the Near East*, ed. J. W. Drijvers and A. A. MacDonald. Leiden, 1995, 217–28.

THOMPSON, P., 'The Disease that We Call Cancer', in S. Campbell *et al.* (ed.), *Health, Disease and Healing*, 1–11.

THORNDIKE, L., *A History of Magic and Experimental Science.* 8 vols., New York and London, 1923–58.

TOEWS, J. E., 'Intellectual History after the Linguistic Turn: The Autonomy of Meaning and the Irreducibility of Experience', *American Historical Review*, 92 (1987), 879–907.

TSCHACKERT, P., *Peter von Ailli.* Gotha, 1877.

TURNER, B. S., *The Body and Society: Explorations in Social Theory.* Oxford, 1984.

TURNER, B. S., *Medical Power and Social Knowledge*. London, 1987.

—— 'The Discourse of Diet', in *The Body: Social Process and Cultural Theory*, ed. M. Featherstone, M. Hepsworth, and B. S. Turner. London, 1991, 157–69; also in *Theory, Culture and Society*, 1 (1982), 23–32.

VAUCHEZ, A., *La Sainteté en Occident aux derniers siècles du Moyen Âge*. Rome and Paris, 1981.

—— *The Laity in the Middle Ages: Religious Beliefs and Devotional Practices*. Notre Dame and London, 1993.

VIEILLARD, C., *Gilles de Corbeil*. Paris, 1909.

VOLLMANN, B. K. (ed.), *Geistliche Aspekte mittelalterlicher Naturlehre*. Wiesbaden, 1993.

WAKEFIELD, W. K., 'Heretics as Physicians in the Thirteenth Century', *Speculum*, 57 (1982), 328–31.

WALZ, A., *Compendium Historiae Ordinis Praedicatorum*. Rome, 1948.

WEBSTER, C., 'Paracelsus: Medicine as Popular Protest', in *Medicine and the Reformation*, 57–77.

WELTER, J.-TH., *L'Exemplum dans la littérature religieuse et didactique du Moyen Âge*. Paris, 1927.

WENZEL, S., *The Sin of Sloth*. Chapel Hill, 1967.

—— *Verses in Sermon: Fasciculus Morum and its Middle English Poems*. Cambridge, Mass., 1978.

—— 'Academic Sermons at Oxford in the Early Fifteenth Century', *Speculum*, 70 (1995), 305–29.

WESTERNIK, L. G., 'Philosophy and Medicine in the Late Antiquity', *Janus*, 51 (1964), 169–77.

WICKERSHEIMER, E., *Dictionnaire biographique des médecins en France au Moyen Âge*. Geneva, 1936.

WINKLER, E., 'Scholastische Leichenpredigten: die *sermones funebres* des Johannes von St. Geminiano', in *Kirche, Theologie, Frömmigkeit*. Festgabe für D. Gottfried Holtz. Berlin, 1965, 177–86.

YATES, F. A., 'The Art of Ramon Lull', *Journal of the Warburg and Courtauld Institutes*, 17 (1954), 115–73.

ZIEGLER, J., 'Arnau de Vilanova: A Case-Study of a Theologizing Physician', *ATCA* 14 (1995), 249–303.

—— 'Medical Similes in Religious Discourse: The Case of Giovanni da San Gimignano OP (ca. 1260–ca. 1333)', *Science in Context*, 8/1 (1995), 103–31.

—— 'Steinschneider (1816–1907) Revised : On the Translation of Medical Writings from Latin into Hebrew', *Medieval Encounters*, 3 (1997), 94–102.

INDEX

Index